Cattle and Buffalo Genetic Resources in India

Cattle and Buffalo Genetic Resources in India

Dr. Subhash Taraphder
Associate Professor
Department of Animal Genetics and Breeding
Faculty of Veterinary and Animal Sciences
West Bengal University of Animal and Fishery Sciences
37 KB Sarani, Belgachia, Kolkata 700 037, West Bengal, India

Prof. Ajit Kumar Sahoo
Dean
Faculty of Veterinary and Animal Sciences
West Bengal University of Animal and Fishery Sciences
Mohanpur, Nadia, West Bengal, India

Dr. Rajesh Paul
Head
Department of Animal Genetics and Breeding
College of Veterinary Sciences and Animal Husbandry
R.K. Nagar, West Tripura, India

SATISH SERIAL PUBLISHING HOUSE
403, Express Tower, Commercial Complex
Azadpur, Delhi-110033 (India)
Phone : 011-27672852, Fax : 91-11-27672046
e-mail : info@satishserial.com, hkjain1975@yahoo.com
Website : www.satishserial.com

Published by :

SATISH SERIAL PUBLISHING HOUSE

403, Express Tower, Commercial Complex, Azadpur, Delhi-110033 (INDIA)
Phone : 011-27672852 Fax : 91-11-27672046
E-mail : info@satishserial.com, hkjain1975@yahoo.com

ISBN 978-93-86200-61-7

Composed, Designed & Printed in India

Dedicated

to

My Reverend Father

Late Kalidas Taraphder

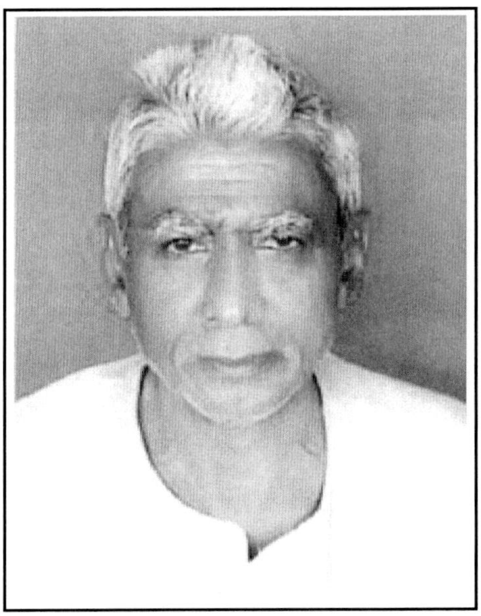

Whose Innumerable Hardship and Sacrifices Brought Me to This Level

...... My Best Regards: Your Subhash

WEST BENGAL UNIVERSITY OF ANIMAL AND FISHERY SCIENCES
68, Kshudirom Bose Sorani, Belgachia, Kolkata - 700 037,
Phone : 2556 3450, Resi. : (033) 2550 2229, Fax: 91-33-2557-1986
Web : www.wbuafscl.ac.in, E-mail : drpbiswos56@gmail.com / drpbiswas1956@gmail.com

Prof Purnendu Biswas Ph.D.
Vice Chancellor

No. VCS/WBUAFS/M-5/1013
Date: December 12, 2017

FOREWORD

It gives me immense pleasure to write this foreword for the book entitled *"Cattle and Buffalo Genetic Resources in India"* co-authored by Dr. Subhash Taraphder, Prof. Ajit Kumar Sahoo and Dr. Rajesh Paul. In this Book, the authors have attempted to cover all the aspects of cattle and buffalo genetic resources in India in simple understandable language with illustrations. The authors have tried to cover all basic and fundamental information related to cattle and buffalo breeds available in India in the three sections of this Book. The Book will be beneficial for the graduate and post graduate students studying at State Agricultural and Veterinary Universities. The Book will also serve as a reference book for the candidates appearing for the Agricultural Research Service Examinations, National Eligibility Tests as well as Civil Services Examinations.

The authors have rich experience in teaching and research in the discipline of Animal Genetics & Breeding and are currently engaged in the teaching of graduate and postgraduate students of Veterinary and Animal Sciences. They have also published a number of research articles in reputed scientific journals.

It is my belief that the Book written by the authors will be useful and will serve as a Standard Reference Book on Cattle and Buffalo Genetic Resources in India.

I hope that the authors will make continuous endeavour in the field of Animal Genetics and Breeding and come with such publications in future.

I conclude by wishing Dr. Subhash Taraphder, Prof. Ajit Kumar Sahoo and Dr. Rajesh Paul, the co-authors of this book all the very best.

12/12/17

(Prof. Purnendu Biswas)
Vice Chancellor

Preface

India is a gold mine and vast reservoir of the domestic animal germplasm. Bovine is an integral part of it. The genetic diversity in the bovines of India is reflected by a large number of breeds of cattle and buffaloes. Most of the cows of India are poor milkers no-doubt, but they are gifted with excellent draft prowess. Buffalo plays a pivotal role through contribution of milk, meat, hides and draft power for agricultural operations in our country. The Cattle and Buffalo populations are available throughout the country having its own special features and well adapted to their respective agro-climatic and eco-geographical conditions. Some of Indian Cattle and Buffalo breeds are well known in the world for their best performance. It is very difficult to identify and ascertain the total number of animals of specified breeds because of inter-mating among breeds located in adjoining areas. In the process of inter-mating and crossbreeding, it is possible that some of the important breeds may be at the point of extinction. It is, therefore, necessary to take urgent steps for awareness regarding these valuable genetic resources and their sustainable improvement with proper conservation. Keeping these aspects in view, this book entitled on 'Cattle and Buffalo Genetic Resources in India' has prepared on the subject especially meant for the students of Veterinary and Animal Sciences.

This Book is compilation of details information on Cattle and Buffalo Genetic Resources available in India along with its morphological characteristics and genetic diversity. The content of this book is an abstract science of Cattle and Buffalo Genetic Resources. The fruit-bearing research on cattle and buffalo at different Research Institutes are presented in concise manner in this book. Authors have also attempted to introduce each topic in precise and concise manner to make the book more understandable and useful to its users. The present book has been prepared keeping in mind the easy mode of teaching also. Authors hope and trust that this book will be useful to the Teachers and Students in getting glimpses of these important species of cattle and buffalo available in India. As such, we feel that this book would be of great help to the concerned students as well as the persons engaged in this field especially for offering teaching in Cattle and Buffalo Genetic Resources in India.

This book is assembled of different valuable information on cattle and buffalo species. In this book, authors do not claim any originality as this is a compilation work. Rather, it should be viewed as a concise collection of various important topics from various published sources which we prepared as teacher of the discipline of Animal Genetics and Breeding. Authors thank all researchers who have worked and contributed valuable information on these species.

Authors are very much grateful to the great many people who extended their wholehearted support, co-operation and contribution in compilation of this book. The resource persons who have contributed information for this book are people of outstanding merit with immense teaching and research experience. The information received from all other sources is greatly acknowledged. We abide by our appreciative acknowledgement to all those who helped us in bringing out the present form of this book. Authors are also grateful to the different resource persons and organization for providing photographs (NBAGR, CIRC, CIRB etc.) on website from which necessary photographs of different breeds along with information were taken for compilation of this work.

At this adjacent moment, we would like to extend our sincere thanks to Satish Serial Publishing House, 403, Express Tower, Commercial Complex, Azadpur, Delhi-110 033 (India) for publishing this book. Their strenuous allegiance and sincere efforts in preparation of this book are incredible and deserves special appreciation.

We shall be grateful for any suggestion and observation from readers and actual users (both students and teachers) which would help in bringing out a revised and improved version of this title. Any suggestions for correction and valuable suggestion for its further improvement will also be highly appreciated.

Finally, we are very much grateful to our families for constant support without which the work could not have been completed.

Kolkata, West Bengal **Authors**
1St January 2017

About the Authors

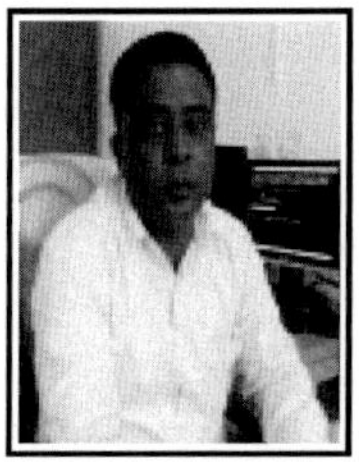

Dr. Subhash Taraphder, Head, Department of Animal Genetics and Breeding, Faculty of Veterinary and Animal Sciences, West Bengal University of Animal and Fishery Sciences, 37 & 68 KB Sarani, Belgachia, Kolkatta-700 037 (West Bengal), India, graduated in B.V.Sc. & A.H. from West Bengal University of Animal and Fishery Sciences. Subsequently, Dr. Taraphder completed Master and Doctorate Degree in Animal Genetics and Breeding from National Dairy Research Institute (NDRI), Karnal, Haryana, India. Dr. Taraphder has published numerous research papers in reputed academic journals.

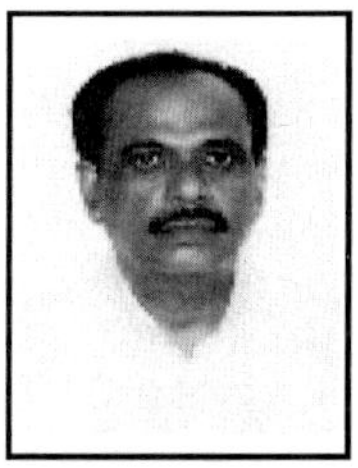

Prof. Ajit Kumar Sahoo, Dean of the Faculty of Veterinary and Animal Sciences, West Bengal University of Animal and Fishery Sciences, Mohanpur, Nadia, West Bengal, India, graduated in B.V.Sc. & A.H. from B.C.K.V.V, Mohanpur, Nadia, West Bengal. Prof. Sahoo completed Master and Doctorate Degree in Animal Genetics and Breeding from the same University. He was the former Head of the Department of Animal Genetics and Breeding, West Bengal University of Animal and Fishery Sciences, Mohanpur, Nadia, West Bengal, India. He has completed more than 28 years of teaching and research experiences in the Animal Genetics and Breeding.

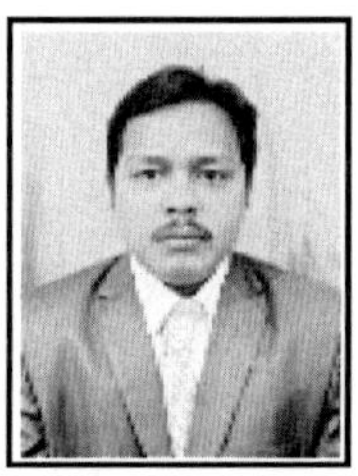

Dr. Rajesh Paul, Head of the Department of Animal Genetics and Breeding, College of Veterinary Sciences and Animal Husbandry, R.K. Nagar, West Tripura, India, graduated in B.V.Sc. & A.H. from West Bengal University of Animal and Fishery Sciences, Kolkata, West Bengal. Dr. Paul completed Master and Doctorate Degree in Animal Genetics and Breeding from same University. He has published numerous research papers in reputed academic journals.

Contents

Preface .... *vii*

UNIT-1: Cattle Genetic Resources in India

1.0 Introduction 1
2.0 History 2
3.0 Origin of Indian Cattle 2
4.0 Domestication of Indian Cattle 4
5.0 Bos taurus and Bos indicus Cattle 5
6.0 Scientific Classification 7
7.0 Current Scenario of Indian Cattle 7
8.0 State wise Indigenous Cattle Population 9
9.0 Trend of Cattle Population 10
10.0 Distribution of Indian Cattle 12
11.0 Salient Feature of Indian Cattle 14
12.0 Importance of Indigenous Cattle Breeds 15
13.0 Characteristics of Indigenous Cow 15
14.0 Classification of Indian Cattle 17
15.0 Indian Cattle Breed 19
16.0 Registered Breeds of Indian Cattle 20
17.0 Breed wise Cattle Population 22
18.0 Estimated Number of Animals Under Indigenous Cattle Breed 23
19.0 Indian Cattle Breed Based on Coat Colour 26
20.0 Breed Description of Indian Cattle 28
21.0 Morphological Feature of Indian Cattle for Identification 80
22.0 Unique Features of Indigenous Cattle Breed 85
23.0 Cattle Breed with Medicinal Properties 85
24.0 A1 versus A2 Type Milk 86
25.0 Crossbred Strains/Breeds Evolved 87

26.0 Dwarf Cows found in India 87
27.0 Indian Cattle Breed at Risk 88
28.0 Productive and Reproductive Performance of Cattle 88
29.0 Cattle Breeding Farm in India 89
30.0 Indigenous Cattle Improvement Programme 94
31.0 AICRP on Cattle 96
32.0 Crossbreeding Programme 97
33.0 Cattle Breeding Programme 99
34.0 Breeding Strategies for Genetic Improvement of Cattle 99
35.0 Cattle Breeding Policy 100
36.0 Present Breeding Policy 102
37.0 Main Features of Present Cattle Breeding Policy 102
38.0 Cattle Breeding Policy in Different States of India 103
39.0 Cattle Breeding Policy of West Bengal 105
40.0 Schemes for Development of Indigenous Cattle 107
41.0 Rashtriya Gokul Mission 115
42.0 Advanced Technologies for Genetic Improvement 117
43.0 Constraints in Cattle Improvement 117
44.0 India Risks Losing Indigenous Native Cattle Breeds 119
45.0 Need for Conservation of Indigenous Cattle Breed 120
46.0 Conservation of Indigenous Cattle Breed 122
47.0 Development and Conservation of Recognised Cattle Breed 125
48.0 Economics of Milch Animal 126
49.0 Central Institute for Research on Cattle (CIRC) 127
50.0 Overview 130

UNIT-2: Buffalo Genetic Resources in India

1.0 Introduction 133
2.0 History 134
3.0 Origin and Domestication 135
4.0 Evolution and Domestication 136
5.0 Scientific Classification of Wild Water Buffalo 137

6.0 Water Buffalo Fact 138
7.0 Interesting Water Buffalo Fact 139
8.0 Classification of Water Buffalo 140
9.0 Classification of Domestic Buffalo 144
10.0 Phylogenetics of Water Buffalo 151
11.0 Current Scenario of Indian Buffalo 153
12.0 Buffalo Wealth and Growth Rates in India 153
13.0 Scientific Classification of Domestic Buffalo 156
14.0 Salient Feature of Buffalo 157
15.0 Buffalo Statistics in India 158
16.0 State wise Buffalo Population in India 162
17.0 Breed of Indian River Buffalo 163
18.0 Registered Breeds of Buffalo in India 166
19.0 Breed wise Buffalo Population In India 166
20.0 Estimated Number of Animals under Indigenous Buffalo Breed 167
21.0 Characterization of Indian Buffalo 169
22.0 Breed Description of Indian Buffalo 170
23.0 Morphological Feature of Indian Buffalo for Identification 188
24.0 Characteristic Feature of Phenotypic Trait 190
25.0 Average Performance of Buffalo Breed 192
26.0 Present Status of Indian Buffalo Breed 192
27.0 Reasons for Loss of Buffalo Genetic Resources 194
28.0 Buffalo Breeding in India: Present and Future 195
29.0 Buffalo Development Programmes in India 196
30.0 All India Coordinated Research Project on Buffalo 197
31.0 Network Project on Buffalo 198
32.0 Current Priorities of Government of India 199
33.0 Buffalo Breeding Policy 200
34.0 Breeding Strategies for Buffalo in India 201
35.0 Schemes for Development of Buffalo in India 202
36.0 Interventions Towards Genetic Improvement of Buffalo 208

37.0 Buffalo Breeding for Milk Production 209
38.0 Constraints to Buffalo Production and Future Outlook 210
39.0 Genetic Aspects of Some Characteristics of Buffalo 211
40.0 Cattle vs. Buffalo Crossbreds for Dairy Production 212
41.0 Need for Conservation of Buffalo Breed 212
42.0 Strategies for Conservation of Buffalo 215
43.0 Development and Conservation of Recognized Buffalo Breed 221
44.0 Steps for Protection and Conservation of Native Breeds of Cattle and Buffalo 223
45.0 Observation on Buffalo Traits for Future Improvement 224
46.0 Some Considerations for Certain Breeding Strategies for Buffalo 225
47.0 Central Institute for Research on Buffaloes (CIRB) 228
48.0 Cloned Buffalo in India 230
49.0 Buffalo Breeding Farm in India 231
50.0 Overview 234

UNIT-3: Documentation of Cattle and Buffaloes Genetic Resources

1.0 National Bureau of Animal Genetic Resources (NBAGR) 239
2.0 Characterization of Cattle and Buffalo 241
3.0 Registration of Cattle and Buffalo Genetic Resources 244
4.0 Monitoring of Cattle and Buffalo Genetic Resources 247
5.0 Determining Risk Status of Cattle and Buffalo 249

Appendix-I: Questionnaires for Survey of Cattle and Buffaloes Genetic Resources 251
Appendix-II: Application for Registration of Cattle and Buffalo Breeds 259
Appendix-III: Breed Descriptor Format for Cattle and Buffalo Breeds 263

References 267

UNIT-1

Cattle Genetic Resources in India

1.0 Introduction

Cattle, colloquially cows, a prominent modern member of the subfamily Bovinae are the most common type of large domesticated ungulates. They are the most widespread species of the genus *Bos* and are most commonly classified as *Bos taurus* and *Bos indicus.* Over 800 breeds of cattle are well recognized worldwide, some of which adapted to the local climate, others which were bred by humans for specialized uses.

India contributes about 12.5 percent of total world cattle population. About 80 percent of the total cattle population in India is non-descript and rest 20 percent is descript. These altogether contribute the highest number of cattle population and milk production in the world. Thus the number of cattle possessed by India is simply amazing.

The cattle genetic diversity in India is reflected by a large number of breeds of cattle that plays a pivotal role in the farmer's economy and offers strong contribution to the animal husbandry sector of this country. The distinct cattle population are spread out in the length and breadth of the country each having its distinctive features and are also well adapted to their respective agro-climatic and eco-geographical conditions. The indigenous breeds of cattle are essentially the products of long term natural selection and are better adopted to withstand tropical diseases and perform well under low and medium input. Many of these breeds may have useful genes for growth, production, disease resistance, medicinal value and small size body conformation. Such utility genes and breeds shall be identified, conserved and utilized. Inter-mating among cattle breeds located in adjoining areas is very common. So, it is very difficult to identify and ascertain the total number of individuals of specified breeds. In the process of inter-mating and crossbreeding, it is possible that some of the imperative breeds are continuously losing their unique features rendering them toward the point of endangered level. It is, therefore, essential to take up necessary measures for their conservation as well as their overall improvement.

2.0 History

All animals currently used for food and agriculture are the result of domestication from wild progenitor species like their wild relatives. These domestic species are continuously evolving at an accelerated rate due to human activity. In general, the history of cattle follows the history of man, be it either primitive or modern. Man has tended to bring them for his own breeds of cattle. During Vedic period many of the useful animals have been brought under service of man especially for milk and became useful since Rigvedic period. The selected animals' species are having vigor, inborn proximity, social ability and docility. The evolutionary process has been accelerated in the domestic species particularly cattle, as a consequence of 10,000 years of selection by human. During this period within the species genetic variation which is essential for the survival of all species has been partially redistributed in thc formation of the large number ot today's unique cattle breeds.

These breeds have adopted too many environments as the breeds spread and have been used to produce different types and combinations. A major group of mammals to be domesticated after caprinae were the large ruminants (Bovinae) which included the humped (*Bos indicus*) and humpless *(Bos taurus)* cattle, yak, mithun, banteng and buffalo. This range of species in the family Bovidae makes a very large number of important contributions to food and agriculture, providing just under 30% world meat and 87% world milk. Same types of zebu animals are present from the time of Indus Valley civilization dating back to 3000 BC. Indian subcontinent is a treasure house of *Bos indicus* Cattle.

3.0 Origin of Indian Cattle

The Aurochs, also urus, uri, is a grand extinct wild ox that inhabited in Europe, Asia and North Africa. The extinct aurochs is a completely separate species from the European bison. It was a very large animal of the elephant size but of a shape of wild ox of Europe. They were aggressive in nature.

Aurochs developed in India some two million years ago, went to the Middle East and further into Asia, and reached Europe about 2,50,000 years ago. The taming of the Urus began in Southern Caucasus and in Upper Mesopotamia starting from the IV century AD, whilst the genetic appearances suggest that the Uri were tamed independently in North Africa and in India.

Once, there were three subspecies of Urus *(Bos primigenous):* the *Bos primigenius namadicus* living in India, the *Bos primigenius mauretanicus* of North Africa and, of course, the *Bos primigenius primigenius* of Europe and Middle East. Only the European subspecies has survived until more recent times. All the present day's domesticated cattle descended from aurochs or urus.

In modern cattle, numerous breeds share characteristics of the aurochs, such as a dark colour in the bulls with a light eel stripe along the back (the cows being lighter), or a typical aurochs-like horn shape. Modern cattle have become much smaller than their wild ancestors: the height of a large domesticated cow is about 1.5 meters (5 feet), while aurochs were about 1.75 meters (5.75 feet). Aurochs also had several features not often seen in modern cattle, such as lyre-shaped horns set at a forward angle, a pale stripe down the spine, and different color according to the gender. The males were black with a pale grey or brownish stripe along the back bone; whilst the females and the calves were reddish. These colours are still found in a few domesticated cattle breeds, such as Jersey cattle.

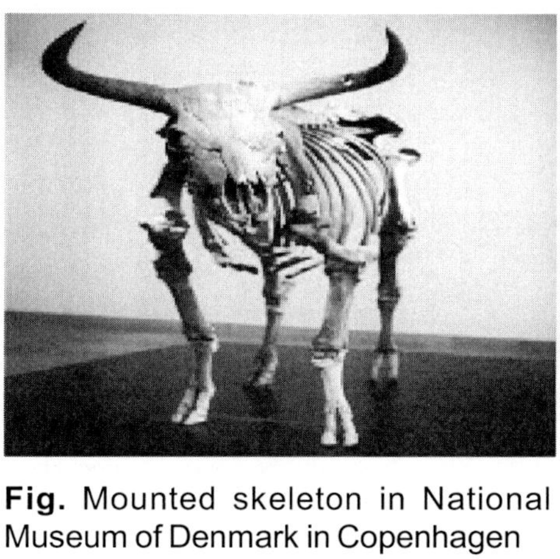

Fig. Mounted skeleton in National Museum of Denmark in Copenhagen

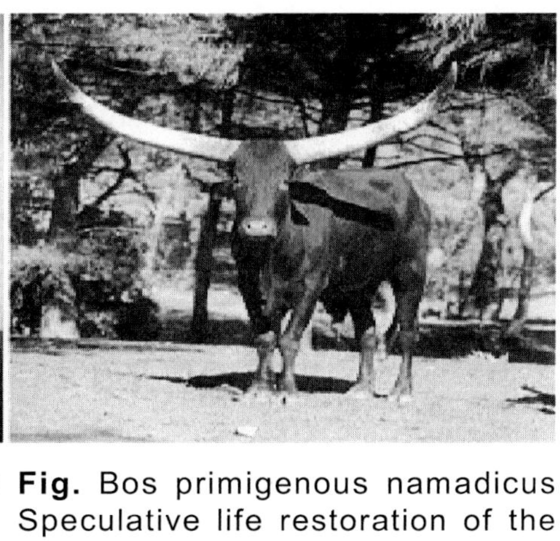

Fig. Bos primigenous namadicus Speculative life restoration of the enigmatic Indian aurochs

In the XIII century A.D., owing to intensive hunting for its flesh, skin and horns, it had limited access to the Polish, Lithuanian, Moldavian meadows and pasturages up to the former Prussia and Transylvania. But, originally, it was present also in Asia, Middle East, North Africa (Egypt, Tunisia, Morocco, Algeria). The species survived in Europe until the last recorded aurochs died in the Jaktorow Forest, Poland in 1627.

Another ancestor of present days breeds of European origin has been developed from *Bos longifrons* which was in Europe as a domesticated animal early in Neolithic. This was comparatively small size animal. The present day European or American breeds of cattle may have been developed as a result of various degrees of crossing between the ancestors.

The Indian breeds of cattle descended from *Bos primigenius* are mostly evolved out of generations of adaptability to the local environment. Often many of them resemble each other with slight morphological changes but because of constant inbreeding in the locality these seem to have been evolved as independent breeds with some distinct features.

4.0 Domestication of Indian Cattle

The cattle were domesticated during The New Stone Age (Neolithic, 8000-6000 BC) both in Europe and Asia. During the Neolithic Revolution, which occurred during the early Holocene, there were at least two aurochs domestication events: one related to the Indian subspecies, leading to zebu cattle; the other one related to the Eurasian subspecies, leading to taurine cattle. Other species of wild bovines were also domesticated, namely the wild water buffalo, gaur, and banteng.

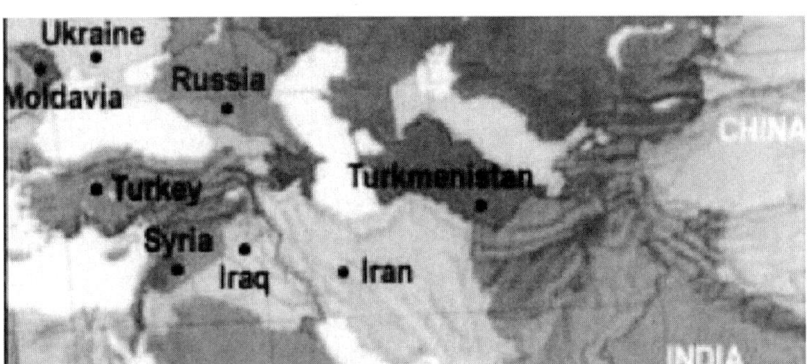

Fig. Domestication area of cattle

The domesticated cattle are of two types living now: *Bos indicus* (humped cattle of tropical countries) and *Bos taurus* (humpless cattle of temperate zones). Breeds fall into two main types, regarded as either two closely related species, or two subspecies of one species. *Bos indicus* cattle, also called zebu, are adapted to hot and humid climates. Zebu cattle or humped cattle are of Asia and Africa. The exotic cattle or humpless cattle are found in Europe, North-eastern Asia, and parts of Africa-they are referred to as taurine cattle, and many are adapted to cooler climates. *Taurus/Indicus* hybrids are widely bred in many warmer regions, combining characteristics of both the ancestral types such as the Sanga cattle of Africa. The cattle of the United States are purely of European origin.

In some parts of the world, further species of cattle are found (both as wild and domesticated animals), and some of these are related so closely to taurine and indicus cattle that interspecies hybrids have been bred. Examples include the Dwarf Lulu cattle of the mountains of Nepal with yak blood, the Beefalo of North America with bison genes, the Selembu breed of India and Bhutan with gayal genes. The Madura breed of Indonesia may have banteng in its parentage. In addition to these fertile hybrids, there are infertile crossings such as the male Dzo of Nepal, a cattle-yak crossing which is bred for agricultural work - like the mule they have to be continually bred from the parent species.

A study done by the University of Missouri researchers reported that ancient domesticated African cattle originated from multiple regions in the middle-east and India. A study on 134 breeds showed that today's cattle were originated from Africa, Asia, North and South America, Australia and Europe.

5.0 Bos taurus and Bos indicus Cattle

Evidence suggests that origin of *Bos taurus* and *Bos indicus* split in two independent events, the first being over 200,000 years ago and the second some 10,000 years ago. Essentially *taurine* cattle were developed in the Fertile Crescent region while the zebu type cattle was domesticated in the Indus Valley region. Since then, many breeds have been developed in both sub-types so that there are now many taurine types and many zebu types throughout the world. The number and variation of the breeds is dependent upon the definition of 'breed' as well as on local activities.

- European breeds are classified as *Bos taurus.* They generally have a small dewlap, little evidence of a hump and more hair to suit the wetter, colder climate. *Bos indicus* cattle are leaner, have looser, thicker skin, larger ears, with a large dewlap and prominent hump suited for dry-tropical climates of Asia/Africa. Zebu cattle are late maturing too.
- *Bos indicus*/zebu cattle have a high degree of heat tolerance, partially resistant to ticks, many tickborne diseases and have low nutritional requirements. Potential for milk production is poorly developed in most zebu cattle and that milk let-down is a problem. Such types of features are rarely found in *Bos taurus.*
- Brahman (zebu known in America) has lower respiratory rates, greater packed cell volume but poorer temperament. The greater skin area also contributes to the heat tolerance in Zebu. *Bos indicus* calves exposed to cold are more susceptible than *Bos taurus* calves. The additional surface area (about 12% over taurine breeds) and the Ongole cattle breed skin secrete sebum which acts as a fly repellent and filters the UV rays of Sun.
- Upper (UCT) and Lower Critical Temperatures (LCT) for different breed types: 38°C and 10°C respectively for Indigenous breeds, 24°C and 2°C for Jersey and crosses, 20°C and 10°C respectively for Holsteins. Temperatures at which milk production starts to reduce is 21°C for Holsteins, 24/27°C for Jersey and Brown Swiss and 32°C for Zebu type.

		Chromosome Morphology					
		Autosomes				Sex Chromosomes	
Cattle	2n	Meta Centric	Sub-Meta Centric	Acro centric	Telo Centric	X	Y
Bos indicus	60	-	-	58	-	Sub Metacentric	Smallest Acrocentric
Bos taurus	60	-	-	58	-	Sub Metacentric	Small Metacentric

6.0 Scientific Classification

Kingdom	:	Animal
Phylum	:	Chordata
Class	:	Mammalia
Order	:	Artiodactyla
Family	:	Bovidae
Subfamily	:	Bovinae
Genus	:	Bos
Species	:	*Bos indicus* : Humped Cattle
		Bos taurus: Humpless Cattle
Binomial Name	:	*Bos indicus:* Indian Cattle
		Bos taurus: Exotic Cattle

Conservation status : Domisticated

7.0 Current Scenerio of Indian Cattle

- India has the largest number of cattle in the world. As per livestock causus report 2012, the total number of cattle in the country is 190.90 million which accounts for about 12.5 percent of the world's total number of cattle and about 37.28 per cent of the total livestock population of India.
- It has already been mentioned that Indian cattle are, by and large, of poor quality. The average yield of milk per cow is just one kg per day whereas this yield is 30-40 kg in some of the advanced countries like New Zealand, Denmark and Holland. This is the reason that Indian cow is often called tea-cup-cow.
- The average annual milk yield of Indian cattle is 1172 kg which is only about half of the global average, and much less than found in New Zealand (3343 kg), Australia (5600 kg), UK (7101 kg), US (9332 kg) and Israel (10214 kg).
- The average milk yield of indigenous breeds of cattle has been around 1.98 kg as compared to crossbreds (6.75 kg) and buffaloes (4.50 kg). The above yield of indigenous cattle may not include the yield of draft breeds and non-descript cows which are hardly

milked due to low yields. Thus, except 15-20% of crossbreds and elite native breeds, about 80-85% of the livestock, particularly the cattle are not contributing to the milk production. However, they compete for fodder and feed, resulting in huge shortage of feed resources.

- Although majority of Indian cattle are of poor quality, there are only 4 well defined excellent breeds of milch cattle and 25 well known draught breeds of cattle, and 12 dual purpose breeds of cattle.
- Some exotic breeds have been crossed with Indian breeds and high milk yielding new breed called cross breed has been developed in India, especially in 20 military farms in hilly areas.
- Madhya Pradesh and Uttar Pradesh shared the largest number of cattle which is about 10.27 and 10.24 per cent of the total cattle population in India. Next in descending order are West Bengal (8.65%), Maharashtra (8.11%), Rajasthan (6.98%), Bihar (6.41%), Orissa (6.09%), Assam (5.40%), Gujarat (5.23%), Chattisgarh (5.14%) and Andhra Pradesh (5.03%). The other states with considerable number of cattle are Karnataka (4.98%), Tamil Nadu (4.62%) and Jharkhand (4.57%).
- As per 19th Livestock Census Report (2012) of Government of India, the population of cattle decreased by 3.14% in rural areas. There is negative growth in cattle with 18.34% in urban areas. The female cattle (cows) population has increased by 6.52% over the previous census (2007) and the total number of female cattle in 2012 is 122.9 million.
- The number of animals in milk in cows and buffaloes has increased from 77.04 million to 80.52 million showing a growth of 4.51%.
- The number of milch animals (in-milk and dry) in cows and buffaloes has increased from 111.09 million to 118.59 million showing an increase of 6.75%.
- The percentage change of in-milk cattle-exotic population during 2007-12 has shown an increase of 10% in rural areas as compared to the percentage change during 2003-07.
- The percentage change in-milch cattle - Indigenous population has decreased by 65% during 2007-12 as compared to 2003-07 in rural areas.

- Crossbreeding of indigenous cattle with exotic stocks to enhance genetic potential of cattle has been successful only to a limited extent. After more than five decades of crossbreeding, the crossbred cattle population is only 20.12% in India.
- The exotic/crossbred milch cattle increased from 14.4 million to 19.42 million, giving rise to an increase of 34.78%, whereas the indigenous milch cattle increased marginally from 48.04 million to 48.12 million, showing an increase of 0.17%.

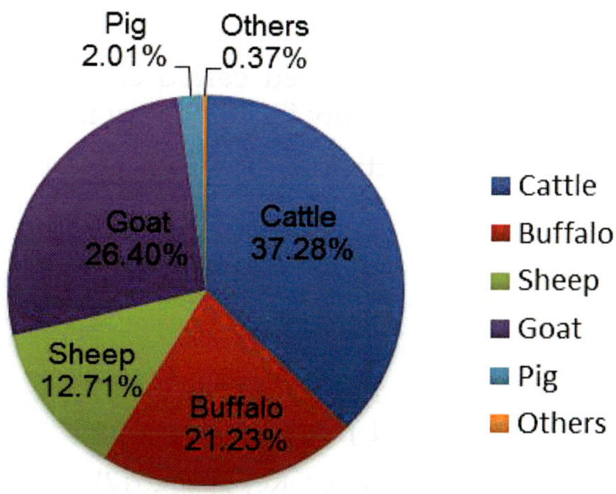

Fig. Distribution of Livestock in India

8.0 State Wise Indigenous Cattle Population [Livestock Census-2012]

S.No.	State	Population
1	Andaman and Nicobar Islands	45625
2	Andhra Pradesh	9595942
3	Arunachal Pradesh	463758
4	Assam	10307604
5	Bihar	12231523
6	Chandigarh	8962
7	Chhattisgarh	9814896
8	Dadra and Nagar Haveli	41870
9	Daman and Diu	2096
10	Goa	57480
11	Gujarat	9983953

12	Haryana	1808116
13	Himachal Pradesh	2149259
14	Jammu and Kashmir	2798326
15	Jharkhand	8730083
16	Karnataka	9516484
17	Kerala	1328627
18	Lakshadweep	3099
19	Madhya Pradesh	19602366
20	Maharashtra	15484207
21	Manipur	263843
22	Meghalaya	896000
23	Mizoram	34573
24	Nagaland	234974
25	NCT of Delhi	86433
26	Odisha	11621272
27	Puducherry	59896
28	Punjab	2427714
29	Rajasthan	13324462
30	Sikkim	140467
31	Tamil Nadu	8814042
32	Tripura	948794
33	Uttar Pradesh	19557067
34	Uttarakhand	2006053
35	West Bengal	16514239
	Total Cattle Population	190,904,105

9.0 Trend of Cattle Population

- Cattle rearing in India has been a traditional practice and intimately linked to agricultural economy. India had 204.58 million cattle in 1992, Between 1987 and 1992 cattle population grows at an annual growth rate of 0.48%.
- Out of the 204.58 million cattle, 15.21 million were crossbreed cattle, which is 7.43% of the total cattle population in 1992. Total crossbred number grew from 8.80 million in 1982 to 11.59 million in 1987 (31.70%), and 15.21 million (31.32%) in 1992 with annual growth rate of 6.25% from 1987 to 1992.

- The changes within the cattle population over the last two decades indicate a radical shift in the priority of the farming community from production of work animals to milk production.
- Between 1972 and 1982, the number of working male in cattle population declined sharply (by 12 million) and among females the proportion of adult females increased (63% in desi and 61% in crossbred) gradually. However, the proportion of desi cows steadily declined and a phenomenal growth in the number of crossbred was marked.
- The variations in Indigenous in-milk cattle population has decreased drastically during 2007-12 as compared to 2003-07.
- Further the cattle have registered an increase of 28 per cent from 155.3 million in 1951 to 198.9 million in 1997 but decrease about 4.52% in 2012 compared to 2007 livestock census.

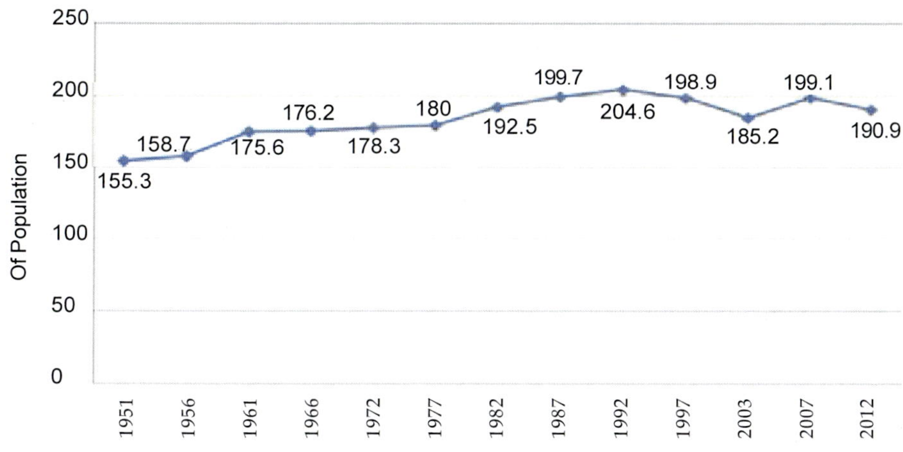

Fig. Cattle Population in India (in million)

- An increasing trend of cattle population in India was observed from 1951 to 1992. Maximum number cattle population was observed in the year 1992. It is about 204.6 million. Then the cattle population was declined upto the 2003. Although an increasing trend was again observed in the year 2007 but it again declined in the year 2012.

10.0 Distribution of Indian Cattle

Agro-Ecological Zones | Cattle/Sq Km

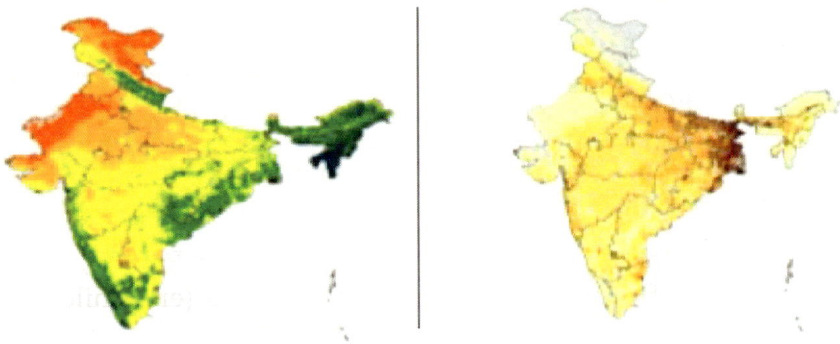

Agro-Ecological Zones	Cattle/Sq Km
Desert	< 50
Arid	50-100
Semi arid	100-150
Dry sub-humid	150-200
Moist sub-humid	< 200
Humid	Unsuitable

Fig. Agro-ecological Zones and Densities of Cattle Population

- The cattle population in India is so diverse in structure and body conformation as to suit the different climatic conditions available in the country. They are either adapted to the prevalent conditions and climatic factors in different parts of the country or thrive only on the particular environments in which they are bred and reared.
- In India, there are forty one distinct breeds of cattle in addition to a large number of non-descripts, which are small in size and of low productivity.
- Most of the good milch, draught or dual purpose breeds are found in dry northern, north-western and southern parts of the country. The humid regions generally do not support good breeds of cattle.
- Indian cattle do well in dry areas, whereas other breeds require suitable temperature and humidity. In general, the cattle from

the drier regions are well built, and those from the heavy rainfall areas, coastal regions and hilly regions are comparatively smaller in built.

- In the eastern parts of the country and in the coastal areas, the animals are non-descriptive and are poor milk producers. Thus, inferior stock is found in Assam, West Bengal, Orissa and Kerala. In hilly areas, where rainfall is heavy, cattle are of a poor breed. The quality of cattle in other parts of the country is intermediate between these two classes.
- The best Indian cattle breeds are found in Punjab, Haryana, Rajasthan, Saurashtra, parts of Maharashtra (erstwhile Bombay State), Madras, Mysore and Andhra Pradesh. Gujarat can boast of some of the excellent breeds of cattle such as Gir and Kankrej.
- In the northern region desi cow population has declined substantially and the region now accounts for 40% of all crossbreds in the country. The South has the second largest population of crossbred cattle (34%) followed by west - some 15% of the crossbred. Eastern region has the highest proportion of desi cows and lowest percent of cross breds (11%).
- Among the States, Uttar Pradesh, Tamil Nadu, Maharashtra, Kerala and Punjab have the largest number of crossbred cattle and together they account for nearly 65% of all the crossbred cattle population in the country.

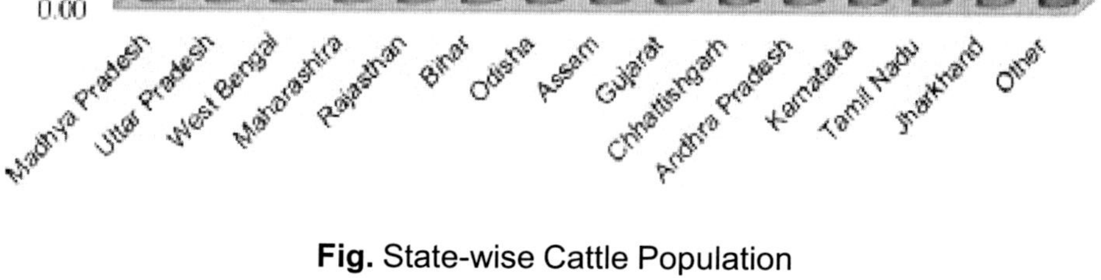

Fig. State-wise Cattle Population

Percentage share of Cattle Population 2012

11.0 Salient Feature of Indian Cattle

The Indian cattle is also called 'the humped cattle'. The size and shape of the hump vary by breed, sex and age of animals. Other external features common to most zebu cattle are narrow body, rather long legs and well developed brisket and dewlap, particularly in the males. The most important characteristic of this group is its adaptation to the tropical environment. This adaptation may derive from first three main aspects:

- In indigenous cattle, high degree of heat tolerance partly due to low heat production (associated with low metabolic rate and low productivity) and partly due to a high capacity to dissipate heat.
- Low nutritional requirements of Indian cattle mainly due to low metabolic rate and small size and also possibly due to more efficient digestion at low feeding level.
- Indigenous cattle are sturdy, endowed with quality of heat tolerance, partially resistant to ticks and many tickborne diseases and ability to thrive under extreme nutritional stress.
- Indian cattle have considerable degree of resistance to ticks and also to many tick-borne diseases prevalent in tropical countries.
- Indian cattle are generally leaner, with a large dewlap and prominent hump suited for dry-tropical climates. *Bos indicus* cattle have looser, thicker skin, larger ears, a prominent hump, and live in the more hotter, humid climates. Most of the Indian cattle are white to light grey in body colour.
- Most of the Indian cattle reflect the low productivity of their milk yield and that milk let-down is a problem. This is mainly due to poor plane of nutrition as well as low genetic potential for milk production and health care. Zebu cattle are late maturing too.
- About 80 percent of our indigenous cattle are non-descriptive and only remaining 20 percent are descriptive. The cattle genetic resources of India are represented by 41 well recognized breeds.
- Most of the cattle breeds (about 62 percent) are suited for draught power but produce little milk. About 28 percent Indian cattle breeds are dual purpose and remaining only about 10 percent cattle breeds are milch purpose cattle.

12.0 Importance of Indigenous Cattle Breeds

- During 2012-2013, about 45 million cattle were 'in milk'and contributed around 59 million tonnes of milk. Cattle not only contribute substantially to milk production but are also used as draught animals for agricultural operations and transport in rural areas. Most of the agricultural operations by small farmers are performed by bullocks. Indigenous cattle are categorized as Zebu and are suited for draught power because of the presence of a hump.
- Indigenous cattle are well known for their quality of heat tolerance and ability to withstand extreme climatic conditions. Studies of impact of climate change and effect of temperature rise on milk production of dairy animals indicate that temperature rise due to global warming will negatively impact milk production. The annual loss in milk production of cattle and buffaloes due to thermal stress in 2020 will be about 3.2 million tonnes of milk costing more than Rs 5000 crore at current price rates. The decline in milk production and reproductive efficiency will be highest in crossbred cattle followed by buffaloes. Indigenous cattle breeds will be least affected by climate change as they are more hardy and robust.
- Due to their unique characteristics of heat tolerance, tick and pest resistance, resistance to diseases and the ability to thrive under extreme climatic conditions, these animals have been imported by several countries including USA, Brazil and Australia for development of heat tolerant disease resistant stock.
- Most of the indigenous cattle breeds possess A_2 allele of beta casein as compared to exotic cattle, known to possess higher frequency of A_1 type allele. Reportedly, A_1 milk is possibly associated with some metabolic disorders like diabetes, heart diseases etc. and A_2 milk produced by indigenous breeds does not have any such association.

13.0 Characteristics of Indigenous Cow

- **Hump:** For cows hump is not very prominent but in bulls it is huge and clearly visible just after their birth.
- **Dewlap**: Larger dewlap, better resistance power of the cow towards parasites and diseases.

- **Skin color**: Most Indian breeds have by default uniform color.
- **Forehead:** Forehead of Indian cows bulges out slightly on the eye area. It will be narrow and furrowed in the middle. It is clearly visible in bulls. Gir cow is the only exception; it has a massive convex forehead.
- **Hooves:** Hooves are small in size and the rear hooves split very close to each other. It should not be wide open. Indian cattle have developed strong hooves to walk on uneven and rocky terrain.
- **Tail:** Tail should almost touch the ground, however if it is a calf then the tail will be small but should be at least below the knee.
- **Dung:** All Indigenous Indian cows have semi solid form of dung. Dung will be covered by thin mucous which makes the dung not to stick on the skin of cows and even human hands when handling. It should have a pleasant smell and not foul odour.
- **Oily appearance and not fury texture:** Cows skin should have short glossy hair with greasy appearance which acts as an insect repellent. When we rub our hands on the cow, oil should stick to our hands. It should not have fur like texture on the skin, it is a sign of western breed from cooler climate.
- **Horn:** All cows have horns and it keeps growing as they gain age, there may be some exceptional case. Some people state Vechur cows have very small or almost negligible horn, but that is not true.
- **Round Back:** All well fed Indian cows will have round back. Western or crossbred cows have different bone structure. They tend to have huge stomach with never ending appetite. Some lactating Indian cows do not have round back, however, they gain weight once lactation stop.
- **Surya Ketu Nadi**: This is not visible through naked eyes, but one can feel it on the backbone of any pure zebu cattle (Indian Holy Cow). When we move our fingers through the backbone starting from the hump we should be able to feel a small cavity on the backbone denoting the nerve. This nerve is said to give urine, milk, dung etc. of pure quality. It helps in absorbing energy from sun, moon and universe as per ayurvedic texts. On a western or hybrid cow backbone will be visible through naked eyes and no nerve can be felt even after touching.

14.0 Classification of Indian Cattle

About 20 percent of Indian cattle are descript and classified into three distinct categories as milch breed, draught breed and general utility breed of India. These cattle genetic resources of India are represented by 41 well recognized breeds. Remaining 80 percent of the total indigenous cattle are non-descriptive and hence remain undocumented.

14.1 Milch Breed

These breeds are generally ponderous in built with pendulous dewlap and sheath, and have lateral and often curved horns. Cows are high yielders, bullocks are of poor quality. The Sahiwal, Red Sindhi, Gir and Tharparkar are some of the outstanding breeds of milch cattle. About 10 percent cattle breed in India comes under milch purpose cattle breed. These milch breeds' cattle first calves between 40 to 50 months and produce 1000 to 2000 kg milk in a lactation with a calving interval of 15 to 18 months.

14.2 Draught Breed

Cows of these breeds are poor milk-yielders, but the bullocks are excellent draught animals. More than 80 percent of the cultivators in India depend upon bullocks for motive power in the farms. About 62 percent breed of the cattle in India are draught animals. The idle time of the bullocks on the farms is economically used in farm transport and village industries. Among the important draught breeds are included the Nagori, Bachaur, Kenkatha, Malvi, Kherigarh, Hallikar, Khillari, Amritmahal, Kangayam, Ponwar, Bargur and Siri. These draught breeds cattle first calves between 48 to 56 months and produce 600 to 800 kg milk in a lactation with a calving interval of 18 to 22 months.

14.2.1 Draught breeds are of four types

1. Short-horned, white or light grey cattle with long coffin shaped skull and face, slightly convex in profile. The Nagori and Bachaur breeds are excellent examples of the first type of draught cattle.
2. Lyre-horned grey cattle with wide forehead, prominent orbital arches, flat or dished in profile, deep body and powerful draught

capacity. Kenkatha, Malvi and Kherigarh breeds belong to the second category of draught cattle.

3. Mysore type, characterized by prominent forehead with long and pointed horns which rise close together. Hallikar, Amritmahal, Khillari, Bargur and Kangayam breeds are Mysore type of draught cattle which are very hardy and suitable for fast road work.
4. Small black, red or dun cattle, often with large patches of white markings, either short-horned or slightly lyre-horned. Ponwar and Siri are notable draught breeds of this group.

14.3 General Utility Breed

These cattle breeds are dual purpose animals. The cows are fairly good milk-yielders and the bullocks are good for draught purposes. So, animals have characteristics intermediate between the strictly milch and draught breeds. The proportion of country's total cattle population accounted for specialized purposes is relatively small.

About 28 percent of the cattle breed are dual purpose breed in India. Cultivators prefer cattle for their draught power, while milch cattle are meant more useful for breeding bullocks than for producing milk.

Cattle of these breeds are used both for milk and for draught purposes. Hariana, Mewati, Kankrej, Rathi, Dangi, Gaolao, Krishna Valley and Ongole are important breeds of this category.

14.3.1 General Utility Breeds are of two types

1. Short-horned, white or light grey cattle with long coffin shaped skull and face, slightly convex in profile. Dangi, Hariana, Mewati (Koshi), Ongole, Gaolao, Lakhimi and Krishna Valley are good examples of first type of general utility breeds.
2. Lyre-horned, grey cattle, deep bodied with wide forehead, prominent orbital arches, flat or dished in profile and good draught capacity. Kankrej and Rathi are two important dual purpose breeds of Indian depicting characters of the second type of cattle.

Dual purpose breeds like Hariana, Kankrej, Rathi, Ongole, Deoni and Gaolao first calve between 45 to 55 months, produce between

600 to 1500 kg of milk and have a calving interval between 15 to 20 months.

The remaining 80 percent of the cattle are non descript which first calve descriptive at an age of 60 months, and produce about 500 kgs in a lactation and have a calving interval between 20 to 24 months.

15.0 Indian Cattle Breed

Milch Breed	Draught Breed	Dual Breed
1. Sahiwal	1. Hallikar	1. Hariana
2. Gir	2. Amritmahal	2. Kankrej
3. Red Sindhi	3. Khillari	3. Ongole
4. Tharparkar	4. Kherigarh	4. Deoni
	5. Kenkatha	5. Rathi
	6. Kangayam	6. Dangi
	7. Khariar	7. Krishna Valley
	8. Malvi	8. Gaolao
	9. Nimari	9. Mewati
	10. Nagori	10. Belahi
	11. Siri	11. Gangatiri
	12. Ponwar	12. Lakhimi
	13. Bargur	
	14. Bachaur	
	15. Punganur	
	16. Vechur	
	17. Umblachery	
	18. Pullikulam	
	19. Red Kandhari	
	20. Motu	
	21. Kosali	
	22. Malnad Gidda	
	23. Binjarpuri	
	24. Ghumusari	
	25. Badri	

16.0 Registered Breeds of Indian Cattle

S.No.	Breed	State	Purpose	Accession Number
1	Gir	Gujarat	Milch	INDIA_CATTLE_0400_GIR_03007
2	Red Sindhi	On organized farms only	Milch	INDIA_CATTLE_0000_REDSINDHI_03025
3	Sahiwal	Punjab and Rajasthan	Milch	INDIA_CATTLE_1617_SAHIWAL_03026
4	Tharparkar	Rajasthan	Milch	INDIA_CATTLE_1700_THARPARKAR_03028
5	Amritmahal	Karnataka	Draught	INDIA_CATTLE_0800_AMRITMAHAL_03001
6	Bachaur	Bihar	Draught	INDIA_CATTLE_0300_BACHAUR_03002
7	Bargur	Tamil Nadu	Draught	INDIA_CATTLE_1800_BARGUR_03003
8	Binjharpuri	Orissa	Draught	INDIA_CATTLE_1500_BINJHARPURI _03033
9	Ghumusari	Orissa	Draught	INDIA_CATTLE_1500_GHUMUSARI _03032
10	Hallikar	Karnataka	Draught	INDIA_CATTLE_0800_HALLIKAR_03008
11	Kangayam	Tamil Nadu	Draught	INDIA_CATTLE_1800_KANGAYAM_03010
12	Kenkatha	Uttar Pradesh and Madhya Pradesh	Draught	INDIA_CATTLE_2010_KENKATHA_03012
13	Kherigarh	Uttar Pradesh	Draught	INDIA_CATTLE_2000_KHERIGARH_03013
14	Khariar	Orissa	Draught	INDIA_CATTLE_1500_KHARIAR _03034
15	Khillari	Maharashtra and Karnataka	Draught	INDIA_CATTLE_1108_KHILLAR_03014
16	Kosali	Chhattisgarh	Draught	INDIA_CATTLE_2600_KOSALI _03036
17	Malvi	Madhya Pradesh	Draught	INDIA_CATTLE_1000_MALVI_03016

18	Motu	Orissa, Chhattisgarh	Draught	INDIA_CATTLE_1526_ MOTU _03031
19	Nagori	Rajasthan	Draught	INDIA_CATTLE_1700_ NAGORI_03018
20	Nimari	Madhya Pradesh	Draught	INDIA_CATTLE_1000_ NIMARI_03019
21	Ponwar	Uttar Pradesh	Draught	INDIA_CATTLE_2000_ PONWAR_03021
22	Pullikulam	Tamil Nadu	Draught	INDIA_CATTLE_1800_ PULIKULAM_03035
23	Punganur	Andhra Pradesh	Draught	INDIA_CATTLE_0100_ PUNGANUR_03022
24	Red Kandhari	Maharashtra	Draught	INDIA_CATTLE_1100_ REDKANDHARI_03024
25	Siri	Sikkim and West Bengal	Draught	INDIA_CATTLE_2221 _SIRI_03027
26	Umblachery	Tamil Nadu	Draught	INDIA_CATTLE_1800_ UMBLACHERY_03029
27	Vechur	Kerala	Draught	INDIA_CATTLE_0900_ VECHUR_03030
28	Dangi	Maharashtra and Madhya Pradesh	Dual	INDIA_CATTLE_1104_ DANGI_03004
29	Deoni	Maharashtra and Karnataka	Dual	INDIA_CATTLE_1108_ DEONI_03005
30	Gangatiri	Uttar Pradesh and Bihar	Dual	INDIA_CATTLE_2003_ GANGATIRI_03039
31	Gaolao	Maharashtra and Madhya Pradesh	Dual	INDIA_CATTLE_1110_ GAOLAO_03006
32	Hariana	Haryana, Uttar Pradesh and Rajasthan	Dual	INDIA_CATTLE_0520_ HARIANA_03009
33	Kankrej	Gujarat and Rajasthan	Dual	INDIA_CATTLE_0417_ KANKREJ_03011
34	Mewati	Rajasthan, Haryana and Uttar Pradesh	Dual	INDIA_CATTLE_1705_ MEWATI_03017
35	Krishna Valley	Karnataka	Dual	INDIA_CATTLE_0800_ KRISHNAVALLEY_03015

36	Ongole	Andhra Pradesh	Dual	INDIA_CATTLE_0100_ ONGOLE_03020
37	Rathi	Rajasthan	Dual	INDIA_CATTLE_1700_ RATHI_03023
38	Malnad Gidda	Karnataka	Draught	INDIA_CATTLE_0800_ MALNADGIDDA_03037
39	Belahi	Haryana and Chandigarh	Dual	INDIA_CATTLE_0532_ BELAHI _03038
40	Badri *	Hilly areas of Uttarakhand	Draught	INDIA_CATTLE_2400_ BADRI_03040
41	Lakhimi*	Assam		INDIA_CATTLE_0200_ LAKHIMI_03041

*India has registered first ever indigenous cattle breed from hilly areas of Uttarakhand State and North Eastern State of Assam in the year 2017, taking the number of "desi" cattle breeds to 41 of cow.

17.0 Breed wise Cattle Population

According to the 19th Livestock census report (2012), cattle contributed about 37.28 percent of the total livestock population in India, which is the highest contribution among the livestock species available in the country. As per Breed Survey Report (2013), cattle population in India is broadly categorized into indigenous, exotic and crossbred cattle. Cattle originated in the country are known as indigenous cattle. They belong to descript (identified) or non-descript (non-identified) animals. Cattle which have their origin in other countries are considered as exotic cattle. The most important exotic dairy cattle breeds available in India are Jersey (J) and Holstein Friesian (HF). Cattle which are produced by crossing of indigenous cattle with exotic breeds and have exotic inheritance, are described as crossbred cattle while cattle which are produced by using indigenous non-descript cattle with indigenous descript breed are called as graded cattle.

18.0 Estimated Number of Animals Under Indigenous Cattle Breed

S. No.	Breed Name	Pure (number)	Graded (number)	Total (number)	Percentage share with respect to total
1	Hariana	16,39,181	46,40,782	62,79,963	4.15
2	Gir	13,80,208	37,32,786	51,12,994	3.38
3	Sahiwal	10,92,459	37,89,835	48,82,294	3.23
4	Kankrej	19,45,094	10,83,185	30,28,279	2.00
5	Kosali	24,31,859	377	24,32,236	1.61
6	Khillari	11,02,359	9,11,993	20,14,352	1.33
7	Hallikar	12,11,242	5,96,690	18,07,932	1.20
8	Malvi	11,58,172	5,52,293	17,10,465	1.13
9	Bachaur	7,41,432	8,05,056	15,46,488	1.02
10	Rathi	8,65,921	3,71,588	12,37,509	0.82
11	Malnad Gidda	8,99,091	1,50,452	10,49,543	0.69
12	Tharparkar	1,97,291	5,35,182	7,32,473	0.48
13	Kenkatha	3,93,291	2,77,109	6,70,400	0.44
14	Ongole	1,15,905	5,18,621	6,34,526	0.42
15	Red Sindhi	59,642	4,97,744	5,57,386	0.37
16	Motu	4,69,320	67,438	5,36,758	0.36
17	Nagori	3,73,224	1,35,474	5,08,698	0.34
18	Red Kandhari	2,35,058	2,22,982	4,58,040	0.30
19	Nimari	3,41,828	1,11,805	4,53,633	0.30
20	Khariar	2,90,015	93,809	3,83,824	0.25
21	Deoni	1,51,236	2,00,364	3,51,600	0.23
22	Gaolao	1,21,538	2,01,145	3,22,683	0.21
23	Amritmahal	1,05,343	1,23,720	2,29,063	0.15
24	Kherigarh	75,116	1,24,135	1,99,251	0.13
25	Dangi	1,19,373	74,407	1,93,780	0.13
26	Kangayam	80,620	1,12,825	1,93,445	0.13
27	Binjharpuri	79,428	31,129	1,10,557	0.07
28	Ghumsuri	58,855	24,959	83,814	0.06
29	Umblachery	39,050	33,460	72,510	0.05
30	Mewati	14,773	18,167	32,940	0.02
31	Ponwar	20,067	7,900	27,967	0.02
32	Siri	12,171	5,578	17,749	0.01
33	Bargur	14,154	2,153	16,307	0.01
34	Krishna Valley	3,462	10,919	14,381	0.01
35	Pullikulum	7,352	2,733	10,085	0.01
36	Punganur	2,772	56	2,828	0.00
37	Vechur	1,065	1,414	2,479	0.00
	Descript/Breed	**1,78,48,967**	**2,00,70,265**	**3,79,19,232**	**25.08**
	Non-Descript	11,32,53,063	---	--	74.92
	Total Indigenous Cattle	**15,11,72,295**			

18.1 Indigenous Cattle: Descript and Non-descript

Besides the pure breeds, Breed Survey also considered estimation of total number of animals in specific breeds which have more than 50 percent phenotypic characteristics of a particular breed under the definition of graded breed of that particular indigenous breed. The above table shows the number of animals in various indigenous cattle breeds.

According to Breed Survey Report (2013), the highest contribution is from non-descript category of cattle which is about 74.92 percent of the total Indigenous cattle and rest 25.08 percent comes under descript indigenous cattle breed. Out of the remaining 25.08 percent, the highest contribution of about 4.15 percent is from Hariana Breed following which Gir and Sahiwal contribute over 3 percent each of total indigenous cattle. Besides, Kankrej breed contributes 2 percent of indigenous cattle, other breeds such as Kosali, Khillar, Hallikar, Malvi and Bachaur are also contributed over 1 percent each of the total indigenous cattle. The percentage contributions of top ten breeds in terms of their number in the indigenous cattle based on the estimation are depicted in the following graphical presentation. All other recognized breeds of cattle contribute less than 1 percent each of the total indigenous cattle.

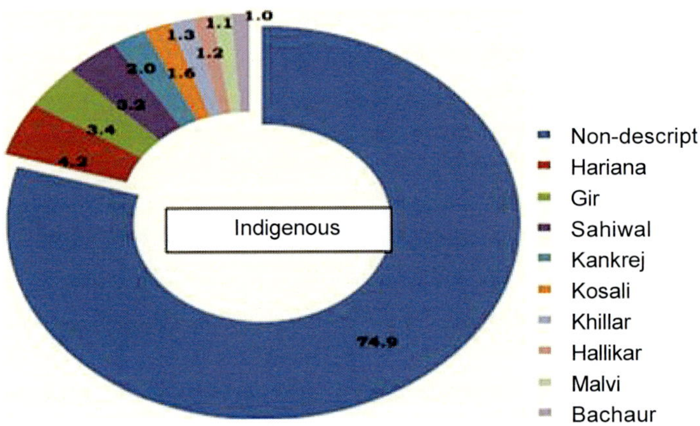

Fig. Percentage contribution of various major Indigenous breeds including non-descript cattle

The Following Graph gives a picture on the percentage share of 37 (Pure and graded) breeds excluding non-descript category. Among the individual breeds it shows that only 18 breeds are having their pure breeds more than 60 percent in number. In all other breeds (rest 19 breed) major contributions is from graded breeds.

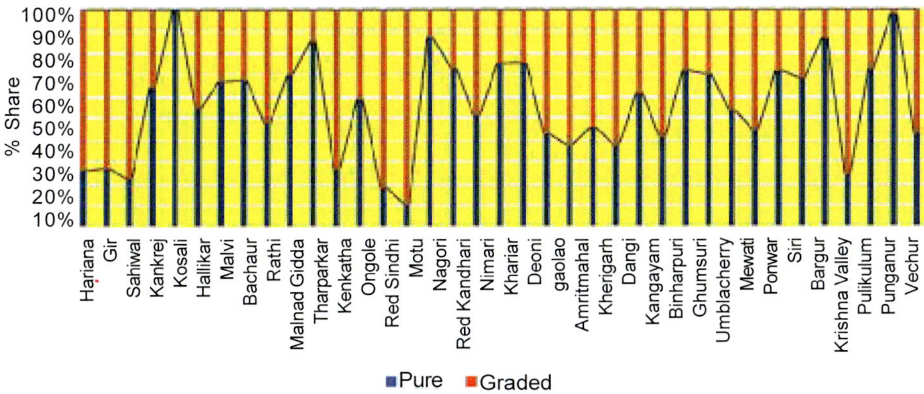

Fig. Percentage share between pure and graded cattle

At present in a total of 41 cattle breed available in India, out of these number, 37 breed were registered at NBAGR upto 2012 and rest four cattle breed got their registration after completing the last livestock census-2012. There are plenty amount of indigenous cattle remain undocumented. Therefore, extensive study needs to be conducted for their characterization as well as for their registration as new breeds in the cattle breed list of India.

18.2 Cattle Exotic and Crossbred

To enhance the milk production of the country, crossbreeding of our indigenous cattle is extensively practiced with the exotic cattle. The exotic and crossbred category is one of the high yielding categories of animals in cattle. According to the 19th Livestock Census Report, the exotic and crossbred animals contribute nearly 21 percent of the total cattle population. In the Breed Survey, the breeds namely Jersey, Crossbred Jersey, Holstein Friesian (HF) and Crossbred HF are considered under exotic and crossbred category. The following table shows the breed-wise number of animals.

18.2.1 Breed wise estimated number of animals under exotic and crossbred cattle

S.No.	Breed Name	No. of Animals
1	Jersey	
	Pure	6,75,647
	Crossbred	2,29,54,211
	Total Jersey	**2,36,29,858**
2	Holstein Friesian	
	Pure	6,43,859
	Crossbred	1,54,58,093
	Total Holstein Friesian	**1,61,01,952**
	Total number of Exotic and Crossbred cattle	**3,97,31,810**

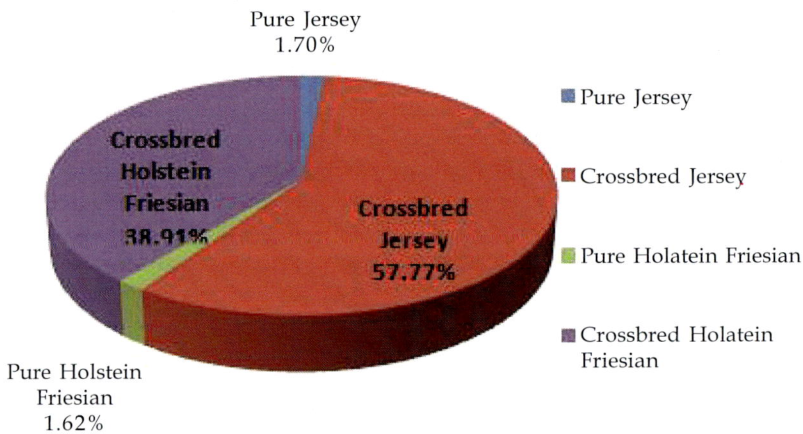

Fig. Percentage share of various breeds in exotic/crossbred cattle

It is observed from the graph that the crossbred Jersey has the highest share of 57.77 percent as compared to 38.91 percent of crossbred Holstein Friesian. The pure exotic category has a share with 1.70 percent in Jersey and 1.62 percent in Holstein Friesian. Hence, crossbreeding of our indigenous cattle with exotic Jersey cattle is more predominant than exotic Holstein cattle owing to their small body size for which they need less amount of food.

19.0 Indian Cattle Breed Based on Coat Colour

Based on coat colour characteristics the Indigenous cattle genetic resources can be grouped as follows:

1. **Red / Dark Red / Pale Red / Fawn / Brown / Chocolate-Brown Colour**

   About 29% Indian cattle breeds comes under this coat colour. The indigenous cattle come under this coat colour are Gir, Red Sindhi, Sahiwal, Red Kandhari, Vechur, Motu, Kosali, Malnad Gidda, Nimari, Belahi, Badri and Lakshimi.

2. **Spotted Colour**

   About 10% of Indian cattle breeds comes under this coat colour. Deoni, Dangi, Bargur and Rathi are the Indigenous cattle having such type of coat colour.

3. **Black and White Colour**

   Only 5% cattle breed of India having such coat colour. Coat colour of Siri and Ponwar cattle are Black and White.

4. **Grey / Dark Grey/ Silver Grey/ Iron Grey Colour**

   About 17% cattle breed of India having this type of coat colour. Kankrej, Kenkatha, Kangayam, Hallikar, Amritmahal, Pullikulam/Alambadi, Umblachery having such coat colour.

5. **White/Grey Colour**

   Maximum Indian cattle breed are in this colour. It is about 39%. Hariana, Tharparkar, Ongole, Nagori, Gangatri, Binjharpuri, Khillari, KrishnaValley, Bachaur, Ghumusari, Malvi, Khariar, Gaolao, Mewati, Punganur, Kherigarh are main bearers of such type coat colour.

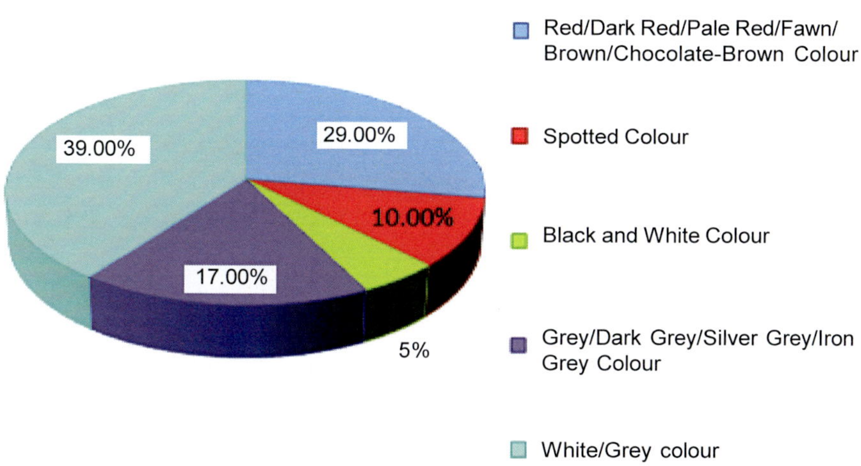

Fig. Colourwise Indian Cattle Breed

20.0 Breed Description of Indian Cattle

The description especially for Origin, Breeding tract, Distinguish Feature and Performance of the Forty One distinct Indigenous cattle breed are emphatically described in details as follows:

1. Sahiwal

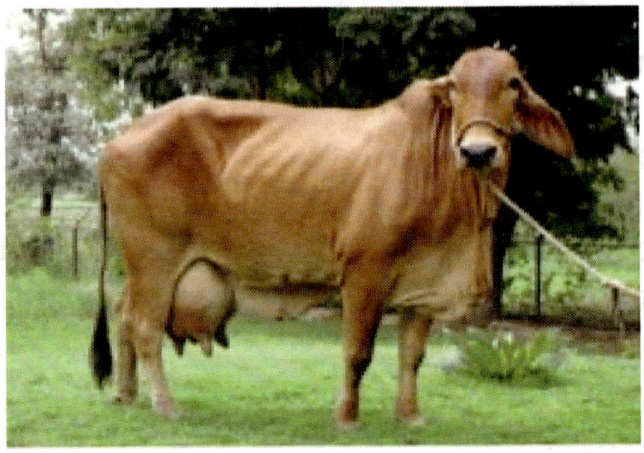

Synonym: Lola, Montgomery, Lambi-Bar, Multani, Teli

Origin and Distribution: The Sahiwal breed has its origin in the Montogomery district of Pakistan which is now named as Sahiwal district of Pakistan and is widely raised in Punjab, Haryana, Rajasthan, Uttar Pradesh and Delhi. This breed derives its name from Sahiwal area in Mantogomery district of Punjab (Pakistan). A few herds of pure Sahiwal cattle are available around Fazilka and Abohar towns of Ferozepur district.

Morphological Characteristics: It is comparatively a heavy breed with symmetrical body and loose skin (hence the name lola), when compared with Red Sindhi with which it closely resembles. The animals are usually long, fleshy with heavier body built but lethargic. Navel flap is prominent in female. Broad head, prominent foreheads, voluminous dewlaps, short legs. Lateral and even-curled short thick stumpy horns, do not exceed 3 inches. Long whip like tail almost reaching the ground, tapering to a good black switch. The general colour is reddish dun or pale red, sometimes flashed with patches. They are usually spotted either red or white, or are of various shades of red and white or solid red dun or brown. The distinguishing feature between Sahiwal and Red Sindhi is muzzle. Red Sindhi has dark-coloured muzzle whereas Sahiwal has lighter coloured muzzle. Sahiwal has also a whitish ring along the eyes. Muzzle and eye-lashes are light in colour. Male weighs on an averge 540 kgs while female 327 kgs.

Performances: The milk yield ranges from 1400 to 2500 kg In village the average milk yield is 2150 kg in 300 days lactation while at some of the farmers the herd average has gone up to four to five thousand kilogrammes. The fat percentage ranges from 4.9 to 5.1 percent with average 4.9 percent. The age at first calving ranges from 37 to 48 months and the calving interval is from 430 to 580 days. The bullocks of this breed are lethergic but useful for slow work.

Remarks: Sahiwal is one of the most popular dairy breeds of the sub-continent. This breed thrives well in all parts of India, and high milk yields have been achieved. This cattle breed has been extensively used for breed improvement programme in India. It is used both as a pure breed, for upgrading of unimproved cattle and for crossbreeding with European breeds. Sahiwal has made important contributions to most of the new breeds of Zebu x Temperate cattle. Pedigree Sahiwal bulls are in great demand in other tropical countries of the world for breeding purposes. It has been exported to Sri Lanka, Kenya, many countries in Latin America and West Indies where a new breed called Jamaica Hope has been evolved out of Sahiwal and Jersey crossbreeds.

2. Red Sindhi

Synonym: Red Karachi, Sindhi, Malir.

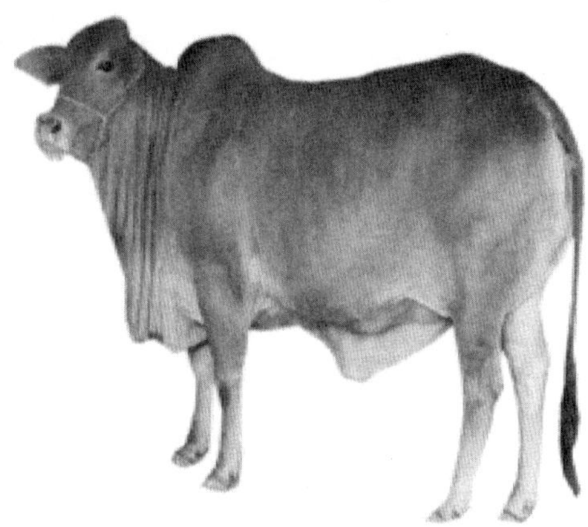

Origin and Distribution: This breed is one of the most distinct cattle breeds of India. Red Sindhi is considered to have originated from Las Bela cattle found in the state of Bela, Baluchistan. They originated from the Kohistan, Sindh Province presently in Pakistan. The home tract of this breed is in Karachi and Hyderabad districts of Pakistan. Red Sindhi are found over a fairly large area of Sindh Province, and in the border districts of India. It is found in pure form only in the areas of its origin and elsewhere in an impure state due to infusion of their blood with the grey colour breeds. The Sindhi breed is mainly raised in Gujarat, Rajasthan and Maharashtra although it can be raised in several other parts of the country due to its disease resistant quality.

Morphological Characteristics: Medium size and well-proportioned compact body frame. Pendulous dewlap with round drooping quarters. Thick horns emerging laterally and end in blunt point. They are extremely docile and intelligent facial expression is a notable characteristic of this breed. The colour is red with the shades varying from dark red to brown. Specks of white colour are sometimes seen on the dewlap and occasionally on the forehead. Male weighs, on an average 450 kg while female 295 kg.

Performances: They are fairly regular breeders. Milk production in the herds maintained in the institutions ranges from 1250 to 1800 kg. Age at first calving is between 39 to 50 months and the calving interval is of 425 to 540 days. Red Sindhi bullocks are medium sized, compact animals with good bone and muscle. They are steady workers, useful for field operations and for working on the roads.

Remarks: Red Sindhi cows are high milk-yielders and are perhaps the most economical milk producers among the Indian breeds of cattle and are second only to that of Sahiwal. Owing to their small size, adaptability to varying climatic conditions and capacity to resist common diseases, Red Sindhi cattle are extensively used in India for grading up local stock in some parts of the country, particularly Assam, Orissa, Kerala, and parts of Madras. This cattle breed had also been used for crossbreeding purposes to develop new breeds such as Karan Swiss at NDRI, Karnal, Haryana. Red Sindhi has also been exported out of its native tract to many other parts of the world including Sri Lanka, Tanzania, Philippines, USA, Malaysia, Iraq, Cuba, Korea, Japan, Burma and Indo-China.

3. Gir

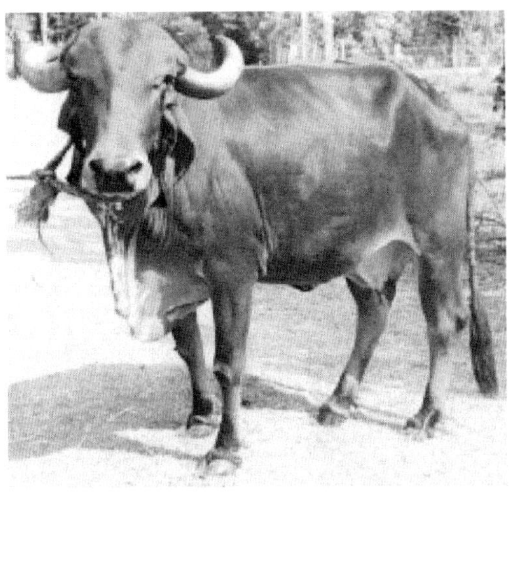

Synonym: Kathiawarhi, Surati, Desan, Sorthi, Gujarati.

Origin and Distribution: Gir cattle breed is originated from Gir forest in the State of Gujarat. They are mainly found in Junagarh of south Khathiawar of Gujarat and western part of Rajasthan. Gir blood can be detected in various breeds in the surrounding areas on account of their habit of covering a wide area in search of suitable grazing. This breed of cattle named after the Gir forest, the geographical/origin of the breed. Gir cattle are largely reared by professional breeders known as Rabaris, Bhanoads, Maldharis, Ahirs and Charans.

Morphological Characteristics: Appearance of Gir cattle is strikingly impressive. They have well-proportioned ponderous body built with heavy dewlap. The head is moderately long but massive in appearance with prominent bony forehead, straight and leveled back are the most marking characters of this breed. Eyes are partially close in appearance. Ears are long pendulous frontward turned, folded like leaf, notch at the tip. Tail is long, whip-like with a black switch at the end. Horns are even-curled lateral horns, starting at the base of crown, downward, upward and again upward, half-moon in appearance. The popular colour is dark red/brown or chocolate-brown patches distributed all over the body. Its peculiar features are prominent protruding-broad and convex-long forehead and markedly pendulous frontwards turned ears resembling a tiny curled leaf. Adult body weight of male cattle is about 544 kg while female is about 310 kg.

Performances: Gir cows are good milker. The milk yield ranges from 1200 to 1800 kg. The average milk fat % is 4.6 and varies from 3.9 to 5.1%.The age at first calving varies from 45 to 54 months and the intercalving period from 515 to 600 days. The bullocks of this breed are heavy, powerful animals but are medium paced in movement. They are extensively used as draught animals. They are known for its tolerance to stress condition.

Remarks: This is one of the best known dairy breed of cattle in India. Gir is world-renowned breed known for its tolerance to stress condition. This cattle breed is extensively used for breeding in different coastal parts of India for genetic improvement of our non descriptive indigenous cattle. They are exported to other countries, particularly to the tropical countries, for grading up purposes. The Gir breed has been most popular for export to the other parts of the world. In Brazil where large herds are found, it is known as Gyr. Brazil has also evolved a strain called InduBrasil which is a cross between Gir and Kankrej. Gir animals are highly prized by Brazilian breeders and they have a Breed Society. Gir has also been exported to the USA, especially to Texas, Florida and Lousiana states.

4. Red Kandhari

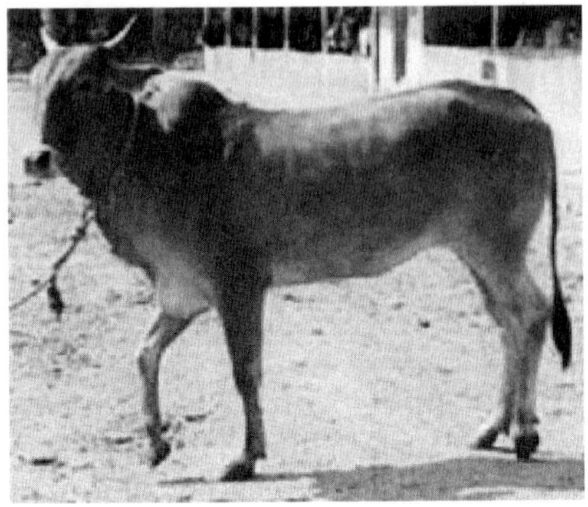

Synonym: Lal Kandhari, Lakhalbunda

Origin and Distribution: Red Kandhari cattle breed is known to have originated from Kandhar Taluk of Nanded district of Maharashtra state. The breeding tract of Red Kandhari cattle breed comprises of Latur, Parbahni, Nanded and Hingoli districts of Maharashtra. They are also commonly found in adjoining North Karnataka region. The breed is known to have got royal patronage from King Somadevaraya who ruled over Kandhar in 4 A.D. The climate of the breeding tract is dry and semiarid.

This breed having red colour and common Kandhar tehsil of Nanded district also naturally acquires the name Red Kandhari.

Morphological Characteristics: Red Kandhari cattle breed is of medium size, strong and compact body and good looking, robust in appearance. On an average, cows have 109 cm body length, 128 cm height at wither, 150 cm heart girth, 46 cm face length, 24 cm ear length, 16 cm long horn and 75 cm long tail up to the switch. The corresponding figures in bullocks are 118, 131, 109, 48, 24, 21 and 85 cm, respectively. Horns are evenly curved and medium in length.

The eyes are having black coloured rings around it. The black ring encircles around the coronet forming a ring. Navel flap is very small in cows. Sheath is very much tucked-up to the body. Tail is well set on the body and fairly broad, tapering, moderately long with a black switch which extends below hocks and coronet. Udder is small and tucked up. Teats are small but squarely placed.

The colour is uniform deep dark red, but variations from a dull red to almost dark brown are also found. Red Kandhari is locally known as Lal Kandhari. They are named so because of their almost universal deep red coloured skin. Skin is tightly drawn over the body with small short glossy hair. The breeding bulls are shade darker than cow. The adult body weight is 430 kg for male and 340 kg for female.

Performances: The lactation milk yield, fat percent, lactation length and dry period range from 400-600 kg, 4.5%, 230-270 days and 130-190 days, respectively. The age at first calving, service period and calving interval range from 30-45 months, 120-170 days and 360-700 days, respectively. Cows are low milk producers and bullocks of the breed are preferred over the Deoni breed for better draught ability and smaller size. The bullocks are used for heavy agricultural work like ploughing and carting as well as for transportation.

Remarks: Kandhari cattle are widely used for draught purposes, mainly for heavy works. The animals are maintained under extensive management system on grazing only in small herds. The survey conducted revealed that animals of this breed are sufficient in number and needs immediate attention to improve milk yield and draught ability.

5. Vechur

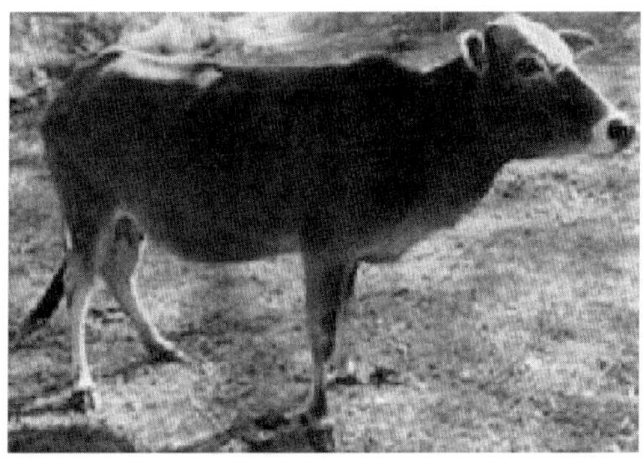

Synonym: Dwarf cattle

Origin and Distribution: The home tract of this breed is Vechur of Kerala. The Vechur cattle is a rare breed of *Bos indicus* cattle named after the village Vechur in Kottayam district of the state of Kerala in India. Vechur cow got its ancient name from the village where it is supposed to have evolved. The Vechur cow was popular in Kerala until the 1960s, but became rare when native cattle were crossbred with exotic varieties. As a result of crossbreeding, the number of indigenous cattle gradually dwindled and by the 1980's the Vechur cattle became almost extinct. In 2000, the Vechur cow was listed on the FAO's World Watch List of Domestic Animal Diversity, in its 'Critical-Maintained Breeds List', as the number of breeding females and males fall to very low level.

The Vechur animals were saved from extinction due to conservation efforts by Dr. Sosamma Iype, Professor of Animal Breeding and Genetics along with a team of her students. In 1989, a conservation unit was started. A conservation trust was formed in 1998 to continue the work with farmer participation. Kerala Agricultural University had taken a project to conserve this breed. The number of cows with the farmers has increased and they find it very suitable and sustainable to raise them. About 200 cows are supposed to exist today, nearly 100 of them with the Veterinary College of KAU, Kerela, India.

Morphological Characteristics: This breed of cattle is extremely small and compact body size. Head is long and narrow. Horms are small, curving forward and downdard. Tail is long. The breed has average body length of 124 cm and height of 87 cm. The coat colour of Vechur cattle is light red, black, fawn and white. The adult body weight of this cattle is around 130 kg.

Performances: This breed of cattle is very poor in milk production. Their average lactational yield is about 561 kg. Fat% ranges from 4.7 to 5.8%. Age at first calving and calving interval, on an average is 36 and 14 months, respectively. Cow yields up to 3 kgs of milk in a day. This is much less than that of the hybrid varieties but, unlike them, the Vechur cow requires little feed or maintenance.

The milk is believed to have medicinal qualities and easy digestibility due to smaller fat globule size. A recent report claims that the milk of the Vechur cow has more of the beta casein variety A_2, rather than the variety A_1 which is implicated in conditions like diabetes, ischaemic heart disease and autism.

The medicinal property of the Vechur cow's milk has been documented traditionally by Ayurveda and recent scientific studies have substantiated this. The protein component of the Vechur cow's milk has an improved antimicrobial property. As per recent findings, the anti-bacterial property of the lactoferrin protein present in the Vechur Cow milk is more than that of the antibiotic ampicillin. Although lactoferrin, present in the milk of all mammals, is found to have antimicrobial, antiviral, antitumor, immunodefence and anti-inflammatory properties, recent studies prove that in the case of the lactoferrin protein in the Vechur Cow milk, these properties are much more enhanced. The Vechur Ghee (clarified butter) produced from Vechur cow's milk, is famous for its high medicinal values due to the presence of A_2 beta-lactalbumin protein and higher arginine content which is good for the health of convalescing people.

Remarks: It is the smallest cattle breed in the world according to the Guinness Book of Records and is valued for the larger amount of milk it produces relative to the amount of food it requires. A controversy arose in 1997 when environmentalist Vandana Shiva alleged that a Scottish company, The Roslin Institute was trying to patent the cow's genetic code. Shiva described the action as piracy. The Roslin Institute denied the charge which was subsequently proved to be baseless.

6. Motu

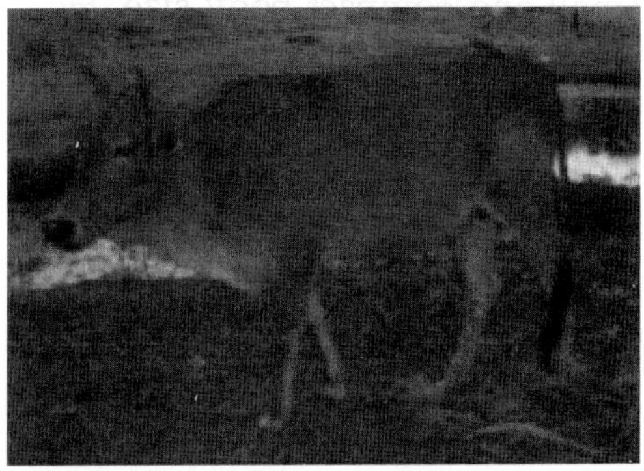

Synonym: Deshi

Origin and Distribution: The breed is named after local area "Motu" of Malkangiri district in Orissa. Sandy and clay type soil is predominant in this area. The common breeding tracts of this breed are southern part of Malkangiri district and adjoining area of Chhattisgarh and Andhra Pradesh. Heavy concentration is in Motu, Kalimela, Podia and Malkangiri area of Malgangiri district in Orissa. Most of the area is covered with forest. This breed are generally reared by Koya tribes of Orissa.

Morphological Characteristics: Coat colour is mainly brown (reddish) and sometimes grey. Few animals are white in colour also. Though the breed is small sized but they are strong in built. Horms are straight, upward with rounded tip. Animals are mostly polled. The average height(cm), body length(cm), heart girth(cm) and adult weight(kg) are 102, 107, 128 and 172 kg for male. The respective figures for female are 99, 104, 116 and 137 kg.

Performances: Milk production of these cattle is low. These dwarf cattle are used for draught purpose in hilly and undulated terrain. The average age at first calving is 53 months and calving interval is 14 months. The cows are very poor milker and their milk yield varies from 100 to 140 kg per lactation.

Remarks: They are fairly regular breeders. Small separate milk and drought breed live on scanty grazing under the open air condition throughout the year.

7. Kosali

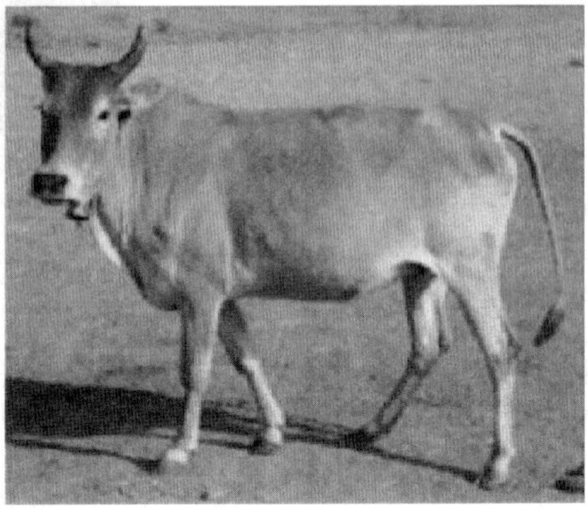

Synonym: Nil

Origin and Distribution: The breed is predominantly seen in the plains of Chhattisgarh and the breeding tract includes Raipur, Durg, Bilaspur and Janjgir districts. The ancient name of this region was 'Kowshal' named after the maternal uncle house of Lord Ram. So the name of this cattle breed is Kosali. Farmers particularly of Yadava/Rawuth community are keeping this breed of cattle, generation after generation.

Morphological Characteristics: Kosali is small sized cattle breed. Horns are stumpy, emerging straight, then going outward, upward, and inward from the polls. Muzzle, eyelids, tail switch and hooves are black. Broad head with flat and straight forehead. Hump is small to medium in size. Udder is small and bowl shaped. Most predominant colour is light red, followed by whitish grey. Few animals having black coat colour or red with white patches are also seen. Mature body weight of male and female is 260 and 160 kg, respectively.

Performances: The lactation yield ranges from 200 to 250 kg with average fat % from 3 to 4.5. The average age at first calving is 53 months that ranges from 48 to 60 months. Calving interval ranges from 18 to 24 months. These are mainly reared for manure, draught and milk. Bullocks of this breed are very efficient for ploughing and other operations in the paddy fields. Farmers prefer bullocks of this breed for cleaning of weeds from paddy field.

Remarks: Animals are known for very efficient working ability and high disease resistance. They are draft purpose cattle breed of Chhattisgarh.

8. Malnad Gidda

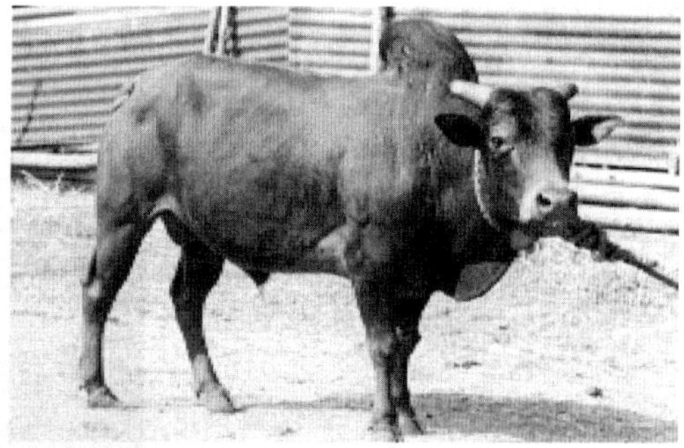

Synonym: Uradana, Varshagandhi, Malenadu Gidda.

Origin and Distribution: 'Malnad' means a hilly region receiving heavy rainfall, where these cattle are inhabited and 'Gidda' means small or dwarf. Malnad Gidda is a short statured dwarf breed of cattle native to the hilly, rainy and densely forested Malnad region of the Western Ghats in the state of Karnataka in India. The breeding tract of this breed includes Chikmagalur, Dakshin Kannada, Hassan, Kodagu, Shimoga, Uttar Kannada and Udupi districts of Karnataka.

Morphological Characteristics: Malnad Gidda cattle are small sized compact body frame animals. Average body length, height at withers and chest girth are 87, 90, and 118 cm for female and 86, 91 and 118 cm for adult male, respectively, indicate the small size of Malnad Gidda breed among all the known cattle breeds of India. Horns are generally small, straight, outward, upward and inward. Tail switch is black in color, hump is small, udder is also small and bowl shaped. The predominant coat colour is black with light shades of fawn on thigh and shoulder region. There are 5 coat colours found in these animals (black, brown, red, fawn and white, sometimes mixture of any two colour) but black colour is predominant.

Performances: The age at first calving of cows, service period, dry period and calving interval are 38 months, 45 months, 8 months, 7 months and 17 months, respectively. Elite cows give 3-5 kg of milk per day and the average lactation yield is around 220 kg.

Remarks: Animals of this breed are playing a significant role in the rural livelihood of Malnad area of Karnataka in terms of draught, milk and manure with negligible inputs. The population of the breed is about 7-8 lakh in Karnataka but is showing a declining trend. There is a need to take up systematic genetic improvement programme and sustainable measures for the conservation of population of this breed. They have excellent endurance power and resistance to diseases.

They are well adapted to the local agro-ecological systems of Western Ghats. Malnad Gidda cattle are reared under low input system. In some areas, it is zero input system where animals sustain solely on grazing. These animals are highly adapted to harsh climate including heavy rainfall.

Malnad Gidda, the dwarf variety of cattle native to Malnad region known for their extreme shyness, has got national recognition now.

9. Nimari

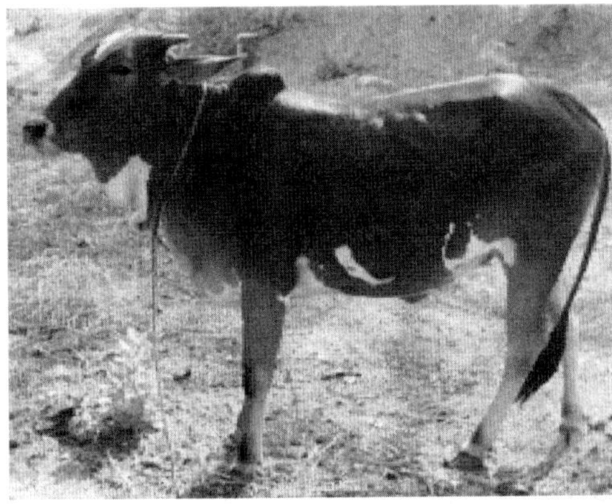

Synonym: Khargaon, Khargoni, Khurgoni, Biological Engine of Nimari, Chitkabri

Origin and Distribution: Nimari breed is believed to be originated from the cross of Gir and Khillari breeds along the Narmada valley around Maheshwar and Barwani region of West Nimar tract of the Madhya Pradesh. The home tract is concentrated in central part of Khargone and Barwani district. The border of Kharone district towards Khandwa, Indore and Dewas has also thin population of Nimari breed of cattle. Gir blood has contributed to its coat colour, massive body structure and convexity of forehead, and Khillari blood to its hardiness, agility and temper. This breed named after place of its origin i.e. Nimari region.

Morphological Characteristics: Nimari breed of cattle have long ponderous body built with pendulous dewlap. The body is long with straight back. The head is moderately long with a somewhat bulging prominent flat forehead, long and narrow face. Skin is fine and slightly loose. Eye canthus is pink in color. Horns are generally medium in size having pinkish brown color which emerge from outer angles of poll in outwards direction and carried upwards with a gentle curve to turn at points. The horns are similar to that in the Gir breed. The peculiarity of the animals lies in their hooves; they can withstand rough wear and tear on stony ground. The breed is hence popular on account of its working capacity in rough areas. Nimari cattle are usually red dun or brown in colour with white patches on various parts of the body. Due to spots or patches they are also called as Chitkabri in local Nimari language. Adult body weight is 390 kg for male and 339 kg for female.

Performances: The average daily milk yield is around 2.5 kg. The annual milk yield is 600 to 954 kg, and they are more of draft type animals. The average lactation and dry period are 298 and 221 days, respectively. The average age at maturity and age at first calving are 44 and 54 months, respectively. The average service period and calving interval are 235 and 552 days, respectively. The average gestation period is 271 days.

Remarks: Nimari cattle are efficient both as draught animals and milk producers. Animals are energetic and vigorous but nervous with strangers.

10. Belahi

Synonym: Morni, Desi

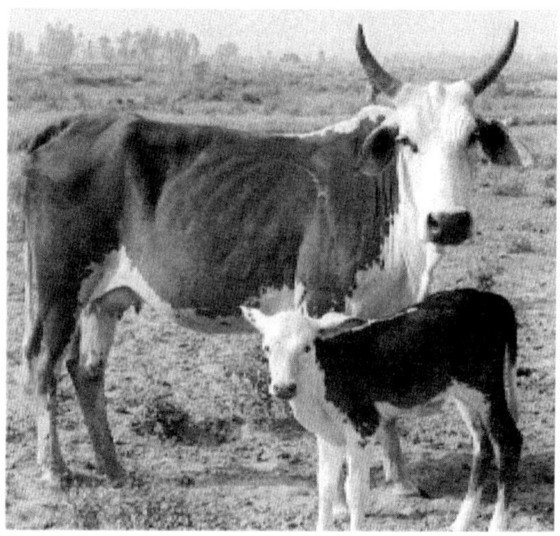

Origin and Distribution: Its home tract is Panchkula and Chandigarh of Haryana. The main breeding tract of this cattle is Ambala, Panchkula, Yamunagar and Chandigarh district of Haryana State. Breeding tract lies in the foot hills of Shivalik in Haryana. The Gujjars of Shivalik known as Langarias are rearing and improving this particular breed from decades. This breed got registered in January, 2016. Belahi is 39th registered indigenous cow breed of our country. The name derived from Belaha means mixture of colors. Belahi cattle are migratory in nature and are maintained on low input cost. Migration starts in February-March and ends in October-November, every year.

Morphological Characteristics: Medium size body with coffin-shaped skull. Prominent orbital arches and erect ears. Black coloured muzzle. Tail reaching upto hock joint and switch is white in colour. Short stumpy horns curving upward and inward in direction like sickle shape. They are red dun/fawn in colour but their head is white in colour. White patches are also seen at belly and legs. Head is straight and broad with prominent poll. The average adult body weight is 305 kg for male and 267 kg for female.

Morphometric measurements of adult cattle from its breeding tract reveal that average face length is 43 cm, face width 14 cm, horn length 25 cm, horn circumference 14 cm, ear length 27 cm, body height 120 cm, body length 116 cm, chest girth 157 cm, pouch girth 159 cm, hip bone 34 cm, pin bone 15 cm, tail length 110 cm and tail length up to switch 93 cm.

Performances: On an average, lactional yield of the cattle is 1014 kg. It varies from 182 to 2092 kg. The Fat% is on an average 5.25% varies from 2.37 to 7.89%. The age at first calving ranges from 30 to 46 months and calving interval ranges from 12 to 15 months. They are mainly used for milk, draught and manure.

Remarks: Belahi cattle are unique but distinct germplasm under migration in Shivalik region of Haryana. According to rough estimation, the population of Belahi cattle is 20 to 25 thousand in the region with herd size ranging from 20 to 90 cows and 2–3 bulls.

11. Deoni

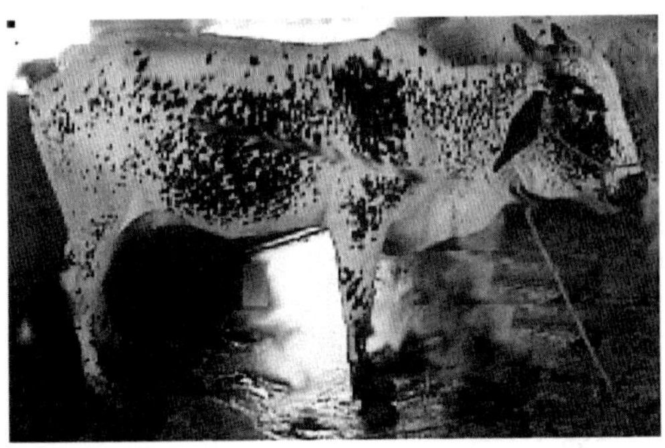

Synonym: Dongarpatti, Dangari (which means 'of the hill')

Origin and Distribution: The actual place of origin is Deoni, Udgir and Ahmadpur Taluk of Latur district of Maharashtra. Its native tract is in the western Andhra Pradesh and Bidar district of Karnataka. The Deoni breed is widely raised in north-western and western parts of Andhra Pradesh, Parbhni, Nanded, Osmanabad and Latur district or Maharashtra. The Deoni breed of cattle has been evolved from the mixture of Gir, Dangi and local cattle about 500 years back. It resembles Gir in size and spotted body and may possess an admixture of other blood. Contribution from the Gir type of the cattle is quite evident in formation of the head and ears, and also of the horns to a certain extent. The breed also shows a great similarity in general conformation and ruggedness to the Dangi cattle breed of Maharastra state. The breed derived its name from Deoni Taluk of Latur district.

Morphological Characteristics: They are more ponderous (heavy) in body built and have pendulous dewlap. Forehead: Prominent, slight bulged. Ears: Grey white with black inside, drooping. Ears unlike Gir breed have no notch near the tip. Horns: Emerge from side of poll behind and above the eyes in upward, outward and backward direction.

They are usually spotted and either red or white, or are of various shades of red and white or solid red dun or brown. Colour is black and white or red and white with irregular patches or spots.

It is found in three colour variations viz. Wannera, Balankya and Shevera. Clear white in Wannera and Balankya strains, whereas irregular black spots are there on all over the white body in Shevera. The head is partially white in Wannera. It is black in colour at the sides i.e. on the cheek and behind the eyes. Sometimes complete black coloured head is observed. In Balankya complete white body and head is observed except black coloured spots are seen on lower side of body or in between hind legs and on the fore or hind legs (knee joint, hock joint and cannon). The three strains are more or less similar in general appearance but comparatively the Wannera and Balankya are completely similar in body conformation and size and the Shevera is slightly smaller in size. Hence, these three strains are Shevera (Black and white spotted), Balankya (White, without spot) and Wannera (White, partial black face). Complete white head is observed at birth in all the strains and it appears slightly black in Wannera and Shevera after 2-3 months.

Performances: The lactational milk yield varies from 638 to 1229 kg with average 868 kg. Fat% averages 4.3% ranges from 2.5 to 5.3%. Age at first calving avarages 45 months and varies from 42 to 48 months. The calving interval is 14 months ranges from 13 to 17 months. The adult body weight of this cattle is 590 kg and 340 kg for male and female, respectively. Male calves are nursed better. Calves are not weaned. The bullocks are good for heavy work and are particularly suitable for intensive cultivation. Certain farmers have selected cows for high milk production.

Remarks: They are popular in the tracts of former Hyderabad state which now forms parts of Andhra Pradesh and adjoining Karnataka. Pure strains of this breed are being evolved in the farms at Udgir, Maharashtra State.

12. Dangi

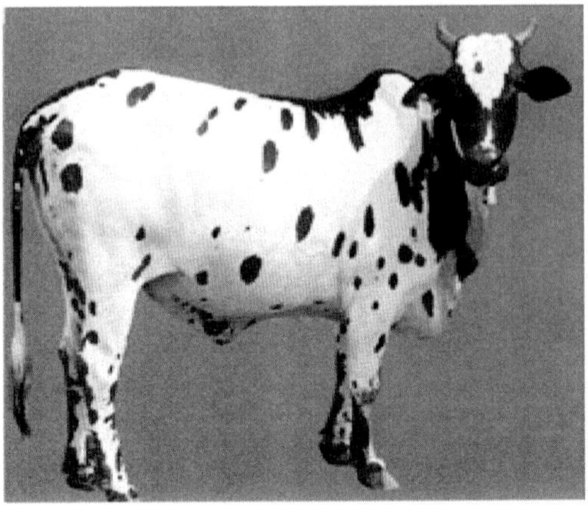

Synonym: Kandadi

Origin and Distribution: This breed is probably evolved from a cross between Gir and local cattle. The home tract of this breed is Ahmednagar, Thane and Nasik districts of Maharashtra called as Dangs Ghat. Generally these animals are found near the hilly tract where forest is available in the ranges of Sahyadri. In Marathi Dang means mountains and these animals are living in mountains. Hence, these are called Dangi. Some believe that this originated from the Dangs deistrict in Gujarat. The synomym name Kandadi suggests the origin of the breed from Karnataka.

Dangi breeders are semi-nomadie, belongs to Kandli, Mahadeo Kali, Konkana, Thakar and Maratha communities.

Morphological Characteristics: The Animals are medium in size with deep body built. They have pendulous dewlap. The head is usually small with prominent protruding forehead. The muzzle is large, the ears are small, and the horns are short and thick. Lateral and even-curled horn. Hooves are black, flint like, very hard. They have usually white with brown or black spots all over the body and shining coat. Skin exudes oil secretion which protect, them from rain. Mature body weight is 317 kg for male and 228 kg for female.

Performances: On an average milk yield is 430 kg varies from 175 to 800 kg per lactation. Fat% is 4.3 ranges for 3.8 to 4.5%. Age at first calving average 53 months varies from 46 to 56 months. Calving interval ranges from 17 to 21 months and average is 19 months. Though the cows are not good milkers, the bullocks are popular in heavy rainfall tracts.

Remarks: Draught, medium to heavy size, known for excellent working qualities in heavy rainfall areas.

13. Bargur

Synonym: Nil

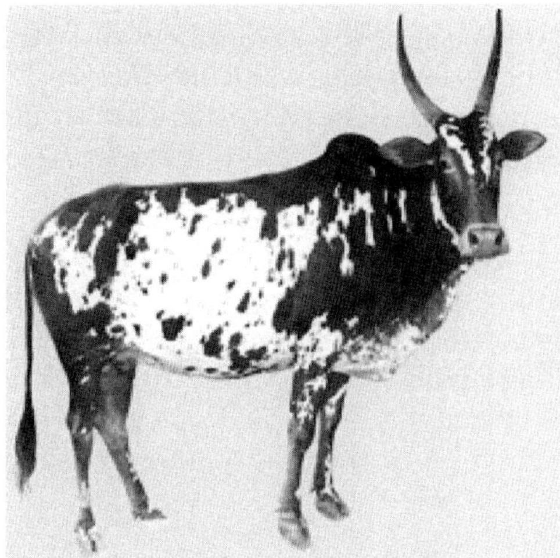

Origin and Distribution: Bargur, the hilly cattle of Tamil Nadu, India is reared mostly inside the forests and is surviving under zero-input condition. Home Tract of this breed is Bargur hill forest in Bhavani taluk in district of Tamil Nadu. Their home tract is restricted to a narrow geographical area in and around Bargur hill at an elevation of about 1000 m above the sea level. The appearance of these cattle resembles Hallikar cattle. The Bargur cattle are tended by hired local tribal labours called lingaiys.

Morphological Characteristics: This is medium-sized, well built compact and attractive animals, having powerful quarters and tight sheaths. Limbs are thin and bony. The most striking characteristics are the formation of head and horns. Forehead is slightly prominent and has a deep furrow between the roots of the horns. The horns emerge from the top of the poll fairly close together in an upward and backward direction. Horns are light brown in colour, closer at roots, sharp at the tip. The distinguishing morphological features of these cattle include its typical brown colour with white patches and being compact in size. The average body length, height at withers and heart girth are 99 cm, 108 cm and 139 cm in cows and 109 cm, 117 cm and 152 cm for adult males, respectively. The mature weight is 340 kg for male and 295 kg for female.

Performances: The average daily milk yield of Bargur cattle is 468 g with a range of 330 g to 790 g. The average milk yield per lactation of Bargur cattle is reported as 350 kg and ranges from 250-1300 kg. The daily milk yield in Bargur cattle is lower compared to other draught breeds of Tamil Nadu. The overall milk fat, solid not fat and total solids content are 5.65, 8.06, and 13.99 percent, respectively. The average age at first estrus is 30 months. The average age at first calving is 40 months. Average calving interval for Bargur cows is 12 to 18 months. Animals are mostly maintained for dung and draft in the breeding tract. Bullocks are unsurpassable in hardiness, spirit and speed and endurance in trotting which inturn mainly used for work in uneven hilly terrains. This cattle are very sensitive and fiery in disposition and are difficult to train. They are light in built and are developed mainly for carrying out agricultural operations in the uneven and hilly terrain.

Remarks: Bargur, fiery hilly drought cattle breed is cautious in behaviour and tend to remain away from strangers. In the last three decades, the population of these animals has declined drastically by about 90% (to less than 10,000) due to various reasons. There is a strong and urgent need to make efforts for conservation so that the extinction of this valuable germplasm may be avoided.

14. Rathi

Synonym: Rath

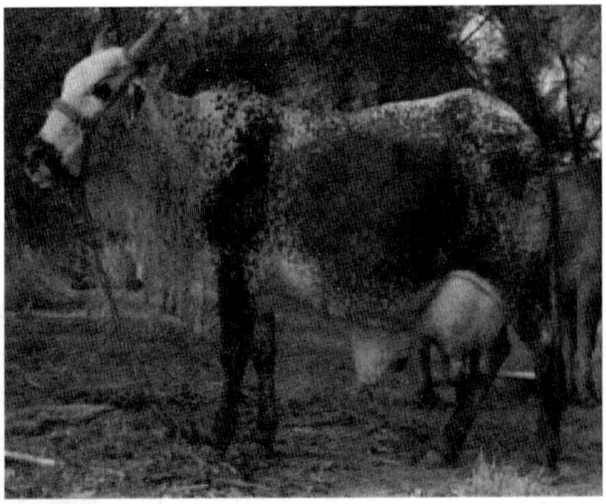

Origin and Distribution: Rathi is an important milch breed of cattle found in the arid regions of Rajasthan. The animals are mostly localized in Alwar district of Rajasthan. Good specimens are also found in and around Bikaner district. Rathi animals are particularly concentrated in Loonkaransar tehsil of Bikaner district, which is also known as Rathi tract. The Breeding tract of this breed lies in the heart of Thar Desert consisting of Bikaner, Ganganagar and Jaisalmer districts of Rajasthan. Rathi cattle are thought to have evolved from intermixing of Sahiwal, Red Sindhi, Tharparkar and Dhanni breeds with a preponderance of Sahiwal blood. It takes its name from a pastoral tribe called Raths who are Muslims of Rajput extraction and lead a nomadic life.

The eco system in its native tract is fragile and the lands are less fertile with very low productivity. Scorching summer (50 degree Celsius), chilly winter (2 degree Celsius), dry monsoon (less than 200 mm rainfall in a year) and dust storms are the characteristics of the region.

Morphological Characteristics: They are medium- sized dual purpose powerful cattle. They are short horned, white or light grey with coffin-shaped skulls, and orbital arches and faces that are slightly convex in profile. It is somewhat similar in appearance of Hariana breed.

The animals are usually brown with white patches all over the body, but animals having completely brown or black coat with white patches are also seen.

Performances: Rathi cows are efficient and good milkers. The cows on an average produce 1560 kg of milk. The lactation milk yield ranges from 1062 to 2810 kg. Selected cows have been reported to produce around 4800 kg at farmer's doorstep. Age at first calving is 47 months ranges frm 36 to 52 months. First calving interval is 17 months varies from 14 to 20 months. The bullocks are well adapted for moderately heavy ploughing and work on the road. These cattle are mostly maintained on cultivated land.

Remarks: This is known as dual purpose cattle. This breed functions as a major livelihood source for the farmers in the arid regions of Rajasthan.

15. Siri

Synonym: Trahbum

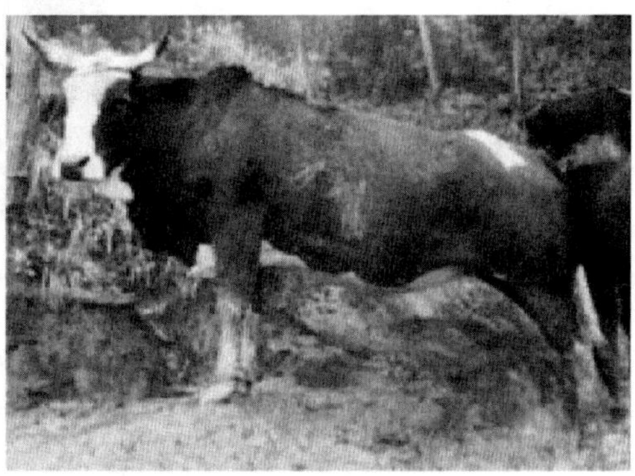

Origin and Distribution: It is found usually in higher altitudes from 1000 to 4000m above the sea-level. Bhutan is said to be the real home of this breed. It is distributed from that area to the various parts of Sikkim and in the hilly tract around Darjeeling in West Bengal. The Siri breed flourishes well in the hilly areas of Darjeeling and Sikkim.

Morphological Characteristics: They are active animals with massive body, square cut small head, wide and flat forehead, presenting convexity. The forehead is white and flat. The horns are sharp and directed forwarded and slightly backward. Well-placed hump covered with a tuft of hair at the top. The position of the hump is slightly forward compared to that in other breeds of zebu cattle. The hooves are broad but strong. They are small, black, red or dun cattle often with large patches and white markings colour patern of this cattle is similar to that of Holstein Friesian cattle. The animals have a thick coat on their body for protection against severe cold and rain. Male weighs is on an average is 454 kg male and female is 363 kg.

Performances: Animals are mostly taken for grazing in the forests. They graze on steep slopes in thick forest. Cows in milk return by the milking time. Average age at first calving is 47 months, calving interval is 17 months, and milk yield per lactation is 425.8 kg. Bullocks are the only source of draught power.

Remarks: They are recognized as a draught breed of cattle in hilly area.

16. Ponwar

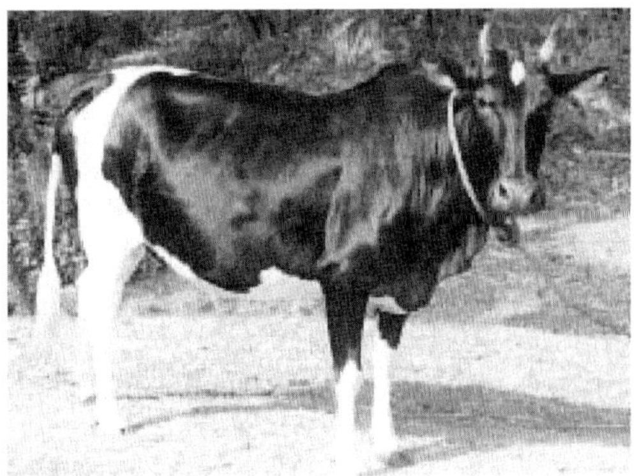

Synonym: Purnea, Kabri (mixture of colour)

Origin and Distribution: Ponwar, a draught breed of cattle from North India, is believed to be evolved from a mixture of hilly cattle (Morang - Nepalese hill cattle) and plain land cattle. It is known to be originated at Ponwar in Puranpur Taluk in Pilibhit district of Uttar Pradesh state and the breed is named after the same place. This cattle breed is restricted to a small geographical area in the foothills Himalayas mainly adjoining Ponwar of Pilibhit district of Uttar Pradesh, India.

Morphological Characteristics: They are active animals with small and compact body size. The animals of this breed possess a small, narrow face, small ears and big, bright eyes. Their body length, height at withers and heart girth in adult cows are 97, 109 and 140 cm, respectively. The neck is short and powerful. The forehead is slightly concave and often has white marking. The tail is long and reaches below the hock tapering with as white switch. The barrel is moderately long. The dewlap is light and thin. The cows have small and poorly developed udders and teats. The hump is well-developed in bulls but is small in cows.

They possess small to medium sized horns, which generally emerge outward, upward and then curve inward with pointed tips. They are either short-horned or slightly lyre-horned cattle. The horns are inclined to be lyre-shaped, which may be due to some mixture of the nearby plains cattle.

Ponwar cattle are usually *black and white* in colour often with large patches and white markings. There are frequent white markings on the forehead, dewlap and limbs. The tail switch is white in black animals and black in those having a greater proportion of white patches. The color markings do not have any particular pattern, but large patches of black and white are intermixed. The adult body weight is 318 kg for male and 295 kg for female.

The animals of this breed possess an aggressive temperament. The animals behave in semi-wild manner and are tough to control. They move in groups putting their heads down in between each other which is a peculiar behavior that has emerged due to fear from predators. The cattle are known to be very active and are of fiery disposition.

Performances: The milk production of the Ponwar cows is low, i.e. about 0.5 to 2.5 kg per day for a lactation period of 8 to 10 (average 8.9) months. Lactation milk yield averages 462.5 kg. The age at first calving ranges from 40 to 60 months and the inter-calving period averages 12 months. The service period in Ponwar cattle varies from 60 to 100 days. The cows remaines dry for average of 110 days. Bullocks of this breed can transport about 800 to 1000 kg load up to 10 kilometres easily. They can plough 0.4 hectares of land in a day working for 6 to 8 hours. Bullocks are fast movers and therefore can use both for agricultural operations and transportation. The cows are poor milkers and are rarely milked even in the flush of their production. It is a draught breed and is mainly used for cart pulling. The bullocks are good for draft purposes. The animals of this breed are observed to mature late.

The animals are maintained in extensive management system, without provision of sheds and are raised entirely on grazing in forestland without feed supplementation. They are observed to thrive well under free grazing conditions.

Remarks: Ponwar is hilly type cattle breed.

17. Kankrej

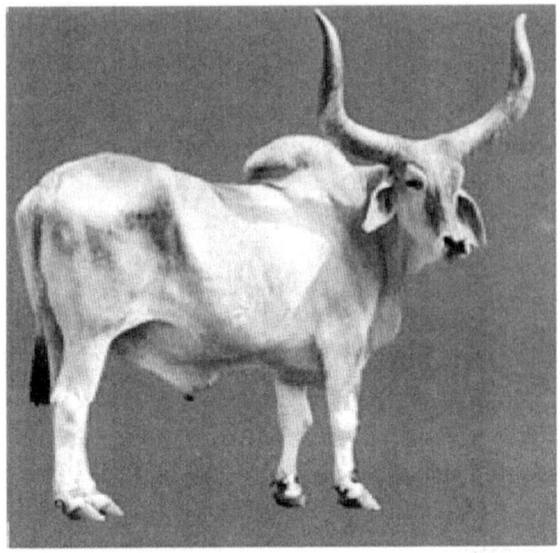

Synonym: Bannai, Vagadia, Wadhair, Nagu, Sanehore, Wadad or Waged, Talabda, Nagar.

Origin and Distribution: The Kankrej breed is indigenous to Gujarat plains. The home tract of this breed is southeast of Rann of Kutch comprising Mehsana, Kutchchh, Ahmedabad, Kheda, Anand, Sabarakantha and Banaskantha districts of Gujarat and Barmer and Jodhpur districts of Rajasthan. It takes its name from the name of geographical area i.e. Kankrej town of Banaskantha district in North Gujarat. Traditionally in the country nomadic breeders, viz. Rabaris, Maldharis, Ahir and Barwars, maintain these cattle. It is also known as Vadhiyari in Kachchh.

Morphological Characteristics: Lyre-Horned *Grey Cattle* with white foreheads dished in the centre, prominent orbital arches and faces with flat or dished profiles. They have broad chest, powerful body, straight back, moderate dewlap, well developed hump and tough skin. The strong lyre-shaped horns are accompanied by skin up to some length than in other breeds. Kankrej cattle have a well built body and are known for their beautiful looks with large half moon shaped horns. Gait is particular to breed known as 1¼ spaces (swai chal) with smooth movements of the body and head noticeably high. It is renowned for its "Swai Chaal", i.e. the back leg reaches further than where the front leg landed, which helps ploughing of fields faster.

The face is short, and the nose looks slightly upturned. The ears are very characteristic, being large, pendulous and open. The legs are particularly well-balanced and the feet small, round and durable. They are active and strong. The hump in the males is well-developed and not so firm as in some breeds. The dewlap is thin but pendulous and males have pendulous sheaths. Pigmentation of the skin is dark and the skin is slightly loose and of medium thickness. Hairs are soft and short.

Coat colour of the animal varies from silver grey to iron grey and steel black. Newly born calves have rust red-colored polls, this color disappears within 6 to 9 months. In males, forequarters, hindquarters, and hump are slightly darker than the rest of the body. Bulls tend to get darker than cows and bullocks. The switch of the tail is black in color. Adult body weight of male and female are 525 and 343 kg respectively.

Performances: They are also fair producers of milk. The cows yield on an average 1400 kg and maximum of 1800 kg of milk in a lactation. The age at first calving in the breed varies from 45 to 47 months and the intercalving period varies from 480 to 510 days. There is scope for improvement in milk production. The cows are good milkers and bullocks are used for agricultural operations and road transport. They are fast, powerful draft cattle. It is adapted to the geo-climatic conditions of Saurashtra and Kachchh, have immense draught power, are resilient to stress conditions and are known for yielding good quantity of milk and good fat content even in stress conditions.

Remarks: The Kankrej cattle are very highly prized as fast, powerful draft cattle breeds in India. It is one of the best dual purpose breeds of India, next only to Hariana. The Kankrej is one of the heaviest of the Indian breeds of cattle. This is an important breed and has been exported abroad widely. Today excellent herds of this breed are found in Brazil. They have been introduced in some other Latin American countries and southern states of the USA. Many local breeds in these countries have some inheritance of Kankrej breed.

The unique characteristics like resistant to tick fever, heat stress, very little incidence of contagious abortion and tuberculosis made Kankrej a very popular one among these foreign countries. Kankrej, famously known as Guzerat in Brazil, is being maintained in large numbers as a pure breed in that country. The Guzerat was the most important breed in the formation of American Brahman.

18. Kenkatha

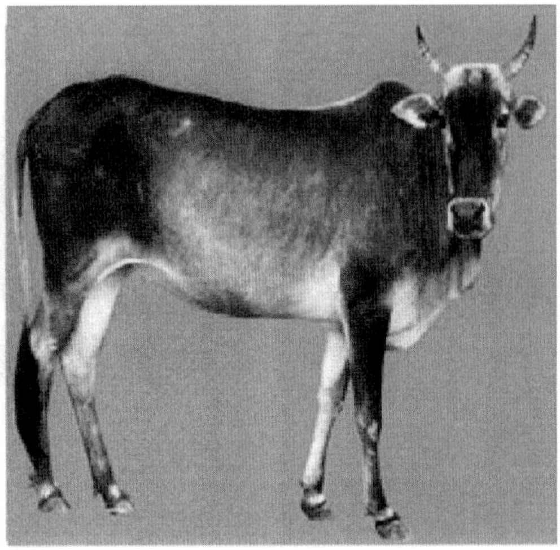

Synonym: Kanwaria

Origin and Distribution: They originated in the provinces of Bundelkhand in the state of Uttar Pradesh along the banks of river Ken and Vindhyas hilly range in Madhya Pradesh. They get their name from the River Ken, as they are bred along the banks of this small river in the hilly area of Bundelkhand. These cattle are also bred in territories of Panna, Charkhari, Bijawar and Ajaigarh which are part of Vindhya Pradesh in India. The Kenkatha or Kenwariya breed hails from Banda district of Uttar Pradesh and neighbouring areas of Madhya Pradesh.

Morphological Characteristics: The Kenkatha cattle are small compact deep built up, sturdy and fairly powerful animals. The head is short and broad and the forehead is dished in shape. Ears are sharply pointed and do not droop. The dewlap is moderately heavy. The hump is well developed. The back is straight but the quarters are drooping. The tail is of medium length with a black switch reaching below the hocks. The limbs are short but powerful and the feet are hard. Horns emerge from the outer angles of the poll in a markedly forward direction and terminate in sharp points. They are varying in color from grey on the barrel to dark grey on the rest of the body. They exhibit different shades of grey and black, rarely white complexions. Adult body weight of male and female is 350 and 300 kg, respectively.

Performances: This cattle is poor milker, gernally used for drought purposes. This breed is very popular for light draft on the road and for cultivation. The cattle is used for draft purposes and is known to have the ability to survive harsh environments and on poor quality forage.

Remarks: They thrive on poor feed and fodder resources.

19. Kangayam

Synonym: Kongu, Kanganad.

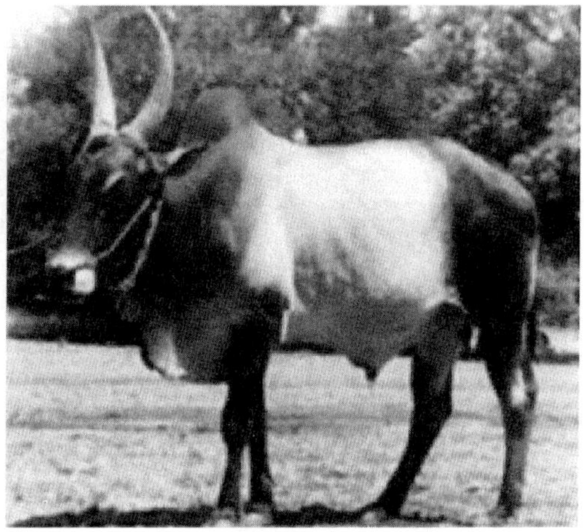

Origin and Distribution: Originated in Kangayam, Dharapuram, Perundurai, Erode, Bhavani and part of Gobichettipalayam taluk of Erode and Coimbatore district of Tamil Nadu State. The home tract of Kangayam breed is Coimbatore district of Tamil Nadu State. The name of this breed was given as it originated from the Kangayam town located in Erode district in the state of Tamil Nadu, India. This breed was developed by Late Pattogar of Palayakottai.

Morphological Characteristics: They are medium-sized compact body animals having powerful quarters. The dewlap is thin. They have short, stout legs with strong hooves. The head is more proportionate to the body. The eyes are dark and prominent with black rings around them. The hump is well developed in the bulls but is firm. The most striking characteristics are the formation of head and horns. The forehead is prominent and the horns emerge from the top of the poll fairly close together in an upward and backward direction. Special points are strong horns with sharp tips. The horns are spread apart, nearly straight with a slight curve backwards. Kangayam cattle are usually grey or white. The colour of the bull is of grey with dark grey to black markings in hump, fore and hind quarters while the cow is white with black markings just in front of the fetlocks on all four legs and sometimes on the knees. This breed is allied to Mysore breeds, and resembles them in appearance. This breed resembles Umblachery breed. Important characteristies feature of this breed is coat colour of calf, red at birth, but charges to grey at about 6 months of age. Adult male body weight is about 540 kgs while female is 380 kg.

Performances: The milk yield ranges from 600 to 700 kg. Although the milk of Kangayam cows has a high nutritious value with no bad fat, the breed is considered as a poor milker. However, in some cases, good milkers are also found, giving 18 to 20 kg per day during the peak milking period. Age at first calving is 40 months varies from 28 to 54 months. Calving interval varies from 12 to 54 months with 16 months average. A large number of bullocks produced in the northern tract are sold to cultivators in other parts for working in the black cotton soils.

Remarks: The animals are considered as good draught breed in South India. This breed of cattle has also been exported to Sri Lanka for draft purposes. The breed is on the wane, due to poor government support for indigenous breeds, although individual conservative efforts are bearing some fruit.

20. Hallikar

Synonym: Mysore

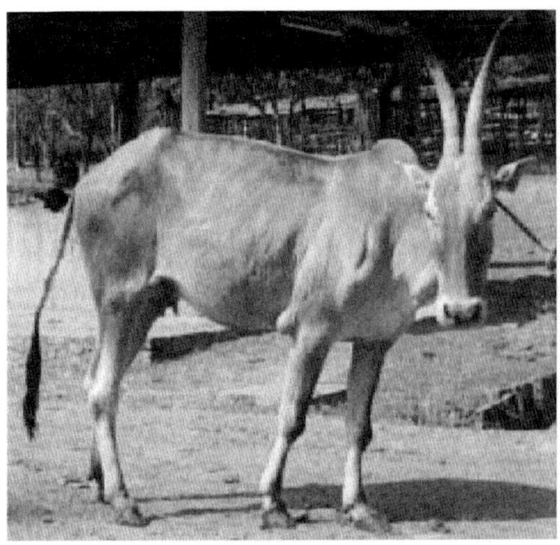

Origin and Distribution: Originated from the former princely state of Vijayanagarm, presently part of Karnataka. The home tract of Hallikar is spread over Chitradurga, Chikamagalur, Tumkur, Mysore, Mandya, Hassan and Bangalore districts of Karnataka. Hallikar breed of cattle is distributed in almost all the districts of south Karnataka and is also found in adjoining areas of Andhra Pradesh and Tamil Nadu States. The name of the breed, Hallikar, has been derived from the name of sub tribe Hallikar of Golla Community.

The responsibility for developing this breed mainly goes to the Gola community and its sub-tribe Hallikar. Hallikar breed is considered as the progenitor of the almost all the cattle breeds of southern India including Amritmahal, Khillari and Kangayam. All these breeds resemble Hallikar with some differences, which might have been the outcome of natural selection reinforced with selective breeding practiced by the farmers within the given ecological niche through generations.

Morphological Characteristics: Compact, muscular and medium sized animal with prominent forehead, long horns, strong legs and tight sheath. The neck is long and thin for the size of the animal. The dewlap is thin and moderately developed. The sheath is very close. The forequarters are well developed and the legs are strong. The hooves are strong, small and tightly set. The back is straight and strong. The face is long with small ears. The hump is moderately developed.

The head and horns are the notable features of the breed. The horns emerge in proximity to each other near the top of the poll and are carried backward, straight for nearly half their length and then with a forward bend. The forehead is prominent. The head is usually long with a bulging forehead, furrowed in the middle.

The coat colour is grey to dark grey with deep shadings on the fore and hind quarters. The colour of these animals varies from white to light grey with slightly darker shoulders and hindquarters. White markings or irregular patches round the eyes and checks, and neck or shoulder region are the distinctive features of this breed. The body length, height at wither and heart girth range from 190 to 200, 132 to 140 and 170 to 200 cm respectively, in males. In females, these average around 170, 188 and 150 cm, respectively. Adult males and females weight are around 340 and 227 kg, respectively.

Performances: Age at first calving ranges from 915 to 1,800 days with an average of about 1,370 days. Lactation milk yield is around 540 kg ranging from 227 to 1,134 kg. Lactation length ranges from 210 to 310 days averaging of about 285 days. Fat is about 5.7%. Average calving interval is 598 days.

Bullocks are strong, well spirited, quick and steady in field as well as on road. A pair of bullocks can pull continuously a maximum draught of 13 to 16 % of their body weight for 6 hr. The average speed and power under average load and climatic conditions are 3 km/hr and 0.91hp/pair.

Remarks: Hallikar is the pride cattle breed of Karnataka. It resembles Amritmahal in some of its features. The breed is best known for its draught capacity and especially for its trotting ability in South India. While rearing the calf, it is difficult to approach the animal. It was used in the war by Tippu Sultan for carrying cannons.

21. Amritmahal

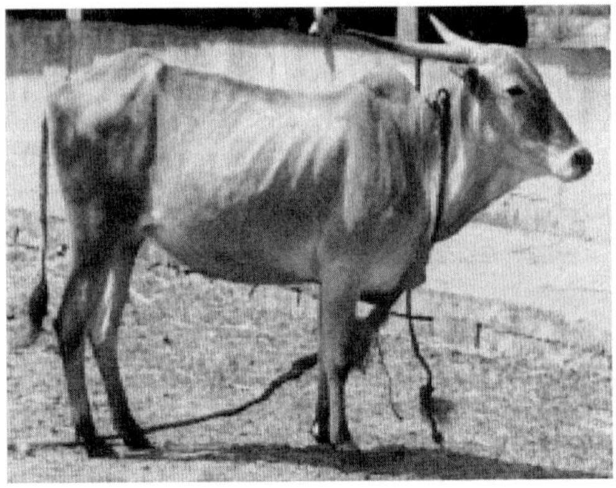

Synonym: Doddadana, Jawari Dana and Number Danal

Origin and Distribution: The breeding tract includes Chikmagalur, Chitradurga, Hassan, Shimoga, Tumkur and Davanagere districts of Karnataka. Its breeding tract stretches from the basin of River Krishna to the River Kaveri. The Amritmahal breed is primarily a draft animal but during the early days it was known for its milch qualities. Maharajas of Mysore had developed large farms called Kavals for developing this breed. The Amritmahal breeds are indigenous to Tumkur, Hassan and Mysore districts of Karnataka but are spread all over the Peninsular India.

Amritmahal literally means the house of milk. "Amrit" means milk and "Mahal" means house. Amritmahal was developed from a herd established by the ruler of Mysore state between 1572 and 1636 A D and was developed from draught breed of southern India with an objective to increase the milk productivity. Originally the rulers of Mysore State had started an establishment of cattle collected from the prevalent types of cattle within the area for the supply of milk and milk products to the palace. At the same time, the bullocks were utilized for the movement of army equipage. The bullocks were regularly classified as gun bullocks, pack bullocks, plow bullocks, etc. They attracted great attention during the nineteenth century on account of their endurance and the speed with which they could move army equipment. It is claimed that they could maneuver a march of 100 miles in 2½ days. The cattle of Amritmahal establishment originally comprised three distinct varieties: Hallikar, Hagalvadi and Chitaldroog. Prior to 1860 it seems that these three varieties were maintained separate from each other. In 1860, the whole establishment was liquidated for reasons of economy. By the year 1866, it was realized that an establishment for the supply of cattle was necessary, and during the year a herd was again established. Thus, the foundation cattle from which the Amrit mahal breed was developed were of the Hallikar and closely related type cattle.

Morphological Characteristics: The body is compact and muscular with well-formed shoulders and hindquarters. The muzzle, feet and tail are usually black. The dewlap is thin and does not extend very far. The naval flap is very small and close to the body. The legs are of medium length and well proportioned. The eyes look bloodshot. The ears are small and taper to a point, being carried in a horizontal position. They are yellow inside. The hump is well-developed and shapely in the bulls, rising to a height of about 8 inches. The neck is strong and fairly long. The back is level, with broad loins and level rump. The fetlocks are short and the hooves are hard, close together and small. The skin is thin, mellow with short glossy hair.

The most striking characteristics are the formation of head and horns. The head is well shaped, long and tapering towards the muzzle. Narrow face and prominent bulges forehead with a furrow in the middle. The horns emerge from the top of the poll fairly close together in an upward and backward direction. Horns are long and end in sharp black points. Long sweeping horns typical of Karnataka type cattle. The formation of head and horns is characteristic; they may be compared to Hallikar, Khillari and Kangayam.

The breed is usually grey in colour but the colour varies from white to almost black. White grey markings are present on face and dewlap in some animals. Dark shades on neck, shoulder, hump and hindquarters. Adult body weight is 500 kg for male and 318 kg for female.

As the cattle are maintained in the pasture areas without any restrictions and handling, they show a very impatient, wild and unruly disposition. They are at time dangerous, particularly to strangers. They need patience and care in training; hard treatment makes them stubborn. Once they are trained they are extremely fine bullocks, particularly for quick transportation. They are observed to have great endurance.

Performances: This is a famous draught breed known for its power and endurance. The animals are fiery and active. The animals are famous for their power of endurance. This breed is pre-eminently suitable for fast work and endurance on the plough or on the road. The animals are, however, apt to be fierce. Bullocks are especially suited for trotting and quick transportation. Cows are very poor milkers. Average milk yield per lactation is 572 kg. The average age at first calving is 50 months with ranges from 36 to 72 months. Calving interval is 14 months which ranges from 12 to 22 months.

Remarks: The features of Amritmahal cattle breed are quite typical of the Mysore cattle. They are closely related to Hallikar. This breed is one of the best known draught breed of India with its home in Mysore.

22. Pullikulam

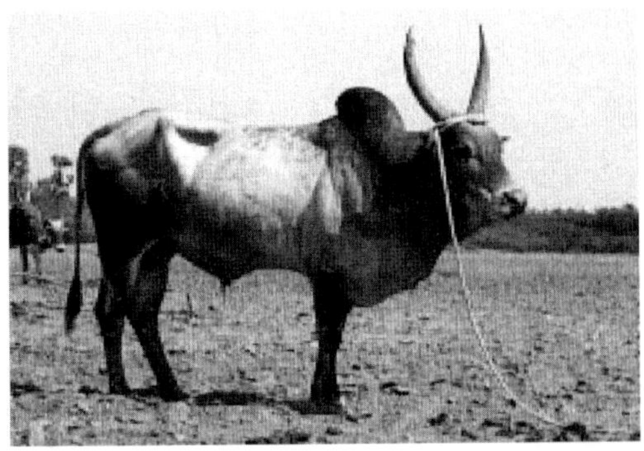

Synonym: Palingu Maadu, Jallikattu Maadu, Kidai Maadu, Mani Maadu, Mattu Maadu and Kilakattu Maadu and Sentharai.

Origin and Distribution: This breed is restricted to Salem and Coimbatore and Cumbum valley of Madurai district in Tamil Nadu State. It is named after its village of origin (Pulikulam in Tamil Nadu). Madurai, Sivaganda and Virudhunagar districts of Tamil Nadu form its breeding tract. This breed of cattle are mostly maintained by Konar and Thevar communities of Tamil Nadu State.

Morphological Characteristics: The animals are small sized with compact body and short legs. Muzzle, eyelids, tail switch and hooves are black. Forehead is broad and has a groove at centre with well-developed hump. Udder is not well developed. Horns are curved outward, upward, backward and then inward, ending with pointed tips spaced wide apart. Typical backward curving horns like Mysore type cattle. They closely resemble Hallikar breed. Usually grey or dark grey in colour. Presence of reddish or brownish spots in muzzle, eyes, switch and back is the characteristic feature of this breed. Males are dark grey in colour while females are white or grey. Adult body weight is 259 kg for male and 208 kg for female.

Performances: Breeds are active, useful draught animals but not fast trotter. Mainly used for penning in the field, useful for ploughing. These cattle are used in games like bull riding (Jallikattu) in local area. The breed is not meant for milk production and only a few animals are milked in large herds for consumption by herdsmen. Generally, milk yield is about 1.25 Kg per day within a range of 0.5 kg to 2 kg. Average age at first calving is 50 months. Calving interval ranges from 17 to 24 months. The animals are also reared for manure purpose.

Remarks: Pullikulam is a popular draught and game breed of Tamil Nadu. Breed is more resistance to communicable and parasitic diseases as compared to crossbreds under hot and wet conditions.

23. Umblachery

Synonym: Jathi Madu, Mottai Madu, Molai Madu, Therkathi Madu.

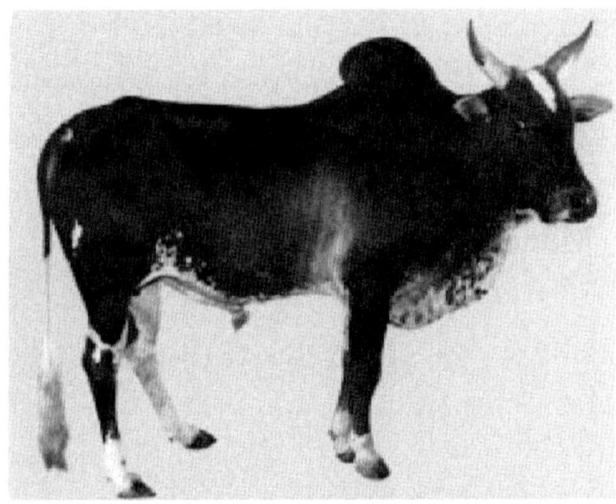

Origin and Distribution: Umblachery is an indigenous breed of cattle in India. It is originated in coastal plains of Thanjavur, Thiruvarur and Nagappattinam districts of Tamil Nadu in South India. It is related to the Kangayam cattle of the same state. It derives its name from its home tract, Umblachery, a small village in Nagapattinam district.

Morphological Characteristics: The predominant coat colour of this adult animal is grey. The intensity of colour varies from grey with a mixture of black to full grey colour. The legs have white markings below the hocks like socks. White markings on face, limbs and tail are also observed. Umblachery calves are generally red or brown at birth which changes to grey at 3 to 4 months of age. Horns are curving outward and inward and sometimes spreading laterally. Horns are very small in size. Male weighs 297 and female weighs 219 kg.

Performances: The cows are poor milkers. The average daily milk yield is 2058 g and it ranges from 400 to 4750 g. The total estimated milk yield for the lactation is 494 kg. The average lactation length is 8 months. The average of milk fat percentage is 4.94 and the average solids-not-fat percentage is 7.80 which ranges from 7.73 to 8.17 percentage. Age at first calving and calving interval of this cattle is about 52 and 15 months, respectively.

Bullocks are small and swift. This breed is noted for its strength and sturdiness especially used in the marshy fields for wet ploughing. The practice of dehorning of bullocks is peculiar in Umblachery cattle.

The milk yield does not show any definite pattern. The milk yield is highly variable with a coefficient of variability of 35%. This suggests the possibility of improving their daily production by genetic means. The milk yield decreases even from first month onwards. The reasons might be due to difference in amount of milk fed to different sexes, allowing growing male calves to suck more milk and milking the animals as to owner's requirement.

Remarks: It is draft purposes breed mainly used for agricultural work.

24. Hariana

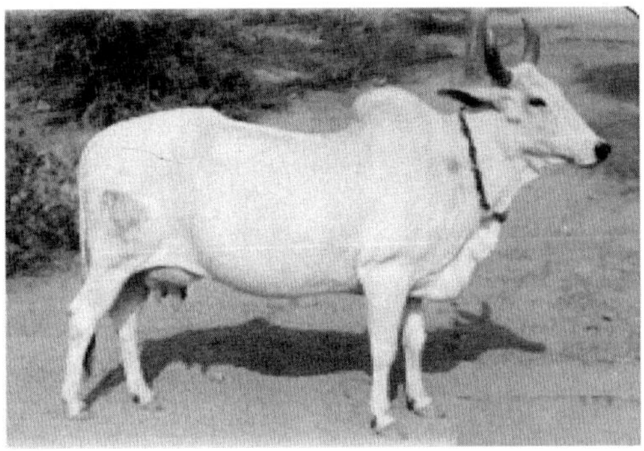

Synonym: Hansi

Origin and Distribution: The main tract of this breed is the Haryana state. The centre of origin is around Rohtak, Hisar and Gurgaon districts of Haryana state. Hariana breed of cattle is widely spread in Punjab, Haryana, Uttar Pradesh and also in parts of Madhya Pradesh. The cattle found in the Hisar district are somewhat different in built from the pure-bred Hariana breed and is named as Hisar breed. This is the most common breed in North India. As its name indicates, the Haryana breed is the much prized cattle of Haryana and is also found in the neighbouring parts of Delhi and Western Uttar Pradesh.

Hariana cattle take their name from the region known as Haryana State in North India. There were two strains of cattle Hisar and Hansi found in this region and known after the name of then native towns. Hariana cattle seems to have originated from these two strains. Hisar and Hansi names do no exist now.

Morphological Characteristics: Proportionately compact body built with coffin-shaped skulls. Orbital arches are long. Long and narrow face, slightly convex in profile. Flat forehead and bony prominence in the centre of the poll. Legs are moderately long and lean. Head is carried high. Short stumpy horns curving upward and inward direction. Short thin tail tapering towards the end with a black switch reaching just below the hocks. Popular colour is white or light grey. The mature body weight of male and female were 499 and 325 kg, respectively.

Performances: Average milk yield is between 600 and 1000 kg. Good specimens of cows yield upto 1500 kg of milk per lactation. Age at first calving ranges from 40 to 60 months depending on management. Intercalving period is of 480 to 630 days. Bullocks are powerful work animals. The bullock is highly recognized for its vigour and persistency for draught.

Remarks: This is the most popular dual-purpose cattle breed in all over the country. Hariana has been the local counterpart in many crossbreeding programmes in India.

25. Tharparkar

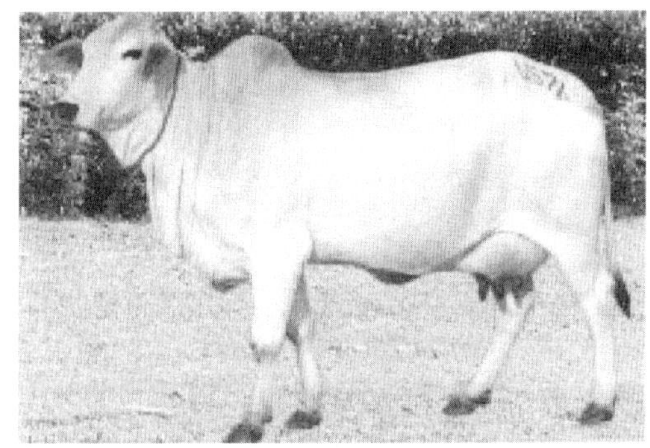

Synonym: Thari, Grey Sindhi, White Sindhi

Origin and Distribution: Tharparkar breed originated in Tharparkar district of southeast Sindh province in Pakistan and is also found along the Indo-Pak border covering western Rajasthan and upto Rann of Kutch in Gujarat. The breed derives its name from its place of origin - The THAR desert. This breed was developed from Kankrej, Red Sindhi, Gir and Nagori Breed.

Morphological Characteristics: The characteristics are majestic built, white in colour, tall, long legged with round barrel. Medium sized well-proportionate compact body frame with straight and long back. Dewlap moderately developed. Prominent orbital arches and faces with flat or dished profiles. Broad poll and forehead is slightly convex with small Lyre-Horns. Long pendulous ears of which inner side is yellowish. The tail is fine with black switch. Short, straight and strong limbs. They are white or light grey in colour. Face and extremities are of darker shade than the body. Adult body weight of male is 475 kg and female is 295 kg.

Performances: Milk yield in cows ranges from 1800 to 2600 kg. Age at first calving ranges from 38 to 42 months and intercalving period from 430 to 460 days. The cows are good milch animals and the bullock are also quite suitable for ploughing and carting. They are resistant to many diseases and are also known for their good reproductive efficiency.

Remarks: Tharparkar has proved to be one of the best milch purpose breed of India and developed primarily for its milking potentiality.

26. Ongole

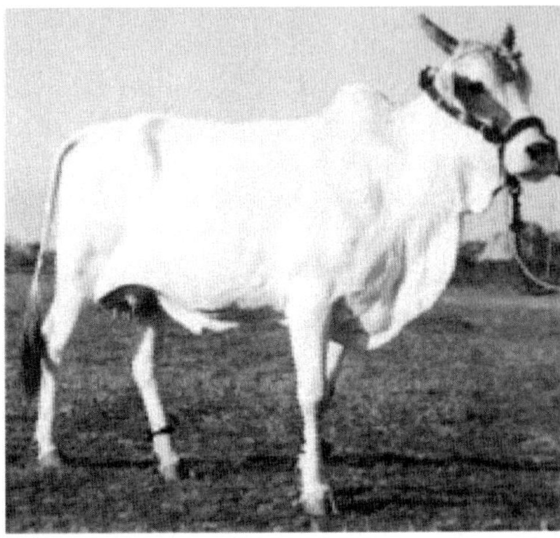

Synonym: Nellore

Origin and Distribution: The native tract of Ongole breed cattle is the Nellore and Guntur district of Andhra Pradesh. The Ongole breed, like other breeds of cattle in India, takes its name from the geographical area in which it is produced. It is also called the Nellore breed for the reason that formerly Ongole Taluk, a division of a district, was included in the Nellore district, but now it is included in the Guntur district. The area is a part of Andhra Pradesh in India.

It is claimed that the finest specimens of the breed are found in the area between the Gundalakama and Alluru rivers in the Ongole and Kandukur taluks, and also in the villages of Karumanchi, Nidamanur, Pondur, Jayavaram, Tungtoor and Karvadi and along the banks of River Musi. They are also famous from the taluks of Vinukonda and Narasraopet.

Morphological Characteristics: The Ongole are large-sized animals with coffin-shaped skulls, large dewlap which are fleshy and hang in folds extending to the navel flap, and slightly pendulous sheaths. They have long bodies and short necks; limbs are long and muscular. The forehead is broad between the eyes and slightly prominent. Eyes are elliptical in shape with black eyelashes and a ring of black skin about ¼ to ½ inch wide around the eyes. Ears are moderately long, measuring on an average 9 to 12 inches, and slightly drooping. Horns are short and stumpy, growing outwards and backwards, thick at the base and firm without cracks. In some animals the horns are loose; this is probably due to poorly grown horn core.

The hump in the males is well-developed and erect and filled up on both sides and not concave. The skin is of medium thickness, mellow and elastic and often shows black mottled markings. The popular color is white. The male has dark grey markings on the head, neck and hump and sometimes black points on the knees and on both fore and hind legs. A red or red and white animal of typical conformation is occasionally seen. They have a white switch of the tail, white eyelashes, a flesh colored muzzle, light colored hooves, dark grey marking on the hindquarters and dark mottle appearance on the body. Animals are greatly alert and docile with good majestic gait. The adult body weight of male is about 434 kg whereas this figure is 382 kg for female.

Ongole cattle skin secretes sebum which filters ultraviolet rays. Due to high vascularity they bleed profusely if punctured and wounds heal quickly. Being black in color, 15% of solar heat is allowed by coat to pass on at once when absorbed by the skin. The Ongole cattle has white external coat and black underlying skin.

It has a great similarity with the Gaolao breed of Madhya Predesh and also has a resemblance to the Bhagnari type of cattle in the north of India. This similarity is not surprising in view of the fact that these breeds lie along the path taken by the Rig Vedic Aryans in their march from the north to the south of India.

Performances: Ongole cattle are efficiently used in their native home for both work and milk production. They are usually docile and the bulls are very powerful, suitable for heavy plowing or cart work but are not considered to be suitable for fast work or trotting purposes. The cows are fair milkers. An average lactation yield of 1000 kg is common. Good specimens have given upto 1500 kg yield per lactation. The age at first calving is between 38 to 45 months with the intercalving period of 470 days. This is essentially a large muscular breed suitable for heavy draft work.

Remarks: It clearly indicates that this breed was originally a dairy breed which was later transformed as dual purpose i.e., dairy and draft animals, presently mostly a draught animal. Ongole is one of the best breeds of cattle in India, highly valued for both work and milk production. They are mostly reputed for their draft traits. Excellent specimen of this breed has been exported to Brazil where large herds are abound. They are known as Nellore breed in Brazil. Specimens of this breed have also been exported in the past to Sri

Lanka, Fiji, Indo-China, Indonesia, Australia, Switzarland, Malayasia and USA. The famous Santa Gertrudis breed evolved in Texas, USA, has the inheritance of Ongole breed in its development.

27. Nagori

Synonym: Nil

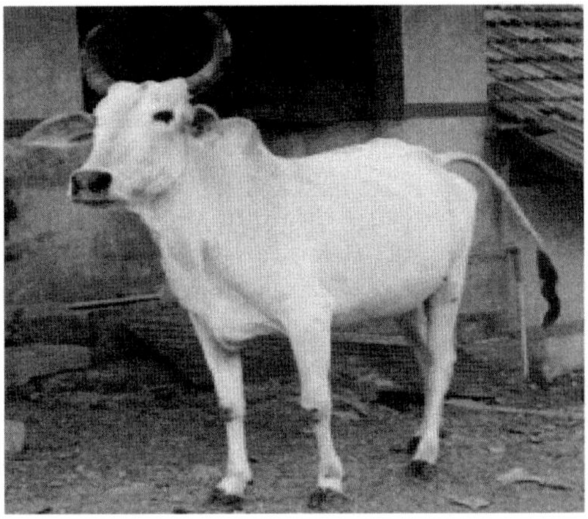

Origin and Distribution: Nagori cattle breed are widespread in the district of Bikaner, Jodhpur and Nagore district of Rajasthan state of India. This breed is supposed to have been evolved from Hariana and Kankrej breeds. There is an admixture of grey blood in this breed. Its name was derived as this breed is available at Nagore district of Rajasthan.

Morphological Characteristics: Long and deep body with coffin-shaped skulls. Narrow face that is slightly convex in profile. Well developed flat forehead. Ears are large and pendulous. Small and fine dewlap. Horns moderately developed emerging from outer angles of poll in outward direction and carried upward with gentle curve to run at points. White or light grey in colour. In same cases head, face and shoulder are slightly greyish.

They are white, upstanding, very alert and agile animal with long and narrow face like that of a horse. Average body weight of adult male is 363 kg and female is 318 kg.

Performances: The average performance for production traits, viz. milk yield, lactation length, milk yield/ day of lactation, milk yield/ day of calving interval and dry period are 535 kg, 267 days, 2.1 kg, 1.3 kg and 154 days, respectively, and for reproduction traits, viz. service period, gestation period and calving interval, are 120, 283 and 423 days, respectively. Average age at first calving is 1503 days and birth weight of calf is 16 kg. In the Barmer district of Rajasthan there are good specimens of milch cows of this breed with yields as high as 900 kg per lactation.

Remarks: This breed is famous for trotting and as draft animal. The bullocks are prized for their fast road work. They are specially suited for deep sandy soils.

28. Gangatiri

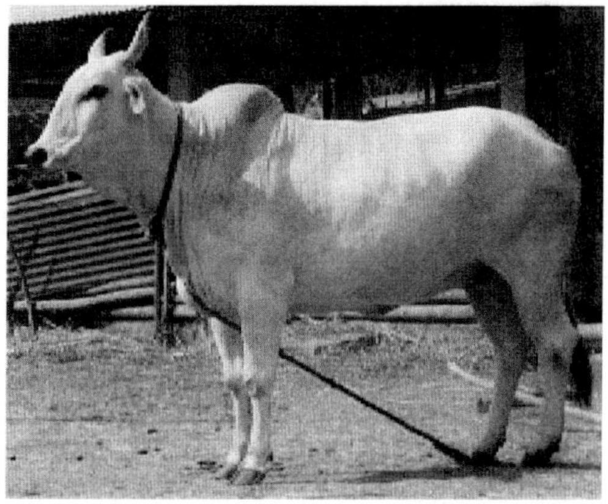

Synonym: Eastern Hariana or Shahabadi

Origin and Distribution: Gangatiri is known to be originated in the region along the banks of Ganga river in eastern Uttar Pradesh and western parts of Bihar state. The breeding tract of this breed includes mainly Balia, Varanasi, Ghazipur and Hazipur districts of Uttar Pradesh and Buxar, Bhabhua, Bhojpur and Sahabad districts of Bihar state. This breed of cattle derived their name from its habitat, in the area nearly river Ganga. This breed are developed by Yadav, Bhumihar and Rajbhor communities of Bihar.

Morphological Characteristics: Well build up stout body. Dewlap and hump are of medium size. Muzzle is black with some spots. Coat colour of Gangatri cow is white with two variant, totally white (Dhawar) and greyish (Sokan). Forehead is prominent, straight and broad with shallow groove in the middle, Eyelids, muzzle, hooves and tail switch are generally black. Horms are medium in size and emerges from side of the poll behind and above eyes in outward and curving upwards and inwards ending with pointed tips. Male adult body weight is 340 kg while female 235 kg.

The average body length, height at withers, chest girth, face length, ear length and tail length are 110, 124, 153, 46, 25 and 85 cm, respectively, in adult cows and 121, 142, 168, 52, 27 and 91 cm, respectively, in bullocks under field condition. Overall body measurement of the breed is lesser than that of Hariana cattle.

Performances: The cows are fairly good milk yielders. These cattle are well adapted to low to medium input production system and produce about 2.5 to 8.0 kg milk in a day. Average lactational yield is 1050 kg varies from 900 to 1200 kg. The average fat % of the milk is

4.33 (range of 3.1 to 6.0%) and SNF contents 8.22% (range of 7.87 to 8.42%). The average lactation period of Gangatiri cows is 339 days. The intercalving period varies between 14 to 24 months. Age at first calving is about 47 months varies from 27 to 82 months. Calving interval, on an average, is 16 months which ranges from 11 to 20 months.

Animals of this breed are reared for milk production as well as agricultural operation. They are fit for ploughing, threashing and power works. These animals are kept in open or Kutcha (Thatched) houses. The animals are sent for grazing for a period of 6-8 hours in a day. The herd size varies from 2-150 animals. Large herds are maintained in the Diyara, the area adjacent to the river Ganga and kept only on grazing i.e. zero input system.

Remarks: Gangatiri is an important dual purpose cattle breed of North India. The breed has been significantly contributing to the livelihood of the people due to its good draught ability and average milk production. Therefore, sincere efforts should immediately be undertaken for its genetic improvement in the breeding tract. Crossbreeding programme with Hariana bulls may be instigated to maintain draught cattle characteristics and increase potential for milk production.

29. Binjharpuri

Synonym: Deshi

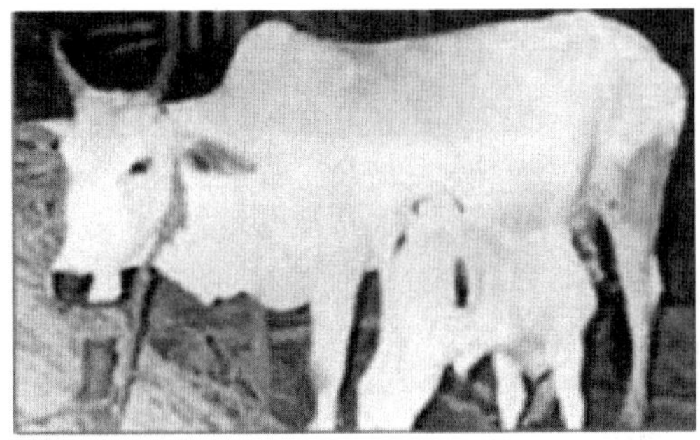

Origin and Distribution: Binjharpuri is a breed of cattle found in Jajpur, Kendrapara and Bhadrak districts of Odisha. Heavy concentration is in Binjharpur area of Jajpur district in Odisha. This breed is named after the local area 'Binjharpur' of Jajpur district of Odisha.

Morphological Characteristics: Medium compact, strong body size. Chiefly white in colour, but some animals are grey, black or brown in colour. In males, the hump, neck and some regions of face and back are black in colour irrespective of their coat color. Mature body weight of this breed is 254 kg for male and 207 kg for female.

Performances: Lactation length: 308 days. Lactation yield: 1338 kg. Calving interval (days): 408 days. Age at first mating (days) 938 days. They are generally reared for draught, manure and milk purpose. Average milk yield is around 4 kg per day in two milking without supplementation of concentrate. Average fat and SNF% of the milk are 4.4 and 8.5%, respectively. Cows are docile and female member of the family usually milks lactating cows.

Remarks: A smaller upgraded Haryana type cattle breed. The draught capacity weighs about 640 kgs. Heat Tolerance capacity is excellent.

30. Khillari

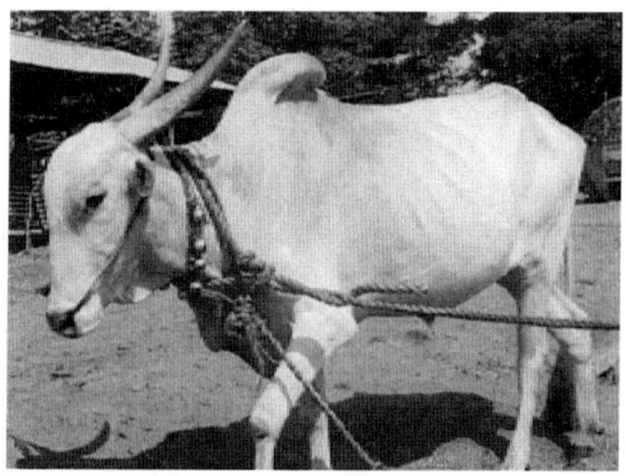

Synonym: Mandeshi, Shikari, Thillar

Origin and Distribution: Originated from Sholapur and Sitapur districts of Maharashtra state. They are at present well distributed throughout the Maharashtra state. This breed of cattle have originated from Hallikar or Amritmahal breed of cattle. Khillari means herds of cattle and herdman is known as Khillari or Thillari. Within this breed, the animals belong to four types, viz. (a). The Atpadi Mahal of Hanam Khillar from the former southern Mahratta state (b) The Mhaswad Khillari from Sholapur and Satara districts (c) The Thillari or Tapi Khillari from Satpura range of hills, and (d) The Nakali, i.e. the imitation Khillar, Solapur and Satara districts comprise the home of the Khillari breed.

Morphological Characteristics: It has a compact body with clear-cut features. They are medium-sized compact animals, having powerful quarters. The breed is having massive head, small eyes and ears, horns are long and pointed, emerging close to each other and follow the backward curve of the forehead. Neck is rather short and firmly set. The forehead of the Khillari is long and with a convex bulge towards the horns with a distinct groove running in the centre of the forehead. The eyes are set in an elongated fashion, are small though prominent and often slightly bulging. Ears are small and pointed, and are always held sideways. The shoulders are tightly muscled. The barrel is long and compact with no loose skin. The legs are straight and strong. The hooves are black with closely set digits. They have strongly set limbs. The gait of Khillari is quick. Hindquarters are well muscled and squarely developed. They are small in comparison with the bulk of the body. They are grey-white in colour.

The most striking characteristics are the formation of head and horns. The forehead is prominent and the horns emerge from the top of the poll fairly close together in an upward and backward direction. The horns are placed close together at the roof. They curve backwards for half the length and then turn forwards in a peculiar fashion. The horns are thick at the base and taper to a fine point. The horns are generally black, sometimes pinkish.

Khillaris of Deccan Plateau - The Mhaswad and Atapadi Khillari is greyish. White Male being darker over the fore-quarters and hind quarters with typical mottled markings on the face. The Tapi Khillari is white with pink nose and pink hoofs. The Nakali Khillari is grey with tawny or brick dust colour over the forequarters.

Khillari breed also closely resembles Hallikar and Amritmahal of Mysore cattle breed. The animals resemble Amritmahal breed of cattle except that Khillari breeds look even more bigger framed. As compared to Hallikar, this has a higher milk potential.

The average adult body weight of Khillari cattle is 271 kg for male and 219 kg for female.

Performances: Excellent cows yield upto 900 to 1000 kg milk. Average age at first calving is 43 months ranging from 37 to 60 months. Calving interval varies from 15 to 21 months and averages 17 months. Khillari bullocks are regarded as fast and powerful draft animals. The bullocks are well known for their strength and are very popular as fast draught animals. They can travel miles without showing any sign of fatigue. It is also accredited with hardiness, ability to endure scarcity of fodder, endurance under the plough or on the road. Animals of this breed thrive under famine conditions and are much valued for this quality.

Remarks: The breed is highly valued as fast paced, powerful draught animals throughout the State of Maharastra. Khillari has been exported to Sri Lanka for crossing with the local cattle for improving their draft qualities.

31. Krishna Valley

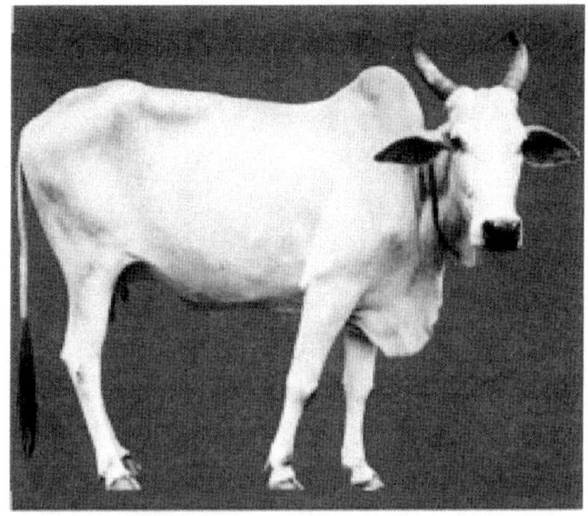

Synonym: Kistna Valley

Origin and Distribution: The breed is of recent origin. It is claimed that during the last two decades of the nineteenth century some of the Rajas of the Southern Mahratta country which lies in the watershed of rivers tried to evolve a powerful bullock for agriculture purposes in the sticky black cotton soil. It is claimed that Gir cattle from Kathiawar, Ongole cattle from Madras, possibly Kankrej from Gujarat, and local cattle having Mysore-type blood in them were used to evolve the Krishna Valley breed. Maharaja Sangli, at one time a well-known breeder of Krishna Valley cattle, contributed substantially in making judicious use of all these strains to produce the desired type of animal which eventually were used for breeding on a wide scale even before the characteristics were fixed to any extent, there is wide variation in the characteristic of the breed. Massiveness in size was the chief dominating factor which attracted the attention of the cultivators.

The home tract of this breed is the black cotton soil along the river Krishna and the adjoining areas of Ghataprabha and Malaprabha in Karnataka. The breed is also found in the districts of Satara, Miraj and Kolhapur of Maharashtra state, and Belgaum, Dharwad and Bijapur districts of Karnataka state. They are also found in certain parts of Andhra Pradesh. The Krishna Valley breed is popular in upper Krishna Valley in Maharashtra and Karnataka.

Morphological Characteristics: Coffin-shaped skull with prominent orbital arches. Face is slightly convex in profile. Distinct bulge forehead. Horns: Small, curved upward and inwards. Ears: Small pointed. Tail: Almost reaches the ground. Colour: white or light grey. Males: Darker shades in fore and hind quarters. Adult body weight of male and female are 550 and 325 kg respectively.

Performances: They are fairly good milkers. The bullocks are massive and powerful, and good for draft in heavy soils. Daily milk yield 3.17 kg; maximum of 8 kg. Milk production per lactation: 960 kg. Age at first calving ranges from 46 to 49 months. On account of contributions form Gir and Ongole, it has also potentialities of milk production. However, the milk-producing capacity is extremely variable in the breed. The bullocks are powerfully built for hauling heavy loads of agricultural production. Due to the softness of the hooves and the heavy weight of the animals they are not generally appreciated by the cultivators in areas other than the native home of the breed.

The Krishna Valley is a heavy draft breed suitable for cultivation purposes in the black cotton soil area which becomes extremely difficult to work during the rainy season, and for hauling heavy loads.

Remarks: The Krishna Valley is triple-purpose cattle that have proved well as draught, milk and meat animals.

Their large size and heavy weight attracted the attention of breeders from Brazil and the United States of America but, though animals of this breed were exported to these countries, they did not retain their identity.

In Brazil, Krishna Valley cow produces 40 liters milk per day. American Brahman influence in the beef industry is felt world-wide, and their genetics are sought by cattlemen in every continent. Brazil has positioned itself as the world newest beef powerhouse. With a national herd of 210 million head and growing, about 80 per cent of the Brazilian herds comprise of Brahman and Krishna Valley/Nellore. The American Brahman is known in the world for their crossbreeding excellence, however many dairy producers in the southern United States and South and Central America also utilize the American Brahman in crossbreeding with dairy breeds. In 2011, 3.6 million doses semen of Krishna Valley/Nellore have been sold in Brazil.

32. Bachaur

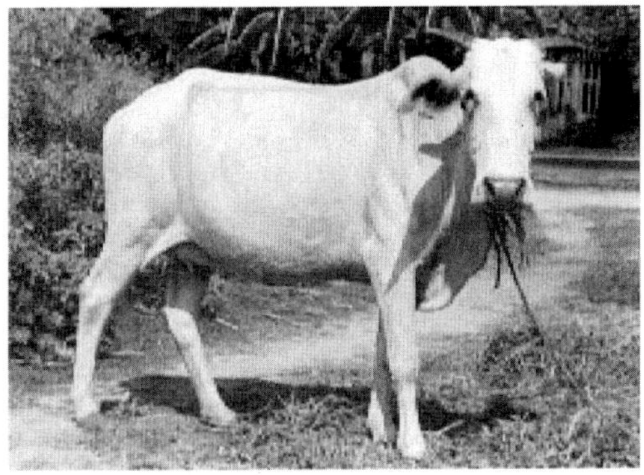

Synonym: Sitamarhi, Bhutia

Origin and Distribution: This breed is mainly found in Sitamarhi, Dharbhanga and Madhubani district of Bihar. It has very close similarity with the Hariana breed. Bachur cattle are now concentrated in the areas adjoining Nepal boarder comprising, Bachaur and Koilpur sub-divisions of Sitamarhi district.

This breed of cattle are maintained by Koir and Ahir Communities of Bihar.

Morphological Characteristics: Bachaur cattle, a small size breed. They have compact body, straight back, well rounded barrel, broad and flat forehead, prominent and large eyes. Ears are of medium size compact and firm hump. Short tail. Grey in colour. The height at withers, body length and chest girth are 119 cm, 116 cm and 150 cm in adult males and 112 cm, 109 cm and 140 cm in adult females, respectively. The estimated body weight of Bachaur cattle is 246 kg in adult male and 200 kg in adult female.

Performances: The cows of this breed are not good milkers. Fat % varies from 4.8 to 7.1 with average 5%. Among the draught breeds of India, the Bachaur cows are reasonably good milkers with an average lactation yield of 752.10 kg and peak yield of 4.70 kg/day. The breed is reported to be regular in reproduction with the age at first calving and calving interval of 31.55 months and 14.44 months, respectively in its breeding tract. The bullocks are well known for the draft capacity and the ability to thrive under poor conditions of feeding.

Remarks: This breed is of only local importance, and is not as well known as the other grey breeds. Bachaur cattle fulfilled the livelihood requirement of cattle farmers in the breeding tract by its draught power to a greater extent and by milk and dung to a smaller extent.

33. Ghumusari

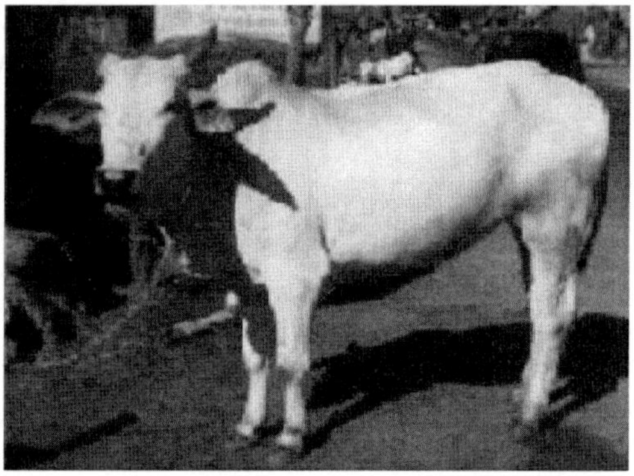

Synonym: Deshi

Origin and Distribution: Ganjam, Phulbani district of Orissa extending upto Srikakulam district of Andhra Pradesh. Heavy concentration is in Ghumusar area of Ganjam and Phulbani districts of Orissa. The Ghumusari breed of cattle is distributed in and around the Bhanjanagar (Ghumusar) sub division of Ganjam. This breed of cattle named after the local area "Ghumusai" of Ganjam and Phulbani district of Orissa.

Morphological Characteristics: The breed with a beautiful look varies from silver grey to white in skin colour body is generally small and compact. Small head with forehead being flat, broad and depressed in between the eyes. Horms curved upward and inward. Some animals have straight horms. Male body weight is about 208 kg and female is about 167 kg.

Performances: The lactation yield is 622 kg and lactation length is 322 days. Fat% is 4.86. Calving interval is 412 days. Average age at first calving is 43 months. They are reared for draught, manure, milk and fuel. Cows are generally docile and the bullocks are good draught animals.

Remarks: Excellent draught and heat tolerance cattle breed.

34. Malvi

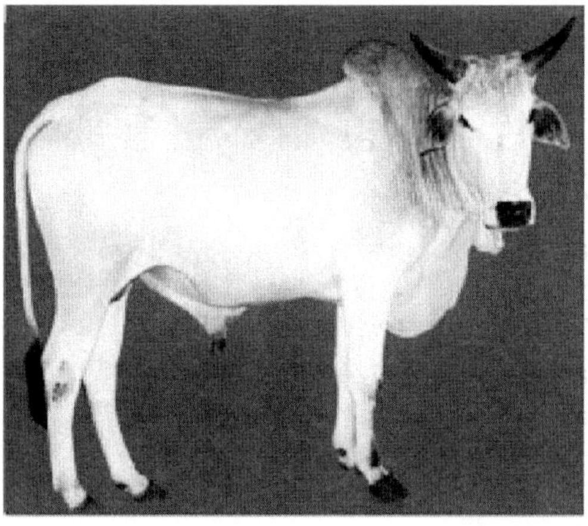

Synonym: Mahadeopuri, Manthani

Origin and Distribution: These are found in Gwalior region of Madhya Pradesh and also in Andhra Pradesh and Rajasthan. The breeding tract includes Rajgarh, Shajapur, Ratlam and Ujjain districts of Madhya Pradesh. The breed takes its name from the Malwa tract, named after the family of kings called Malwa in Madhya Pradesh. Malvi is named after its place of origin viz. 'Malwa' region. The breed is heavily concentrated in Malwa of Madhaya Pradesh and Jhalwar district of Rajasthan. There are two types of Malvi breed which are generally recognized viz. (1) Agar type found around Shajapur disrtrict of Madhya Pradesh and Jhalawar district of Rajasthan (2) Mandsaur of Bhopal type which is comparatively smaller in size and is found in the district of Mandsaur and Bhopal.

Morphological Characteristics: Malvi are of massive built and in some respects resemble the Kankrej. Lyre-horned grey cattle with white foreheads, prominent orbital arches and faces with flat or dished profiles. Deep short and compact body. Ears are alert and short in size. Short neck, thin dewlap, short but straight and strong muscular, proportionate legs. The tail is moderately long with a black switch reaching to the fetlock. Head short, dished forehead. The horns are curved and emerge from the outer angle of the poll in an outward and upward direction and are about 20-25 cm in long. Short but thick horn tapering to a blunt point.

Malvi cattle are white or white greyish - darker in males, with neck, shoulders, hump and quarters almost black. Cows and bullocks become nearly pure white with advancement of their age.

Muzzle and eyelids are black in color. Malvi animals are having medium hump and medium thin dewlap. The animals have a fine bearing and intelligent look. Adult body weight of male and female cattle is 499 and 340 kg, respectively.

Performances: The average daily milk yield is 2.55 kgs. The average lactation and dry period are 260 and 151 days, respectively. The average milk yield in this breed is around 916 kg per lactation with 4.3% fat and ranges from 627 kg to 1227 kg. The average age at maturity and age at first calving are 40 and 49 months, respectively. The calving interval is 480 to 600 days in the farmers' herds. The average service period and calving interval are 116 and 402 days, respectively. The average gestation period is recorded is 271 days. The animals are well known for quick transportation, endurance and ability to carry heavy load on rough roads. The animals of this breed are strong and well-built.

Remarks: They are recognised as draught type cattle breed.

35. Khariar

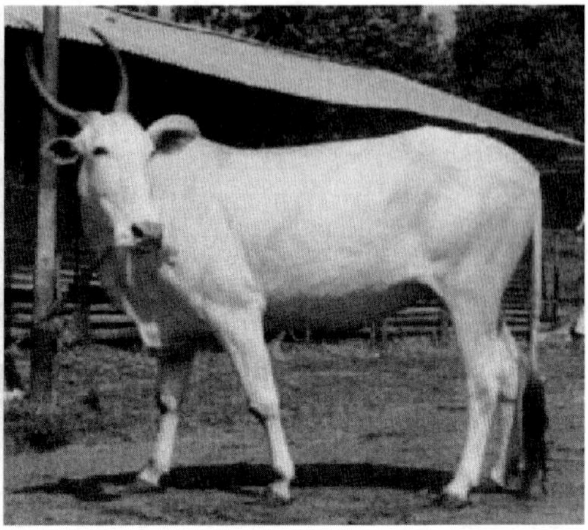

Synonym: Deshi

Origin and Distribution: The name of Khariar breed has been derived from the place of its origin, the Khariar region in Nuapada district in Orissa. Good number of these animals are found in Khariar, Sinapalli and Boden areas in Nuapada district. The adjoining areas in Kalahandi and Bolangir district also harbour a few animals of this breed.

Morphological Characteristics: They are small sized compact body built breed. Hump, neck and some region of face and back are dark in colour. The average height, body length, heart girth and body weight are 106 cm, 114 cm, 113 cm and 195 kg for male. The respective figures for female 102 cm, 106 cm, 123 cm and 156 kg. The coat colour of Khariar cattle ranges from light brown to grey. The breed has unique orientation of horn.

Performances: Kharia r is basically a draft animal. The bullocks are very good draft animals in and around the native tract for agricultural operation and transportation. However, the cows produce considerable quantity of milk, often used for family consumption and even marketed at times. Average lactation milk yield is 366 kg. Average lactation length is 293 days. Average age at first calving is 1522 days. Average calving interval is 512 days.

Remarks: Keeping in view the economic importance, productivity, draft ability, adaptability to low input system of management and the socio-economic status of the farmers in its native tract of Khariar cattle breed, efforts should be made for conservation and improvement of this valuable germplasm through selective breeding.

36. Gaolao

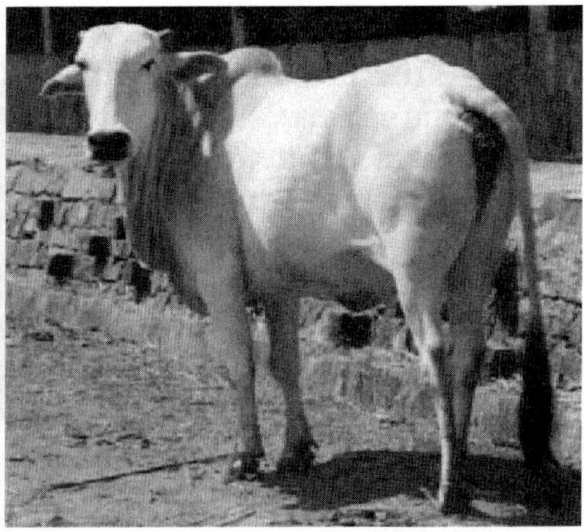

Synonym: Arvi, Gaulgani

Origin and Distribution: In 18th century the Marathas developed this for quick transportation in army. This breed is found in Balaghat, Chhindwara, Rajnandgoan and Seoni districts of Madhya Pradesh, Wardha and Nagpur district of Maharastra. Presently, this breed is restricted to a very small area where it is still popular with the farmers. Nanda Gowali community has developed this breed.

Morphological Characteristics: Medium size body with long coffin-shaped skulls. Face: Slightly convex in profile. Forehead: Slightly convex in appearance. Eyes: Almond shaped, placed slightly at angles, prominent orbital arches. Ears: Medium size, carried high. Horns: short and stumpy, curved slightly backward, blunt at the tip. Skin: White or light grey. Males: Grey on neck, hump and quarters. This breed closely resembles Ongole breed except that it is much lighter and has greater agility. Male body weight is about 430 kg while females weight is 340 kg.

Performances: The animals are essentially draft animals. Milk yield in cows is moderate. Some of the good specimens may yield upto 1,000 kg milk in a lactation of about 400 days. The average daily milk yield and lactation milk yield are 2.9 and 540 kgs, respectively. The average lactation and dry period are 198 and 284 days, respectively. The average age at maturity and age at first calving are 41 and 53 months, respectively. The average service period and calving interval are 192 and 485 days, respectively. The average gestation period recorded is 287 days. The calving interval is about 16 months. This breed reared for draught mainly for fast transportation and milk production.

Remarks: Gaolao is generally considered as a dual purpose cattle in India.

37. Mewati

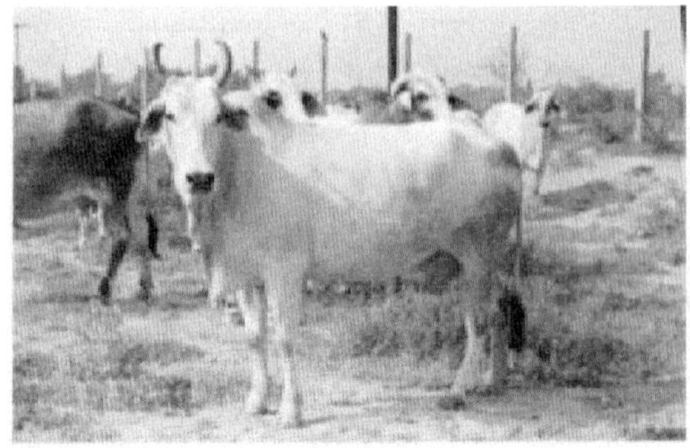

Synonym: Kosi, Mehwati

Origin and Distribution: The Mewati breed is found in Mathura district of Uttar Pradesh and Bharatpur and Alwar districts of Rajasthan. Mewati cattle are found in the tract known as Mewat, but the breed is sometimes called Kosi, due to the large numbers of cattle of this breed are sold from the market at Kosi, a small town in the district of Mathura. Native habitants of Rathi and Nagori cattle being adjacent to Mewat, these two breeds may also have contributed to the formation of the Mewati. They are named after Mewat in Haryana state. They are known to be related to Gir and Hariana cattle breeds.

Morphological characteristics: Coffin-shaped skull with prominent orbital arches. Face is slightly convex in profile. The face is long and narrow with the forehead slightly bulging. Eyes are prominent and surrounded by a very dark rim. The muzzle is wide and square and the upper lip thick and overhanging, giving the upper part of the nose a contracted appearance. The muzzle is pitch black in color. The ears are pendulous but not so long.

The neck and the whole frame is strong but the limbs are light. The legs are relatively long and the frame of the body gives an impressions of being loosely built. The chest is deep but the ribs are flat. The head and neck show an upright carriage. The dewlap, though hanging, is not very loose. The sheath also is loose but not pendulous. The tail is long, the tuft nearly reaching the heels. Cows usually have well-developed udders. Horns are small to medium in size and emerge outwards, upwards and then inwards in majority of animals. However, in some animals the horns emerge outwards and upward. Tips of the horns are pointed. The cattle are almost universally white in colour with the rare occurrence of brown shades. Adult body weight for male is 385 kg while it is 325 kg for female.

Performances: Mewati cattle are in general, sturdy, powerful and docile, and are useful for heavy plowing carting and drawing water from deep wells. The cows are said to be good milkers. The average lactation yield reported is around 958 kg. Daily milk yield (kg): 5 kg per day. The range of age at first calving is from 42 to 54 months and calving interval ranges from 12 to 18 months. It is considered to be a dual purpose breed with good milking and draft prowess. The bulls are known for their strength and endurance, and are employed for agricultural and carting purposes.

Remarks: Mewati is a dual purpose breed. They are similar in stature to Hariana but there are traces of influence of Gir, Kankrej, Rathi, Nagori and Malvi breeds also.

38. Punganur

Synonym: Nil

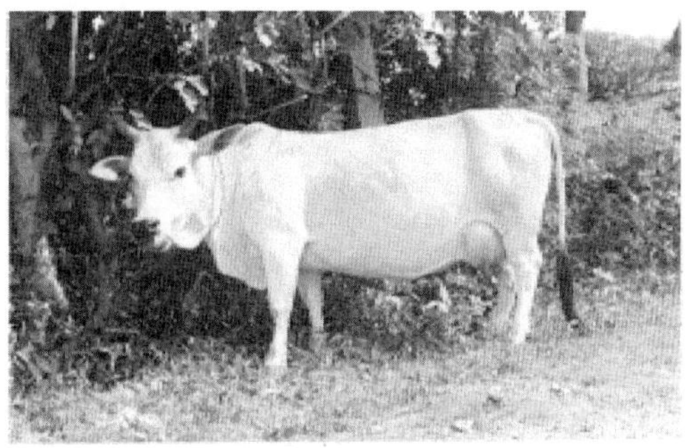

Origin and Distribution: Punganur is a dwarf cattle which originated from the Chitoor District of Andhra Pradesh in southern India. The breed is named after the town of its origin, Punganur in Chittoor district in Andhra Pradesh. The breeding tract is confined to Punganur, Vayalpad, Madna Palli and Palamaner taluk in Chittor district of Andhra Pradesh. This breed was developed by Rulers of Punganur.

Morphological characteristics: Some of the breed characteristics are: broad forehead and short horns. Back sloping downwards from front to hind quarters, tail touching the ground; slight mobile horns, almost flat along the back and normally founds at different heights from each other. Its average height is 70-90 cms and its weight is 115-200 kg. Most of the animals are white and light grey in colour with a broad forehead and short horns.

Performances: The Punganur breed's milk has a high fat content and is rich in medicinal properties. While cow milk normally has a fat content of 3 to 3.5 per cent, the Punganur breed's milk contains 8 per cent. It is highly drought resistant, and able to survive exclusively on dry fodder. The cow is an amazingly efficient milker with an average milk yield of 3-5 kg/day on a daily feed intake of 5 kg. It is known as poorman's cow. Age at first calving is about 37 months. Calving interval varies from 10 to 27 months. Lactational milk yield is 546 kg ranges from 194 to 1100 kg.

Remarks: The Punganur cow is the world's smallest humped cattle breed. Today, Punganur remain while other popular dwarf cow breed has disappeared. Ongole and Punganur cattle breeds are pride of Andhra Pradesh.

The Punganur is on the verge of extinction, with some 60 odd animals remaining. This decline is mainly due to the Indian Government's objective of 'bettering' Indian cattle breeds by crossing with Holstein-Friesian and Jersey cattle from developed countries, and banning the rearing of native bull breeds. The Punganur cattle are being reared mainly on the Government Livestock Farm, Palamaner, Chittoor district, while a small informal group of private breeders are also working on reviving the breed. It is not officially recognized as a breed since there are only a few animals remaining.

The body language of the cow is similar to a deer. The walking style of this cow is beautiful. It is very much auspicious to have this cow. The Punganur breed's milk has a high fat content and is rich in medicinal properties.

The Punganur cows are true Kamadhenu, receives cosmic energy at 64 times higher magnitude than a person who is in deep meditation.

39. Kherigarh

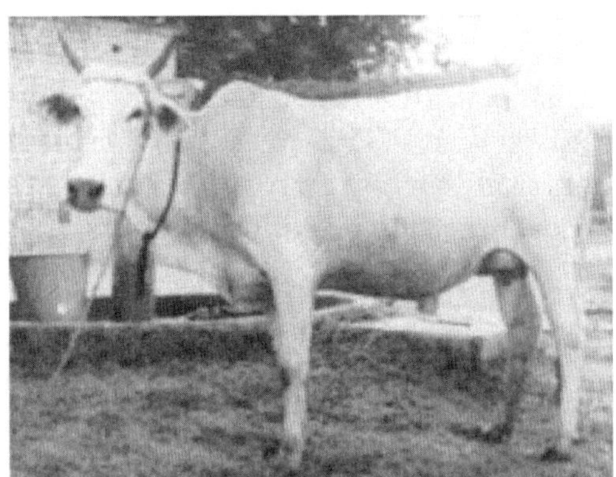

Synonym: Kheri, Khari

Origin and Distribution: These are comparatively obscure breed found in the Kheri district of Uttar Pradesh. They are thriving well on free grazing, and are well suited for the Terai tract. The breeding tract of this breed encompasses Nighasan and Pallia blocks of Lakhimpur Kheri District of Uttar Pradesh. True to the breed animals are available in the interior area of the breeding tract mainly around Sharda and Saryu rivers and around Dudhwa. The breed derives its name from a village 'Kherigarh' situated in the Shinghai area in the Nighasan Tehsil of Lakhimpur Kheri.

Morphological characteristics: The Kherigarh cattle are generally white or grey in color. The face is small and narrow. They have prominent orbital arches. Horns are thin and upstanding and measure 12 to 18 inches in length in bulls; cows usually have smaller horns. The ears are small and the eyes bright. The neck is short and looks powerful. The hump is well-developed in bulls. The dewlap is thin and pendulous and starts from right under the chin and continues right down to the brisket. The barrel is broad and deep. The sheath is short and moderately tight. Limbs are light. The tail is long ending in a white switch. The Kherigarh cattle closely resemble to the Malvi breed and the horn formation is typical of the lyre-horned Malvi type but much lighter in general appearance than the Malvi. Adult body weight for male and female is 476 and 318 kg, respectively.

Performances: *Production traits:* Poor milkers. Daily milk yield: 0.5-2.0 kg; Lactation period: 9-12 months; Milk production per lactation: 300-500 kg; *Reproductive traits:* Age at first calving: 36-54 months; Dry period: 60-120 days; Inter-calving period: 13-15 months; Service period: 90-150 days; *Ability as draught purpose:* The bullocks of this breed are active and have remarkable speed and stamina. Bullocks are good for light draught and quick light transport. A pair of bullocks can haul more than 10 quintals of load in a cart to a distance of 10-15 km without showing signs of much fatigue. The average speed is 4-5 km per hour. A pair of bullocks can plough one acre of land in a day working for 6 to 8 hours.

The animals of this breed are very much active and thrive on grazing only. The breed is primarily employed for agricultural operation, for carrying loads and transportation. These cattle start work when they are about 4 years of age and weigh about 600 pounds.

Remarks: Kherigarh is a draught purpose cattle breed and the bulls are used for light draft works. Animals are resistant to diseases and the expenditure on treatment is almost nil.

40. Badri

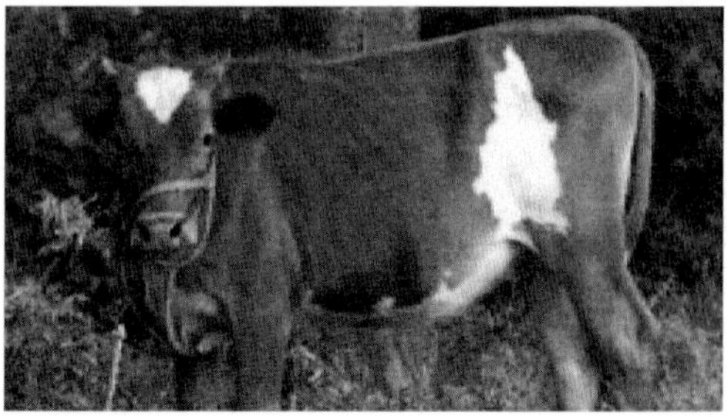

India has registered one new indigenous breed of cattle 'Badri' in 2017, taking the number of "desi" cattle breeds to 40 of cow.

Synonym: Pahadi

Origin and Distribution: Indigenous cattle mainly found in the hilly regions of Uttarakhand. The breeding tract of this breed is Nanital, Almora, Bageswar, Pithoragarh, Champawat, Pauri Garhwal, Rudraprayag Uttarkashi and Chamoli districts of Uttarakhand State. The altitude of this breeding tract ranges from 1200 to 2200 MSL.

Morphological Characteristics: Badri cattle are small in size having long legs and body colours – black, brown, red, white or grey. Hooves and muzzle are black or brown in colour. Straight forehead with prominent poll, medium to large prominent hump. Udder is small in size and tucked up with the body. Horns are curved upward and inward. The height (cm), body length (cm), heart girth (cm), weight (kg) and birth weight (kg), are 110, 115, 145, 257 and 18.7 for male and 108, 116, 140, 238 and 16 for female, respectively.

Performances: They are very poor milker. Average lactational milk yield is 632 kg. The fat% varies from 3.6 to 4.4% and average is 4%. The average age at calving 49 months ranges from 42 to 56 months. The calving interval is on an average 13 months varies from 13 to 15 months.

They are reared mainly for bullock power, milk and manure. These are well adapted to the hilly terrain and climatic conditions and comparatively more resistant to diseases. Balanced gait while walking. Animals are stall fed in the morning and in the night, and grazed from afternoon to evening. These are usually housed at night under the dwelling-house or in separate cowsheds. Fodder consists of mainly of grass carried from hillside by women. Estimated population is approximately 16 lakhs.

Remarks: This breed is mainly used for milk and draught purpose in the hilly area.

41. Lakhimi

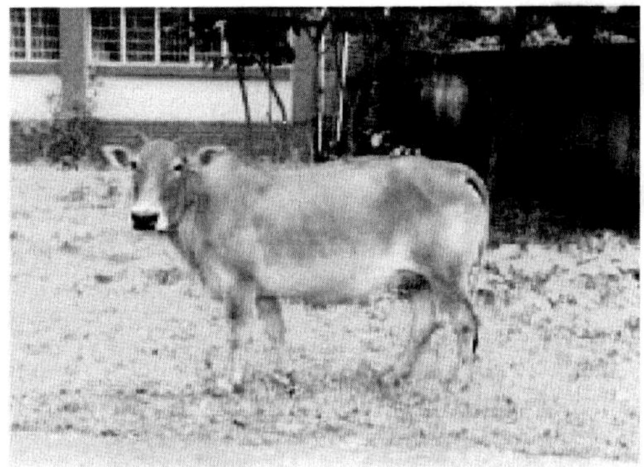

Breed Registration Committee of India in its meeting held on 4th August, 2017 at New Delhi approved registration of one new cattle breed. The institute NBAGR has registered first time indigenous breed of cattle from Assam, northeastern state of India. After including this newly registered breed, total number of indigenous cattle breed now in the country is forty one.

Synonym: Nil

Origin and Distribution: The indigenous cattle of Assam locally called *Lakhimi* are found in the entire state of Assam. These cattle are well adapted to subtropical climatic conditions. They are maintained traditionally under low or zero input system. Animals are let loose in the morning for grazing in nearby areas.

Morphological Characteristics: Animals are small sized and have relatively short legs. Coat colour is variable mainly brown and grey. Hump is medium in size and the backline is slightly curved. Horns are straight and about 17 cm in length. Udder is small and bowel shaped. The average height, body length and heart girth of adult Lakhimi cattle are 101, 92 and 131 cm for male while the respective estimates are 91, 83 and 112 cm for female. The adult body weight was recorded as 240 kg for male and 185 kg for female animal.

Performances: On an average, Lakhimi cow produces 359 kg milk per lactation which ranges between 325 to 375 kg. The fat percentage in milk varies between 4.3 to 6.3 percent with an average 5.3 percent. In general milking is done only once in the morning. Their average age at first calving is 47 months which is varies from 44 to 49 months. Calving interval ranges between 14 to 16 months with an overall average 15 months. Bullocks are excellent draft animals for carting and ploughing especially in the muddy fields for paddy cultivation. The milk produced by Lakhimi cattle is rich in fat for which it fetches a high price.

Remark: They are one and only dual purpose-milk and draught cattle breed of northeastern part of India.

21.0 Morphological Features of Indian Cattle for Identification

S.No.	Breed	Unique Morphological Feature
		1. Colour: Red/Dark Red/ Pale Red/Fawn /Brown/ Chocolate-Brown
1	Sahiwal	• Reddish dun or pale red colour • Symmetrical body and loose skin • Whitish ring along the eyes • Lateral and even-curled short thick stumpy horns • Long whip like tail almost reaching to the ground
2	Red Sindhi	• Red colour with dark red to brown shades • Dark-coloured muzzle • Well-proportioned compact body frame • Pendulous dewlaps with round drooping quarters.
3	Gir	• Dark red/brown or chocolate-brown colour • Ears tiny curled folded leaf, notch at the tip • Eyes partially close in appearance • Horns half-moon in appearance
4	Red Kandhari	• Universal deep red to dark brown colour • Black colour ring around the eyes • Good looking robust in appearance
5	Vechur	• Colour like Jersy cattle (Fawn) • Extremely small size but compact body • Small curving forward, downward horn • Average length: 124 cm, Height: 87 cm, Weighs: 130kg
6	Motu	• Light fawn colour, white speck at legs and dewlap • Small size but strong in built
7	Kosali	• Light fawn colour • Udder small and bowl shaped • Horns outward, upward, and inward from the polls • Muzzle, eyelids, tail switch and hooves black colour
8	Malnad Gidda	• Small size among all known Indian cattle breeds • Light fawn colour shades on thigh and shoulder
9	Nimari	• Reddish colour but white patches on body • Horns similar to that of Gir breed • Heavily built with straight back • Skin fine and slightly loose, pendulous dewlap • Peculiar hooves
10	Belahi	• Light fawn colour • Face white in colour • White patches at belly and legs • Tail upto hock joint and switch white in colour

		• Coffin-shaped skull • Short stumpy horns curving upward and inward
11.	Badri	• Small in size having long legs • Straight forehead with prominent poll • Medium to large prominent hump • Udder small in size and tucked up with the body • Varied body colours- brown, red, black white or grey • Hooves and muzzle black or brown in colour
12.	Lakhimi	• Small sized body with relatively short legs • Medium size hump and slightly curved backline • Mainly brown in colour • Straight horns • Bowel shaped small udder
		2. Colour: Spotted
13	Deoni	• Ears: Grey white with black inside • Ears: Alike Gir but no notch near the tip • Horns: Outward and backward curve • Wannera strain: Clear white with partial black face • Balankya strain: Clear white without spot • Shevera strain: Clear white with irregular black spots • White colour head at birth appears slightly black after 2-3 months
14	Dangi	• White colour with brown or black spots over the shining coat • Slightly protruding forehead • Skin: exudes oily secretion
15	Bargur	• Brown with white markings throughout the body • Horns light brown colour • Horns like Mysore cattle breed • Deep furrow between the roots of the horns
16	Rathi	• White or light grey colour with grey or brown patches • Somewhat similar in appearance with Hariana breed • Short stumpy horn • Coffin-shaped skull
		3. Colour: Black and White
17	Siri	• Black and white colour with large white marking • Hump slightly forward compared to other zebu cattle • Hump covered with a tuft of hair at the top • Thick coat on body

18	Panwar	• Black and white colour with white marking • Horns inclined to be lyre shaped • Switch of the tail white colour
		4. Colour: Grey/Dark Grey/Silver Grey/Iron Grey
19	Kankrej	• Lyre-horned grey colour cattle with white forehead • Strong curved horns accompanied by skin up • Gait 1¼ spaces (swai chal) with smooth movements
20	Kenkatha	• Grey colour barrel, dark grey rest of the body • Different shades of grey and black • Ears sharply pointed and do not droop • Back straight but quarters drooping • Horns forward direction, terminate in sharp point
21	Kangayam	• Grey or white in colour • Eyes dark and prominent with black ring • Strong horns upward, backward direction • Special points are strong horns with sharp tips • Bull grey colour with dark grey markings • Cow white colour with black markings on fetlocks and knees • Resembles Mysore breeds
22	Hallikar	• Light grey with darker shoulders and hindquarters • Long horns backward direction with pointed tip • Bulging forehead, furrowed in the middle
23	Amritmahal	• White to nearly black colour with white grey marking • Long sweeping horns upward and backward direction • Bulge narrow forehead, furrow in middle • Closely related to Halikar, Khillari and Kangayam
24	Pullikulam	• Grey in middle part of body but dark grey at head, neck and hind quarter • Reddish or brownish spots in muzzle, eyes, switch • Typical backward curved horns like Mysore cattle • Closely resemble to Hallikar cattle
25	Umblachery	• Legs white markings below the hocks like socks • Horn grayish white at the base, black at the tip • Switch of the tail grey to white colour • Calves red or brown at birth, in adult turn grey • Related to the Kangayam cattle of the same state

		5. **Colour: White/Light grey**
26	Hariana	• White or light grey colour • Compact body with coffin-shaped skull • Tail with a black switch reaching just below hocks • Orbital arches long • Long, narrow convex face • Flat forehead, bony prominence in centre of poll • Head carried high • Short stumpy horns upward, inward direction
27	Tharparkar	• White or light grey in colour • Long pendulous ears and inner side yellowish • Dewlap well developed • Prominent orbital arches • Medium sized well-proportionate compact body • Broad poll and forehead slightly convex
28	Malvi	• Grey colour, almost black in neck and quarters • Lyre-typed short thick horn • Ears alert and short in size • Resemble to Kankrej
29	Khillari	• Grey-white in colour • Forehead long with a convex bulge • Horns backward for half length then turn forward • Horns generally black, sometimes pinkish • Eyes set in elongated fashion, slightly bulging • Ears small and pointed, always held sideways • Hooves black with closely set digits • Resembles Hallikar and Amritmahal of Mysore cattle
30	Krishna Valley	• White or light grey in colour • Tail: Almost reaches ground • Coffin-shaped skulls with prominent orbital arches • Face: Slightly convex in profile • Horns: Small, curved upward and inwards • Ears: Small pointed
31	Punganur	• White and light grey in colour • Tail touching to the ground • Broad forehead and short horns • Back sloping downwards from front to hind quarters • Curved horns
32	Gaolao	• White or light grey in colour • Eyes: Almond shaped, prominent orbital arches

		• Medium size body with long coffin-shaped skulls
		• Face and forehead slightly convex in profile
		• Horns: Short and stumpy, blunt at the tip
		• Closely resembles Ongole breed
33	Ongole	• White or light grey colour
		• Hump well developed, erect
		• Large, heavy muscular body with coffin-shaped skull
		• Prominent orbital arches
		• Face slightly convex in profile
		• Stumpy short, thick, firm horns without crack
		• Alert and docile with good gait
34	Nagori	• White or light grey in colour
		• Long deep body with coffin-shaped skull
		• Horns outward, upwards, inward curve at tip points
		• Face convex in profile
		• Ears large, pendulous
35	Mewati	• White or light grey colour of skin
		• Coffin-shaped skulls with prominent orbital arches
		• Face slightly convex in profile
		• Similar to Hariana breed with Gir inheritance
		• Admixture of Gir, Rath and Nagori cattle
36	Kherigarh	• White or grey in colour
		• Prominent orbital arches and dished profiles face
		• Small and narrow face with white forehead
		• Resemble Malvi breed
37	Gangatiri	• White with two variant, totally white and grayish
		• Muzzle black with some spots
		• Dewlap and hump are medium size
38	Binjharpuri	• Chiefly white colour, grey, black or brown also found
		• Medium, compact, strong body size
		• In males, the hump, neck black in colour
39	Khariar	• Light grey coat colour
		• Small sized compact body built
40	Bachaur	• Grey in colour
		• Round barrel
		• Tail short in length
41	Ghumusari	• Silver light grey to white in colour
		• Compact small size, hardy draft breed
		• Cows are generally docile

22.0 Unique Features of Indigenous Cattle Breed

Name		Unique Feature
Sahiwal, Red Sindhi, Gir	:	Milch type, heat and draught tolerant
Rathi, Hariana, Ongole	:	Dual purpose, heat tolerance
Nagori	:	Excellent draught animal for hot climate
Vechur	:	Miniature cattle
Punganur	:	Dwarf cattle
Umblachery	:	Excellent for wet ploughing
Siri	:	Dual purpose, high altitude breed
Vechur	:	Medicinal qualities & easy digestibility
Punganur	:	Medicinal properties & high fat%

23.0 Cattle Breed with Medicinal Properties

23.1 Vechur Cattle Breed

The milk is believed to have medicinal qualities and easy digestibility due to smaller fat globule size. A recent report claims that the milk of the Vechur cow has more of the β-casein variety A_2, rather than the variety A_1 which is implicated in conditions like diabetes, ischaemic heart disease and autism.

The protein component of the Vechur cow's milk has an improved antimicrobial property. The anti-bacterial property of the lactoferrin protein present in the Vechur Cow milk is more than that of the antibiotic Ampicillin. Although lactoferrin, present in the milk of all mammals, is found to have antimicrobial, antiviral, antitumor, immunodefence and anti-inflammatory properties recent studies prove that in the case of the lactoferrin protein in the Vechur Cow milk, these properties are much more enhanced.

The Vechur Ghee (clarified butter) produced from Vechur cow's milk, is famous for its high medicinal values due to the presence of A_2 β-lactalbumin protein and higher arginine content which is good for the health of convalescing people.

23.2 Punganur Cattle Breed

The Punganur breed's milk has a high fat content and is rich in medicinal properties. While cow milk normally has a fat content of 3 to 3.5 percent, the Punganur breed's milk contains 8 percent. The cow has an average milk yield of 3-5 kg/day and has a daily feed intake of 5 kg. It is highly drought resistant, and able to survive exclusively on dry fodder.

24.0 A1 versus A2 Type Milk

In July 2007, ***Dr Keith Woodford,*** a professor of farm management at New Zealand's Lincoln University published a paper titled *A2 Milk, Farmer Decisions, and Risk Management* that reported how approximately 500 New Zealand dairy farmers are converting their herds to eliminate production of A1 beta-casein within the milk that is responsible for diabetes, heart disease and autism diseases.

Originally all cow milk was of the A2 type. However, a genetic mutation, probably between 5000 and 10,000 years ago, has resulted in a proportion of cows of European breeds producing a casein variant called A1 beta-casein. A1 beta-casein is absent in the milk of pure Asian and African cattle. The alternative (to A1) is A2 beta-casein, and the associated milk is known as A2 type milk. Milk of European breeds (A1) is addictive and it causes schizophrenia, diabetes and cardiovascular diseases. A1 and A2 beta-casein digest differently and only A1 beta-casein releases beta-casomorphin7 (BCM7) which is a powerful opioid (addictive) and causes diseases and many people who are intolerant to milk are able to drink A2 milk for absence of this. Most consumers and dairy farmers worldwide remained unaware of the issues surrounding A1 and A2 type milk.

Indian scientists of the National Bureau of Animal Genetic Resources (NBAGR) came up with their own study on A1 and A2 type milk. NBAGR scientist screened the status of the A2 allele of the beta-casein gene in 22 indigenous breeds and the two dominant foreign breeds Holstein Friesian and Jersey. While the A2 allele was 100 percent in the top five indigenous milch breeds: Red Sindhi, Sahiwal, Tharparkar, Gir and Rathi and around 94 percent in other indigenous dual and draught breeds, its status was merely 60 percent in Holstein Friesian and Jersey. The A2 allele gene in Indian milk breeds of cows and buffalos are 100 percent, while in foreign breeds, it is around 60 percent.

The major consumer market for A2 milk is in Australia where it is available in some 800 supermarkets and 200 convenience stores. However, overall market share is probably less than 1 percent because of limited publicity. In an increasingly health conscious world, this creates a huge potential for global demand for the A2 milk of Indian cattle breed.

25.0 Crossbred Strains / Breeds Evolved

In India		
Taylor	:	Shorthorn and Jersey with local cows around Patna, Bihar
Jersind	:	Jersey X Red Sindhi at Allahabad, Uttar Pradesh
Sunandini	:	Brown Swiss X Non-descript cattle at Munnar, Kerala
Frieswal	:	3/8 to 5/8 level inheritance of Friesian and rest Sahiwal, at Millitary Dairy Farm, Meerut, Uttar Pradesh
Karan Fries	:	Friesian X Tharparkar at NDRI, Karnal, Haryana
Karan Swiss	:	Brown Swiss X (Sahiwal and Red Sindhi) at NDRI, Karnal, Haryana
Jerther	:	Jersey bull X Tharparkar cows at Bangalore
In abroad		
Australian Milking Zebu	:	20 to 40% Zebu blood (Sahiwal, Red Sindhi) and rest from Jersey at CSIRO
Australian Frisian Sahiwal	:	Sahiwal bulls X Holstein Friesian cows of Queensland Deptt of primary Industry
Jamaica Hope	:	80% Jersey, 15% Sahiwal and 5% Holstein blood in Jamaica of West Indies
Mambi	:	¾ Holstein Friesian and ¼ Zebu in Cuba
Siboney	:	5/8 Holstein Friesian and 3/8 Zebu in Cuba
Pitanquieras	:	5/8 Red Poll and 3/8 Zebu in Brazil
Santa Gertrudis	:	Brahman X Shorthorn at Texas
Brangus	:	Brahman X Angus
Beefmaster	:	Brahman X Shorthorn X Hereford
Charbray	:	Brahman X Charolais
Guernsey	:	Brown and white cattle of Britain X Brindle cattle of Normandy

26.0 Dwarf Cows found in India

There are many dwarf cows in India mostly on the western ghats. They were once upon a time called sahya pashu - cows only found on sahyadri hills. Cows tend to become small in hilly hot and humid areas. Name of the dwarf cows found in India listed below:

1. Puganur (Chittoor district)
2. Vechur (Vaikam)
3. Kasargod Dwarf (Kasargod)
4. Malnad Gidda (Manglore to Kerala border)
5. High Range Dwarf (Idduki)
6. Kuttampuzha Kullan (Ernakulam - Idduki border)
7. Palakad Ottapalam Dwarf (Kanjikode area, Palakad)
8. Coorg Dwarf (Virajpet)
9. Vadakara Dwarf - This cows are not as small as Vechur
10. In Orissa also host small cows

All the above mentioned breeds are on the verge of extinction.

27.0 Indian Cattle Breed at Risk

Red Sindhi, Sahiwal, Tharparkar, Vechur, Punganur, Mewati, Kenkatha, Kherigarh, Bargur, Panwar, Siri and Krishna Valley of Indeginous cattle breeds are now at risk. Hence, immediate attention is utmost necessary for maintaining their identity and availability in future.

28.0 Productive and Reproductive Performance of Cattle

Breed	Age at first calving (month)	First calving interval(days)	First service period (days)	First lactation milk yield(kg)	First lactation length (days)
Hariana	51(41-59)	497(434-523)	214(136-303)	916(730-1170)	267(257-315)
Sahiwal	41(38-48)	443(418-473)	177(136-189)	1907(1597-2125)	314(228-330)
Tharparkar	43(39-53)	437(418-474)	160(130-183)	1877(1326-2139)	300(268-317)
Red Sindhi	44(39-49)	496(436-562)	154(152-158)	1476(1312-1694)	305(284-354)
Gir	53(44-61)	511(456-541)	176(135-259)	1498(1125-1859)	293(230-394)
Ongole	39(36-42)	553(529-637)	226(210-241)	826(658-999)	279(215-301)
Deoni	51(47-55)	466(456-472)	184(173-192)	943(818-1041)	293(282-302)

Figure in parenthesis gives range of the performance of the trait

29.0 Cattle Breeding Farm in India

S. No.	Name of the Breed	Name of the Farm
1	Amritmahal	**Karnataka** • Govt. of Karnataka: Ajjampur, Hessarghatta
2	Deoni	**Andhra Pradesh** • Deoni Cattle Breeding Farm, Gudgaripalli • Govt of Andhra Pradesh, Kampasagar **Karnataka** • Univ. of Agricultural Sci, Dharwad **Maharashtra** • Govt. of Maharashtra, Udgir • Marathwada Agril University, Parbhani
3	Gaolao	**Maharashtra** • Central Breeding Institute, Hetikundi • Govt of Maharashtra: Hetikundi, Pohara, Yeotmal
4	Gir	**Goa** • Govt. of Goa, Copardem **Gujarat** • Akshar Purushottam Mandir Gaushala, Gondal • BAIF-Magazari Farm, Zamp • Bochasanwasi Shree Akshar Purus-hottam Gaushala Trust Bochasan • Govt of Gujarat, Dhoraji • Gujarat Agril University, Junagadh • Lok Bharti Gaushala, Sanosara • Sabarmati Ashram Gaushala, Bidaj **Karnataka** • Govt of Karnataka: Koila **Madhya Pradesh** • Jawaharlal Nehru Krishi Vishwa Vidyalaya, Jabalpur • Kasturbagram Krishi Kshetra, Indore • Raymond's Embryo Research Centre, Gopalnagar **Maharashtra** • Mumbai Gow-Rakshak Mandali, Mumbai • Mumbai Panjrapol, Mumbai • Govt. of Maharashtra: Jath, Kopergaon • Mahatma Phule Krishi Vidyapeeth, Rahuri • Panjrapol Sanstha Sangli, Sangli • Shree Nasik Panchvati Panjrapol, Nasik

		Rajasthan • Govt. of Rajasthan, Dag
5	Hallikar	**Karnataka** • Govt. of Karnataka: Hessarghatta, Koila
6	Hariana	**Assam** • Govt. of Assam: Barpeta, Guwahati, Jagduar, Khanikar, Manja, Pachmile **Bihar** • Birsa Agril Univ, Ranchi, Jharkhand • Govt. of Bihar: Dumraon, Purnea, Sairakela, Jharkhand • Shri Gaushala, Bhagalpur **Haryana** • Government Livestock Farm, Hisar • Haryana Agril University, Hisar • Shri Gaushala Society, Panipat • State Cattle Breeding Farm, Hisar **Madhya Pradesh** • Govt. of Madhya Pradesh: Imlikhera, Kiratpur, Minora, Pakaria **Maharashtra** • Bull Rearing Centre, Nagpur • Govt. of Maharashtra: Hetikundi, Kopergaon • Punjabrao Krishi Vidyapeeth, Warud **Orissa** • Govt. of Orissa: Bolangir, Boudh, Chiplima, Keonjhar **Rajasthan** • Govt. of Rajasthan, Kumher **Uttar Pradesh** • Govt. of Uttar Pradesh: Babugarh, Hastinapur, Neelgaon, Saidpur • Mathura Vrindaban Hasanand Gochar Bhumi Trust, Mathura
7	Kankrej	**Gujarat** • BAIF-Magazari Farm, Zamp • Bidda Pinjrapole & Gaushala, Mandvi • Bochasanwasi Shree Akshar Purush-ottam Gaushala Trust, Bochasan • Govt. of Gujarat: Bhuj, Mandvi, Thara • Gujarat Agricultural University, Anand • Mansa Gaushala Trust, Vijapur

8	Khillari	**Karnataka** • Govt. of Karnataka, Bankapur **Maharashtra** • Govt. of Maharashtra: Hingoli, Jath, Junoni
9	Malvi	**Madhya Pradesh** • Govt. of Madhya Pradesh, Agar **Rajasthan** • Govt. of Rajasthan, Dag
10	Nagori	**Rajasthan** • Govt. of Rajasthan, Nagour
11	Nimari	**Maharashtra** • Govt. of Maharashtra, Bod
12	Ongole	**Andhra Pradesh** • AP Agricultural University, Guntur • Govt. of Andhra Pradesh: Kakinada, Kampasagar, Mahanandi, Vishakhapatnam • Ongole Cattle Breeding Farm, Ramathirtham • Ongole Cattle Breeding Project, Guntur
13	Rathi	**Kerala** • Govt. of Kerala, Maruthamala **Maharashtra** • Govt. of Maharashtra, Hingoli **Rajasthan** • Govt. of Rajasthan, Nohar • SKN College of Agriculture, Jobner • College of Veterinary and Animal Science, Bikaner **Uttar Pradesh** • GB Pant Univ. of Agri & Tech, Pantnagar
14	Red Sindhi	**Assam** • Govt. of Assam: Barpeta, Jagdaur, Silchar • Indo-Australian Cattle Breeding Project, Barpeta **Bihar** • Govt. of Bihar, Gouikarma **Goa** • Govt. of Goa, Dhat **Jammu & Kashmir** • Govt. of Jammu & Kashmir, Beli Charana **Karnataka** • Govt. of Karnataka: Koila **Kerala** • Govt. of Kerala, Kodapanakunnu

		Lakshadweep • Government Dairy Unit, Kavaratti **Maharashtra** • Punjabrao Krishi Vidyapeeth, Warud **Orissa** • Central Cattle Breeding Farm, Basantpur • Govt. of Orissa, Bolangir **Tamil Nadu** • Govt. of Tamil Nadu: Chettinad, Hosur, Orthanad, Pudukkottai, Tirunelveli **Uttar Pradesh** • Govt. of Uttar Pradesh, Kalsi
15	Sahiwal	**Assam** • Govt. of Assam: Jagduar, Pachmile, Silchar **Delhi** • Indian Agricultural Research Institute **Gujarat** • Sabarmati Ashram Gaushala, Bidaj **Haryana** • Government Livestock Farm, Hisar • National Dairy Research Institute, Karnal • Shri Gaushala Society (Regd), Panipat • State Cattle Breeding Farm, Hisar **Jammu & Kashmir** • Govt. of Jammu & Kashmir: Beli Charana **Madhya Pradesh** • Govt. of Madhya Pradesh, Anjora • Raymond's Embryo Research Centre, Goplanagar **Maharashtra** • Govt. of Maharashtra, Bod, Wadsa **Punjab** • Amritsar Pinjrapole Gaushala, Amritsar • Govt. of Punjab: Nabha • Punjab Agricultural University, Ludhiana **Tamil Nadu** • Tamil Nadu Cooperative Milk Producers Federation Ltd, Udhagamandalam **Uttar Pradesh** • GB Pant Univ of Agri & Tech, Pantnagar • Govt. of Uttar Pradesh, Chak-Ganjaria • Military Dairy Farm, Meerut • Project Directorate on Cattle, Meerut

16	Sunandani	**Kerala** • Kerala Livestock Development Board, Mattupatti
17	Tharparkar	**Andhra Pradesh** • Govt. of Andhra Pradesh: Kampasagar, Karimnagar, Mamnoor **Bihar** • Birsa Agril Univ, Ranchi, Jharkhand • Govt. of Bihar: Purnea, Sairakela **Haryana** • Government Livestock Farm, Hisar • National Dairy Research Institute, Karnal **Maharashtra** • Govt. of Maharashtra, Pohara, Yeotmal **Rajasthan** • Central Cattle Breeding Farm, Suratgarh • Govt. of Rajasthan, Chandan **Tamil Nadu** • Govt of Tamil Nadu, Chettinad **Uttar Pradesh** • Central Cattle Breeding Farm, Lakhimpur • Govt of Uttar Pradesh, Bharari

30.0 Indigenous Cattle Improvement Programme

The Government of India had launched a number of cattle improvement programmes from time to time. The brief description of these programmes is given here.

1. Central Herd Registration Scheme

In India the Herd Book was started in 1949 for Sahiwal, Red Sindhi, Gir, Tharparkar, Ongole, Hariana, Kankrej and Kangayam breeds of cattle. This Herd Book contains a list of animals qualifying the breed characteristics and production standard and thus purebred animals of high merit are enlisted in the book. The animals to be registered should meet its breed characteristics. This helps the owners in sale and purchase of the breeding stock.

2. Key Village Scheme

This scheme was launched in 1951 on all India scale taking a key village unit covering an area having a population of 1000 cows. The objectives of this were to use the superior germplasm of bulls. A key village block comprising 6 to 10 key village units was set-up with A.I. station to provide semen to the key village units.

3. Intensive Cattle Development Project

It was started in the year of 1966 for enhancing milk production as an area development approach and taking care of breeding, feeding, health care, extension activities and marketing facilities. It was located in the breeding tract of indigenous breeds of cattle with its coverage upto one lakh breedable cows.

4. Progeny Testing Schemes

This was started with the objective to identify and to produce the outstanding bulls on the basis of their progeny performance in the third Five Year Plan (1961-66). It was first implemented on Hariana cattle at Government Livestock Farm, Hisar, Haryana. The scheme was also started for Sahiwal at State Cattle Breeding Farm, Chakgangaria, Lucknow, Uttar Pradesh; SCBF Durg, Madhaya Pradesh; Red Sindhi at SCBF, Hosur, Tamil Nadu; Gir at SCBF, Junagarh, Gujarat; Hariana at SCBF, Bharatpur, Rajasthan in Fourth Five Year Plan (1969-74).

Later on, two projects namely Associated herd progeny Testing Scheme and Field progeny Testing Scheme were started in to overcome the limitation occured in Progeny Testing Program in India.

5. Military Dairy Farms

It was started in 1889 at Allahabad, Uttar Pradesh with the objective to supply the milk to the British troops and their families. The crossbreeding of Zebu cattle with European breeds was started on large scale in Military Dairy Farm. Ayrshire an exotic cattle breed was used first in this improvement programme. Later on other exotic breeds were also imported. The cows of Sahiwal, Red Sindhi, Gir, Tharparkar and Hariana breeds were used in Military Dairy Farm. The main objective was to evolve a strain of Holstein - Sahiwal crossbred cattle.

6. Project Directorate on Cattle

The PDC Meerut came into existence in November, 1987 with the objective to evolve a new catle breed 'Frieswal' and other crossbred genotypes for high milk production. Ongole and Hariana breeds were taken up for improvement of indigenous breeds in their breeding tracts.

7. Operation Flood

National Dairy Development Board (NDDB), Anand, Gujarat formulated the programme of Operation Flood for the development of Indian Dairy Industry in the year 1969. The Operation Flood was implemented in three phases as Operation Flood-I (1970-80), Operation Flood-II (1980-85) and Operation Flood-III (1985-96). The Operation Flood had contributed for sustained increase in milk production of our country owing to assured market of milk with remunerative price along with Artificial Insemination support.

8. Nucleus Breeding Schemes

Under this scheme, a breed is structured in such a way that all the animals are not allowed to make contribution for genetic improvement but very few are given this opportunity. A nucleus herd is created which is used entirely for production of males for breeding in the population. It may be closed or open depending on the direction of gene flow. An organized herd under conventional Progeny Testing is treated as single herd but under Nucleus Breeding Scheme the herd is divided in two groups i.e. Nucleus herd and Test herd.

31.0 AICRP on Cattle

An ad-hoc scheme entitled 'Behaviour Pattern of Zebu crossbred' was started in 1968 at the Indian Veterinary Research Institute and the Haryana Agricultural University, Hisar, for crossbreeding of Hariana breed with Jersey, Brown Swiss and Holstein-Friesian semen. Subsequently, this was expanded into an All-India Co-ordinated Research Project on Cattle with 5 centres in 1970. The above two at Izatnagar and Hisar used Hariana as zebu breed; the Mahatma Phule University of Agricultural Science at Rahuri and the Jawaharlal Nehru Krish Vishwa Vidyalaya at Jabalpur used Gir breed as the foundation base; the cattle-breeding farm at Lam attached to the Andhra Pradesh Agricultural University used Ongole as the zebu base. In 1973 the crossbreeding experiment at Haringhata (CBP) was merged with AICRP, thus briging the number of the centres was to six. The temperate breeds used were those mentioned above. Preferably frozen semen dosses from the same bulls were randomly distributed in all these farms to mate the cows and heifers of the local breeds. The halfbred exotic heifers were mated to another exotic breed to produce 3-breed genetic groups with ¾ th temperate dairy breed inheritance. The original mating plan was to produce four types of crossbreds for each of the three exotic breeds.

1. First crossbred generation (F_1)
2. Backcross to the parental breed
3. F_2 by mating males and females from the same F_1 cross interse
4. Three-breed crosses by mating mates and females from two different F_1 crosses in all six possible combinations.

The Indian Council of Agricultural Research (ICAR) was started a coordinated research project with the objective of evolving high yielding breeds of cattle and buffalo for different utility. The AICRP on cattle involved the crossing of indigenous cattle breeds (Hariana, Ongole, Gir, Tharparkar, Sahiwal, Red Sindhi and local cattle) with superior exotic breeds (HF, Jersey, Brown Swiss). The objective of AICRP on cattle was to know the optimum combination and level of exotic inheritance based on assessing the production and reproduction performance of the crossbreds in different agro-climatic regions. A control frozen semen bank was also established at Hessarghata (Karnataka) for collection, processing, storage and distribution of frozen semen. On the basis of the results obtained it was found that crossbreds with ¾th exotic inheritance did not do better than half breds due to disease problem, availability of required input and management problems. The better performance had been of those having 50 to 62.50% level of exotic inheritance than all other crossbreds.

In 1963, the Indian Council of Agricultural Research in collaboration with the FAO and PL-480 assistance started a large-scale crossbreeding programme at Haringhata in West Bengal for breeding Hariana type cows with exotic breeds Holstein-Friesian, Brown Swiss and Jersey. The programme was very well laid down. The objectives were to evolve a suitable breed for the warm humid regions. However, due to improper inputs provided and other lack of infrastructural facilities, the programme failed to give the desired results and was finally wound up.

32.0 Crossbreeding Programme

Crossbreeding programme for genetic development of cattle in India was started as early as 1875 near Patna using Shorthorn bull on local cows and the 'Taylor' breed of cattle was evolved. Crossbreeding work on more scientific lines was started between 1910 and 1932 at the Imperial Dairy Research Institute at Bangalore, Agricultural Institute at Pusa, Livestock Research Station at Hosur and Military Dairy Farms at Allahabad. During 1924-1934, the crossbreeding work was started at Allahabad Agricultural Institute using indigenous stocks of Sahiwal, Gir, Hariana, Kankrej and Red Sindhi cows with exotic breeds of Holestein Friesian, Jersey and Brown Swiss sires. Since 1934, the crossbreeding work was limited to Red Sindhi and Jersey having 3/8 to 5/8 Jersey inheritances and a new breed of cattle 'Jersindh' was developed. At Bangluru, Tharparkar cows were crossed with Jersey bulls and a new strain named as 'Jerthar' was developed.

In 1963, the bilateral project was Indo-Swiss Project now named Kerala Livestock Development Board (KLDB) was started at Kerala using Brown Swiss and Jersey sires on local Non-descript graded cattle and a new breed of cattle 'Sunandini' developed. Sunandini is a multipurpose breed for milk, draft and meat, this breed is now becoming exclusively a milch breed. The overall lactation milk yield was 2435 kg in 280 days with 3.89 % fat. The crossbreeding work was started at NDRI, Karnal in 1963 using milch breed cattle of Sahiwal and Red Sindhi with exotic Brown Swiss. Brown Swiss breed was considered for this crossbreeding for their high milk yield, better heat tolerance and draught capacity. Although a number of crossbred groups were formed but they failed to show any significant evidence of non-additive gene action for growth, milk yield and also for age at first calving. Subsequently, all the various crossbred groups were merged and selective breeding was practiced. The Brown Swiss inheritance varied between 50-75 % and the rest from Sahiwal cattle was the next best crossbred group. The creation of synthetic population following selection resulted into a new breed of cattle named as 'Karan Swiss' in 1980. High producing crossbred females will produce 5000 to 6000 kg milk yield with 4.78 % butterfat during lactation. The Karan Swiss breed is usually light gray to dark brown in color. In 1971 at NDRI, Karnal crossbreeding Holstein Friesian, Jersey and Brown Swiss sires semen was used on Tharparkar cows. The various crossbred groups were formed which had not shown significant effect of non-additive gene action for milk yield. All the various crossbred groups were merged and selective breeding was carried out. The Holstein Friesian inheritance varied between 50-62.5 % and the rest from Tharparkar was the next best crossbred group. The creation of synthetic population following selection resulted into a new breed of cattle 'Karan Fries'. The colour of Karan Fries breed predominantly of black patches and sometimes is completely dark with white patches on forehead and tail. The average first lactation milk yield was 3619 kg in 305 days. The average fat percentage ranged between 4.10 and 4.17% and SNF ranged between 8.58 and 8.75 %. The Project Directorate on Cattle (PDC), Meerut has developed a National crossbred cattle "Frieswal" a Holstein Friesian - Sahiwal cattle cross, yielding 4000 kg of milk with 4% butter fat in a lactation of 300 days. The predominant body colour of Frieswal cattle was black and white. Mahatma Phule Krishi Vidyapeeth (MPKV), Rahuri of district Ahmednagar, Maharashtra has developed a triple crossbred cow breed named 'Phule Triveni' giving milk yield of 3000 to 3500 kg per lactation with 4% of fat. The inheritance pattern of this new breed developed through crossbreeding was ½ Holstein Friesian, ¼ Jersey and ¼ Gir breeds.

Another crossbred cattle developed at IVRI, Izatnagar in India through cross-breeding is 'Vrindavani' whose genetic constitution is about 50–75% inheritance from exotic cattle breeds concerning Holstein-Friesian, Jersey and Brown Swiss and 25–50% from indigenous Hariana breed. This cattle exhibit almost all possible coat colors in addition to roan, light-dark brown, black and white and brown and white. They can able to produce around 3,000 kg milk in 305 days of lactation with 4–4.5% fat.

33.0 Cattle Breeding Programme

- The National Cattle Breeding Policy recommended the optimum level of exotic inheritance to be ranged from 50 percent to 62.5 percent in almost all crossbreeding projects in India. For the crossbreeding programme using the exotic and other indigenous breed, the strategies were as follows involving two or three breed crossing.
- Two Breed Crossing can be achieved through back crossing or Inter-se mating. In back crossing, the cross of *Bos taurus* and *Bos indicus* produces F_1 with 50 percent exotic inheritance. On back crossing of F_1 population to the exotic breed, the exotic level was increased to 75 percent in the next generation. i.e, in F_2. To bring it to 62.5 percent level, the F_2 population was again planned to cross with F_1 having exotic inheritance of 50 percent. The animals were then improved by mass selection.
- In India, the backcrossing was followed extensively by Kerala Livestock Development Board, Kerala. In inter-se mating, the *Bos taurus* and *Bos indicus* produces F_1 population with 50 percent exotic level and subsequently the selective mating among F_1 population continue to maintain the exotic level of about 50 to 62.5 percent This was followed in most of the crossbreeding projects of the country.
- For three breed crossing, the level of 50 percent from one exotic breed, 25 percent exotic level from another breed and 25 percent local or indigenous breed has been advised in some regions.

34.0 Breeding Strategies for Genetic Improvement of Cattle

The current milk yield levels for crossbred and indigenous cows could safely be increased to the targeted levels through increased availability of feeds, culling of low producers, strengthening of field programmes of selection and progeny testing of bulls for milk and providing breeding and other input services at the farmers' door. Keeping in view, the Breeding Starategies for genetic improvement of cattle in India are as follows:

S.No.	Type of Animal	Breeding Strategy	Purpose
1	Indigenous dairy breeds of cattle	Selective breeding	Milk production
2	Indigenous draught breeds of cattle	Selective breeding	Draught power
3	Indigenous dual purpose breeds of cattle	Selective breeding	Milk production and draught power
4	Non-descript cattle	Grading up with improved indigenous cattle breeds.	Milk production/ Draught power
		Crossbreeding with exotic dairy breeds followed by selective breeding	Milk production

Through selective breeding, it is expected that genetic improvement of indigenous cattle can be achieved ranging from 1 to 1.5 percent per annum in organized herds and 8 to 10 percent per annum in farmer's herds in initial generations. The crossbreeding of non-descript zebu cattle with semen of exotic dairy cattle breeds has resulted in enhancing milk production by 5 to 8 times to that of non-descript cattle, reducing age at first calving and shortening calving intervals in first generation crossbred progenies. Proper monitoring of grading up programme of nondescript cattle on regular and long term basis can improve the milk yield by 500 to 800 kg in the first generation. By use of zebu bulls of high transmitting ability for grading up subsequently in initial generations, milk yield can be improved to the extent of 5 to 10 percent per annum. In a period of 5 to 6 generations of continuous grading up, the non-descript stock will also be transformed into well-defined breed.

35.0 Cattle Breeding Policy

The current breeding policy recommended by the National Commission on Agriculture (NCA) and adopted by the Central and State Governments was based on the important considerations which were similar to those of the scientific panel on Animal Husbandry. Consequently, a very large scale crossbreeding programme was launched in the country. However, in view of the changed scenario, it become necessary to review and have a fresh look at the cattle breeding policy keeping in view of the research and field experiences, requirement of milk and milk products for consumption and exports, need of draught power for farm operations and transport, availability of feeds and fodders, existing cattle breeds and their strains, available infra-structure and support systems in different regions of the country.

The All India Coordinated Research Project on Cattle Breeding launched by the ICAR had the objective of evolving high yielding cattle breeds which could suit different agro-climatic conditions. It involved crossing of important indigenous cattle breeds like Hariana, Ongole, Gir, Tharparkar, Sahiwal, Red Sindhi and non-descript (Local) with Holstein Friesion, Jersey or Brown Swiss for assessing the production and reproduction performance of the crossbreds in different regions and ascertaining the effectiveness of the level of exotic inheritance and the impact of inter-se breeding crossbreds at different levels so as to determine the best genetic groups. The results indicated that $3/4^{th}$ breds produced from the different exotic breeds did not perform better than halfbreds due to various disease and management problems.

The crossbreds maintained between 50 to 62.5 percent level of exotic inheritance have been found to perform better than all other exotic crosses. Therefore, it has been recommended that crossbred progeny (F_1) should be covered with crossbred bulls having 50 to 62.5 percent exotic inhertance level under field conditions. Crossbreeding with superior exotic dairy breeds specially Holstein and Jersey is being resorted to for increasing milk production. In Kerala, however, Brown Swiss is also being used. The results from crossbred cows have indicated that these.are superior to non-descript cows as well as buffaloes on research and organised farms. However, selection of exotic breed should be based on agro-climatic, bio-physical and socio-economic factors in the area.

The recommended breeding policy for the development of indigenous breeds and non-descript cattle in different states of India is given in following Table. However, in the absence of information about actual breeding practice being followed and comparative performance of developed breeds under field conditions, it is not feasible and appropriate to recommend or reject the existing breeding policy. For this purpose, comprehensive studies should be initiated by agricultural universities and research institutes in collaboration with

Animal Husbandry Departments in different states so as to have adequate information for future planning.

36.0 Present Breeding Policy

- Grading-up of non-descript cattle with pure-bred bulls of milch, dual purpose or draught breeds.
- Improving the milk yields in the well defined breeds.
- Introducing more milk in dual purpose and draught breeds without impairing their draught capacity to any appreciable extent.

General parameters in the breeding policy formulated by various States are:

- Indigenous milch breeds such as Sahiwal, Red Sindhi and Gir, should be selectively developed for dairy traits in their native tracts.
- Indigenous dual purpose breeds such as Hariana, Rathi, Kankrej, Gaolao, Ongole, Deoni etc. should be developed selectively in their native tracts for dairy and draft traits.
- Indigenous draft breeds like Kangayam, Hallikar, Khillari, Amritmahal etc. should be developed selectively for draft traits in their native tract.
- Non-descript cattle will be bred with exotic semen to produce cross breed with Holstein Friesian or Jersey and maintaining 50 percent exotic inheritance. In some States Red Sindhi, Tharparkar and Hariana have also been used for upgrading non-descript cattle.

37.0 Main Features of Present Cattle Breeding Policy

- Selective breeding in the breeding tracts of established/recognized milch, dual purpose or some important draught breeds of cattle.
- Laying more emphasis on milk production in the breeding tracts of draught breeds/types of cattle and replacing the existing draught breeds/types with dual purpose breeds.
- Grading- up of non-descript cattle with recognised dual purpose or milch breeds in the areas where cattle do not conform to any specific breeds.

- Crossbreeding with exotic breeds in hilly and urban areas and around industrial townships to ensure adequate milk supply where facilities for rearing and maintenance of high yielding milch cattle exist.

38.0 Cattle Breeding Policy in Different States of India

State	Breed	Breeding Policy
Andhra Pradesh	Ongole	Selective breeding in Ongole: grading-up of nondescript with Ongole.
	Malvi	Selective breeding in Malvi in pockets grading-up of Malvi with Thatparkar and Deoni.
	Hallikar	Selective breeding in Hallikar: grading-up of nondescript with Hallikar.
Assam	Local Cattle	Grading-up with Hariana and Red Sindhi Crossbreeding with Jersey.
Arunachal Pradesh	Local Cattle	Grading-up with Red Sindhi and Hariana Crossbreeding with Jersey.
Bihar	Local Cattle	Grading-up with Tharparkar, Hariana and Red Sindhi; Crossbreeding with Jersey.
Delhi	Hariana	Selective breeding.
	Non-descript	Grading-up with Hariana and Tharparkar Crossbreeding with Holstein Friesian.
Gujarat	Gir	Selective breeding in Gir and Kankrej; grading-up of non-descript with Gir and Kankrej; Crossbreeding with Holstein Friesian and Jersey.
Goa	Local Cattle	Grading-up with Red Sindhi; Cross-breeding with Jersey.
Haryana	Hariana	Selective breeding
	Sahiwal	Selective breeding
	Non-descript	Grading-up with Hariana, Tharparkar, Sahiwal Crossbreeding with Jersey & Holstein Friesian.
Himachal Pradesh	Local Cattle	Grading-up with Hariana and Red Sindhi; Crossbreeding with Jersey.
Jammu & Kashmir	Local Cattle	Grading-up with Hariana and Red Sindhi; Crossbreeding with Jersey.
Kerala	Local Cattle	Grading-up with Red Sindhi, Kangayam and Tharparkar Crossbreeding with Jersey and Brown Swiss.

	Crossbred Cattle (Sunandani Breed)	Selective breeding; use of F_1 crossbreed bulls obtained by crossing indigenous cattle with progeny tested Jersey, Brown Swiss and Holstein Friesian bulls.
Karnataka	Deoni	Selective breerding.
	Krishna Valley	Selective breeding.
	Khillari	Selective breeding.
	Amritmahal	Selective breeding.
	Hallikar	Grading-up with Red Sindhi and Crossbreeding with Jersey and Holstein.
	Non-descript	Friesian.
Madhya Pradesh	Nimari	Selective breeding.
	Malvi	Selective breeding.
	Kenkatha	Selective breeding.
	Non-descript	Grading-up with Gir. Tharparkar. Hariana, Sahiwal. Ongole & Crossbreeding with Jersey.
Maharashtra	Khillari	Selective breeding.
	Dangi	Selective breeding.
	Gaolao	Selective breeding.
	Nimari	Grading-up of breeds of the region with Hariana
	Non-descript	Crossbreeding with Jersey.
Manipur	Local Cattle	Grading-up with Red Sindhi and Crossbreeding with Jersey.
Orissa	Local Cattle	Grading-up with Red Sindhi and Hariana and Crossbreeding with Jersey.
Punjab	Local Cattle	Grading-up with Sahiwal and Hariana and Crossbreeding with Holstein Friesian.
Rajasthan	Nagori	Selective breeding.
	Malvi	Selective breeding.
	Rathi	Selective breeding.
	Non-descript	Grading-up with Hariana, Gir. Tharparkar and Crossbreeding with Jersey.
Tamil Nadu	Kangayam	Selective breeding; grading-up with Tharparkar.
	Hallikar	Selective breeding.
	Non-descript	Grading-up with Hallikar; Crossbreeding with Jersey.
Tripura	Local Cattle	Grading-up with Tharparkar; Crossbreeding with Jersey.

Uttar Pradesh	Kenkatha	Selective breeding.
	Non-descript	Grading-up with Sahiwal, Tharparkar, Red Sindhi, Hariana and Crossbreeding with Jersey and Holstein Friesian.
West Bengal	Local Cattle	Grading-up with Hariana, Tharparkar Gir and Sahiwal; Crossbreeding with Jersey.

Thus, based on the above depiction, it may be concluded that the performance of Holstein crosses was found to be the best among all other exotic cattle and breeds of dairy animals in north-western part of the country. However, Jersey crosses showed reasonably good performance in hilly regions of Jammu and Kashmir and Himachal Pradesh along with coastal parts of India.

39.0 Cattle Breeding Policy of West Bengal

Animal husbandry programmes have been running through the State Schemes. Each State has to evolve its own breeding policy deciding on choice of breed, cross breeding strategy, optional mixture of animals of different breeds required, breeding goals in terms of expected genetic progress to be achieved, specific breeding programmes and the control measures that should be adopted to achieve the desired genetic gains in the population.

To be very precise, the state has no defined breeding policy; although crossbreeding has been adopted indiscriminately in all the agro-climatic zones of the state to enhance milk production. The 'key village scheme', which started in West Bengal with very small number of breedable native cows was infact the first breeding programme adopted by the state. In this programme, a dual purpose breed 'Hariana' of North-India was used to upgrade the local stock. This programme was extended subsequently covering a large number of breedable populations under Intensive Cattle Development Project (ICDP). A unit of the All India Coordinated Research Project (AICRP) on cattle was also started at Haringhata for improvement in the milk production of native (Deshi) cows through crossbreeding with exotic breeds. Thus, the crossbreeding programme with Hariana and the grades of Hariana was initiated in the milk shed areas of the state using exotic gcrmplasm in pursuance with the recommendation of National Commission on Agriculture. The basic idea in crossbreeding was to exploit heterosis to improve the productive and reproductive features of the local stock.

Recommendation of National Seminar on Cattle and Buffalo Breeding Policy-Perspective-Indigenous Non-Descriptive Cattle of West Bengal is as follws:

Hilly zone

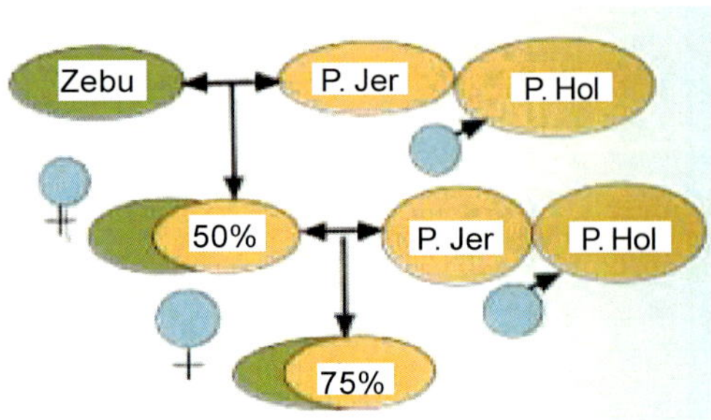

Three hill divisions of Darjeeling

Cross breeding by Holstein Friesian. Farmers' choice for Jersey will also be allowed. Exotic inheritance upto 75% allowed. Inter-se mating amongst the crossbred.

Terai zone

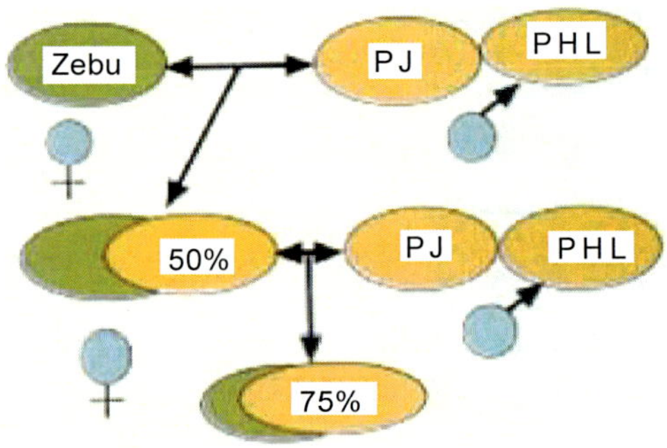

Jalpaiguri district and Siliguri Sub-Division of Darjeeling district

Jersey or Holstein Friesian of exotic inheritance either 50 or 75 percent. Inter-se mating amongst the crossbred.

Costal zone

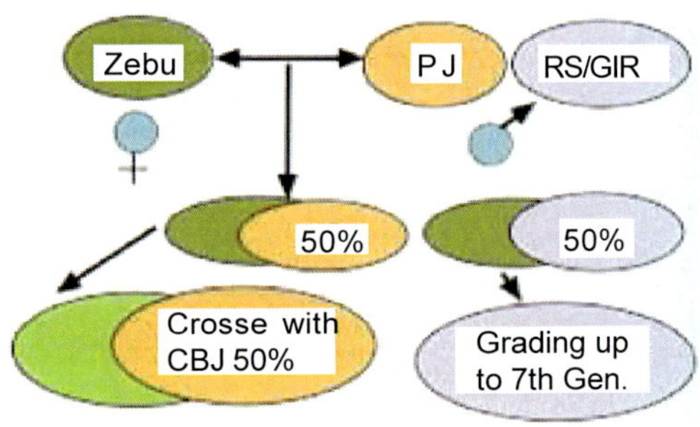

Part of South 24 Parganas, Part of Purba Medinipur and part of North 24 Parganas districrs

Cross breeding using Jersey Exotic inheritance at 50% level. Upgrading with Sahiwal/Gir at certain location.

New and old alluvial zone

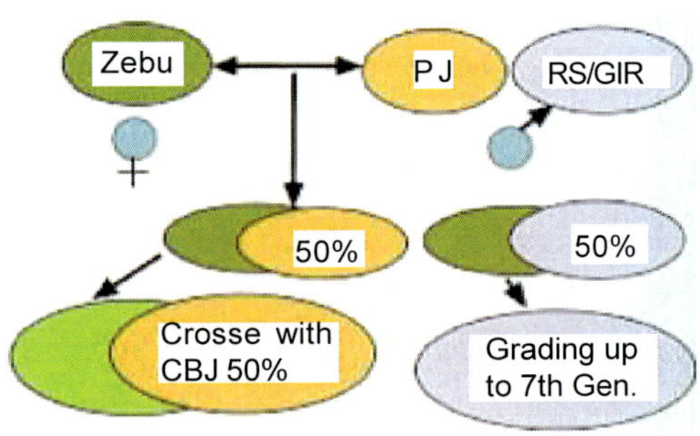

Coochbehar, Maldah, Uttar and Dakshin Dinajpur,

Murshidabad, Nadia, part of North and South 24 Parganas, Hooghly, Howrah, Burdwan and part of Purba and Paschim Medinipur districts.

Cross breeding with Jersey for Non-Descript cows. Grading up with Sahiwal/Red Sindhi/Gir for recognized breeds of Indian Cattle. Exotic Inheritance to be restored to 50 percent. Inter-se mating amongst the crossbred.

Laterite zone

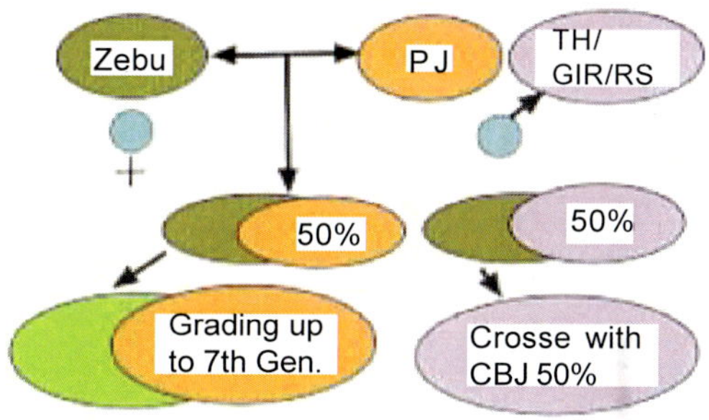

Birbhum, Bankura, Purulia and Jhargram Sub-Division of Paschim Medinipur districts.

Grading up of Indigenous breeds with Tharparkar/Gir/ Red Sindhi. Cross breeding using Jersey Exotic inheritance at 50% level.

Cross breeding programme has greatly influenced the overall dairy economy of the state. The number of animals with superior germplasm has increased. But the crossbreds constitute approximately 7 % of the total breedable female stock which appears to be of low order. However, the production of quality stock has been achieved through the implementation of breeding programme in a systematic manner. The state needs a clearly defined breeding policy which may not be uniform in different agro-climatic zones of the state. The animal feed resources need to be looked into together with the nutritional management of crossbred animals to enhance the milk production.

40.0 Schemes for Development of Indigenous Cattle

To develop indigenous Cattle, Government of India had initiated three schemes namely.

40.1 National Project for Cattle and Buffalo Breeding

40.2 Central Herd Registration Scheme

40.3 Central Cattle Breeding Farms

Now details of the above mentioned schemes are presented below:

40.1 National Project for Cattle and Buffalo Breeding

Genetic improvement in bovine is a long term activity and Government of India had initiated a major programme "National Project for Cattle and Buffalo Breeding" (NPCBB) from October 2000 over a period of ten years, in two phases each of five years, with an allocation of Rs 442 crore for Phase–I. Phase-II of NPCBB was formulated taking into account recommendations of the evaluating agency (NABARD) and was initiated in December 2006 with an allocation of Rs. 775.87 crore for a duration of five years from 2006-07 to 2010-11. A major new component of Phase-II was bull production programme. The project envisaged 100% grant-in-aid to State Implementing Agencies.

The Government of India, in 2000, initiated the above project with the objectives of genetic upgradation on priority basis and also had focus on the development of indigenous cattle and buffaloes so as to improve the genetic makeup as well as their availability in the country. The Project was implemented by State Implementing Agencies (SIA) constituted by the states for implementation of the project with the target of cattle and buffalo breeders of the country and up-gradation of state infrastructure for cattle and buffalo breeding.

Objectives

1. To arrange for delivery of vastly improved artificial insemination service at the farmers door-step.
2. To bring progressively all breedable females among cattle and buffalo under organized breeding through artificial insemination or natural service by high quality bulls within a period of 10 years.
3. To undertake breed improvement programme for indigenous cattle and buffaloes so as to improve their genetic makeup as well as their availability.
4. To provide quality breeding inputs in breeding tracts of important indigenous breeds so as to prevent the breeds from deterioration and extinction.

Components

The project components specially designed to address the existing inadequacies will focus on the hitherto neglected natural mating system as well as the A.I. network with particular attention to:

1. Streamlining storage and supply of Liquid Nitrogen by ensuring supply from industrial gas manufacturers and setting up bulk transport and storage systems for the same.
2. Introduction of quality bulls with high genetic merit.
3. Promotion of private mobile AI service for doorstep delivery of A.I.
4. Conversion of existing stationary government A.I. centres into mobiles centres.
5. Study of breeding systems in areas out of reach of A.I.
6. Quality control and certification of bulls and services at sperm stations, semen banks and training institutions.
7. Induction of breeding bulls for natural service in the areas not under AI coverage.
8. Institutional restructuring by way of entrusting the job of managing production and supply of genetic inputs as well as Liquid Nitrogen to a specialized autonomous and professional State Implementing Agency.

State Implementing Agencies (SIAs)

At the Central Government level a Central Project Management Unit (CPMU) with a core group of professional staff implemented the project. There was a broad based Steering Committee for the project to provide guidance to the CPMU. Since inception of the project in October, 2000, 27 SIAs were constituted under the project in 28 States. These agencies had professional approach in implementing the project. In case of small States, which were unable to constitute viable SIAs, funds were released to the State Governments for implementation of the project.

In a total 28 States and one UT participated in the project. Financial assistance to the tune of Rs 875.72 crore was released to these States/UT upto 2011-12. During the financial year 2012-13 (till 30th September 2012), an amount of Rs 69.52 crore was spent.

Expected benefits

1. By the end of the phase-I it was expected to bring 70% of breedable bovine population under organized breeding programme.
2. Door step delivery of AI services to improve accessibility and conception rate has been adopted in participating States in contrast to the earlier system of taking the animals to stationary AI centres.
3. 14,000 private AI workers were expected to be introduced by the end of the phase-I for door step delivery of AI to generate employment and ensure wider coverage.
4. State Implementing Agencies are managing breeding operations on scientific lines.
5. In order to produce quality-breeding bulls to be used for breeding, large-scale screenings of elite animals from farmers' herds are being conducted.
6. Bulls earlier used for natural service are being gradually phased out and replaced with pedigreed bulls.
7. With the capacity for producing 66 million straws and assured supply of liquid nitrogen, AI network in India will be completely revamped after the phase-I.
8. Specific programmes are being undertaken to make available trained manpower to sustain the extended AI network.
9. Use of quality bulls and semen will result in progressive genetic improvement in the bovine population.
10. Specific action to conserve animal genetic diversity among Indian cattle and buffalo breeds and to promote breeders' organisations is being undertaken in the breeding tracts in most of the States.
11. Although direct benefits will accrue to participating breeders, indirect benefits of breed improvement and higher productivity will percolate to resource-poor rural families at large.

Notable achievements

a) Semen production in the country was increased from 22 million straws (1999-2000) to 44 million straws (2007-2008) and the number of inseminations was increased from 20 million to 41 million. Semen production has increased from 50.5 million to 62 million and AI number from 50 million to 52 million between 2009-10 and 2010-11. Conception rate increased from 20% to 35%.

b) 36000 Government Stationary AI centres were converted into mobile AI centres.

c) 21000 Private AI centres were established or under establishment. 4000 private AI workers were established between 2009-10 and 2010-11.

d) 21700 breeding bulls with high genetic merit were inducted or under induction. 3000 quality breeding bulls have been inducted for natural service between 2009-10 and 2010-11.

e) 50,000 existing AI workers were trained in all the aspects of frozen semen technology (including funds released for training of existing AI workers during current year).

f) 1800 professionals were trained outside the State at reputed training centres.

g) 49 frozen semen bull station were strengthened as per Minimum Standard Protocol (MSP) for semen production.

h) In order to improve quality of semen production in the country MSP for semen production were formulated and implemented at all semen station in the country.

i) Central Monitoring Unit (CMU) were constituted for evaluation of semen stations one in two years and implementation of Minimum Standard Protocol (MSP) for semen production in the country.

j) 22 semen stations was graded as 'A', 17 as 'B' and 3 as 'C' during 2010-11 against 11 as 'A', 16 as 'B' and 7 as 'C' during 2007-08. A and B graded semen station was increased to 39 against 27 in earlier evaluation.

k) 34 semen stations in the country was acquired ISO certification against 3 during 2004.

l) Number of animals in milk was increased from 62 million during 2000 to 77 million during 2008 i.e. about 14 million improved milch animals was added to milch herd of the country.

m) Crossbred cattle population was increased from 20 million (1997) to 33 million (2007)

n) MSP (Minimum Standard Protocol) for progeny testing and standard operating procedures for AI (artificial insemination) technicians was formulated and circulated among all the States.

The National Project for Cattle & Buffalo Breeding were merged in the National Programme for Bovine Breeding and Dairy Development (NPBBDD) on February 2014. This scheme is no more in operation now.

40.2 Central Herd Registration Scheme (CHRS)

Government of India has initiated Central Herd Registration Scheme for identification and location of superior germplasms of cattle and buffaloes, propagation of superior genetic stock, regulating sale and purchase, help in formation of breeders societies and to meet requirement of indigenous bulls in the different parts of the country. Four CHRS units were established in different breeding tracts of the country. For milk recording, 103 milk recording centers were set up. Indigenous cattle breeds covered under the scheme are Gir, Kankrej, Hariana and Ongole. During 2001-2002, final registration for 1795 animals were completed.

Objectives

The scheme aims to, in case of cattle and buffalo, fulfil the following objectives:

- Identification and location of superior germplasm.
- Using data for producing superior germplasm.
- Preservation of indigenous germplasm.
- Introducing Milk recording for further propagation.

Implementing Agencies

- CHRS Unit Rohtak in Haryana
- CHRS Unit Ahmedabad in Gujarat
- CHRS Unit Ajmer in Rajasthan
- CHRS Unit Ongole in Andhra Pradesh.

Target Group/Beneficiaries

The primary aim is to identify elite germplasm for further improvement in milk production. Indigenous breeds covered at present are Gir, Kankrej, Hariana, Ongole of cattle. Under the scheme incentives for rearing of elite cows and their male calves is given to the owners of the elite animals.

Criteria For Registration Under CHRS

The criteria laid down for registration is given in the following table.

Breed	Milk yield in Kg's	
	Category-I	Category-II
Gir	3500 & above	3000 to 3499
Hariana	2700 & above	2500 to 2999
Kankrej	3000 & above	2700 to 2999
Ongole	2500 & above	2250 to 2499

Funding pattern: 100% Central Grant.

40.3 Central Cattle Breeding Farms (CCBF)

India has the largest cattle and buffalo population in the world. Considerable importance was given to the Livestock Development Programme for increasing the production of major products to increase the income of the economically weaker sections of the community i.e. small farmers, marginal farmers and agricultural labourers. One of the field of Animal Husbandry is Cattle Breeding. Keeping in view of the Animal Breeding, seven Cattle Breeding Farms were established throughout India for propagation of recognized cattle and buffalo Breeds.

The seven Cattle Breeding Farms in the Department, are implementing the stated objectives. The Farms are subordinate offices of the Department for implementing the technical programme. There are seven Central Cattle Breeding Farms (CCBFs) located at Alamadhi (Tamil Nadu), Andeshnagar (U.P), Chiplima and Semiliguda (Orissa), Dhamrod (Gujarat), Hesserghatta (Karnataka), and Suratgarh (Rajasthan). These seven Central Cattle Breeding Farms are meant for maintenance/propagation and distribution of pure bred bull calves. They are producing high pedigree bull calves of indigenous and exotic breeds of cattle for distribution to States for use in the cattle development programmes. The bull calves are produced from Tharparkar, Red Sindhi, Jersey, Holstein Friesian and Crossbred cattle, breeds. The Farm at Andeshnagar and Chiplima are producing HF x Tharparkar crossbred and Jersey x Red Sindhi crossbred bulls, respectively. The bulls and bull calves are for sale and distribution to the State Governments.

Objectives

- Progressive genetic improvement of the herd for milk production in important breed/type of cows and buffaloes by scientific selection and mating system.
- Production and distribution of superior pedigreed bulls for breeding programme in the states/country under Cattle and Buffalo Breeding Programmes.
- Conservation of threatened indigenous breeds of national importance.
- Production of upgraded crossbred animals suitable for specified breeding tracts.
- Training/Demonstration of scientific breeding and farm management practices to the farmers.
- Production and supply of seeds, planting materials of high yielding varieties of fodder crops and grasses in areas around the farm.

Seven Breeding Farms

The following seven breeding farms were established in the country for implementing the objectives of this scheme.

S.No.	Name & location of the farm	Breed maintained
1	Suratgarh (Rajasthan)	Tharparkar
2	Dhamrod (Gujarat)	Surti Buffalo
3	Chiplima (Orissa)	Red Sindhi (RS) and RS X Jersey
4	Hessaraghatta (Karnataka)	Holstein Friesian
5	Sunabeda (Orissa)	Jersey
6	Alamadhi (Tamil Nadu)	Murrah Buffalo
7	Andesh Nagar (U.P.)	Holstein Friesian X Tharparkar

The Production of Bull Calves (Nos.) is as under during the 9th Five Year Plan period:

Year	Target	Achievement
1997-1998	330	346
1998-1999	330	321
1999-2000	300	449
2000-2001	350	362
2001-2002	350	370

Target Group / Beneficiaries

Various cattle and buffalo development agencies are benefited from the scheme by way of using high quality bulls produced at the farms. These bulls are used for semen production and natural breeding to help upgrade the animals in the country.

41.0 Rashtriya Gokul Mission

Introduction

Cattle rearing have been a traditional livelihood in India and are closely linked to agricultural economy. India with about 190 million cattle (as per 19th Livestock Census 2012) has 12.5% of the world cattle population. Of this, 79% i.e. 150 million are indigenous. Most of the indigenous cattle (about 80%) are non-descript and only 20% belong to Indigenous Breeds recognized by National Bureau of Animal Genetic Resources. The cattle genetic resources of India is represented by 41 well recognized Indigenous Breeds. Indigenous cattle, in India, are robust and resilient and are particularly suited to the climate and environment of their respective breeding tracts. They are endowed with qualities of heat tolerance, resistance to diseases and the ability to thrive under extreme climatic stress and less than optimal nutrition. The potential to enhance the productivity of the indigenous breeds of India through professional farm management and superior nutrition is immense. For this it is essential to promote conservation and development of indigenous breeds. The Rashtriya Gokul Mission aims to conserve and develop Indigenous Breeds in a focused and scientific manner.

Aim of the Scheme

The "Rashtriya Gokul Mission" has been launched by the Government for conservation and development of indigenous breeds in a focused and scientific manner. The mission also envisages for establishment of integrated cattle development centres Gokul Grams to develop indigenous breeds including upto 40% nondescript breeds.

Rashtriya Gokul Mission is a focussed project under National Programme for Bovine Breeding and Dairy Development, with an outlay of Rs 500 crore for three years from 2014-15 to 2016-17.

Objectives

The Rashtriya Gokul Mission is being implemented with the objectives of: a) development and conservation of indigenous breeds b) breed improvement programme for indigenous cattle breeds to improve their genetic makeup and increase the stock; c) enhancement of milk production and productivity; d) upgradation of nondescript cattle using elite indigenous breeds like Gir, Sahiwal, Rathi, Deoni, Tharparkar, Red Sindhi and e) distribution of disease free high genetic merit bulls for natural service.

Implementing Agency

Rashtriya Gokul Mission is being implemented through "State Implementing Agencies (SIA)" viz. Livestock Development Boards. All Agencies having a role in indigenous cattle development are "Participating Agencies" like CFSPTI, CCBFs, ICAR, Universities, Colleges, NGO's, Cooperative Societies.

Funding Pattern

Scheme is implemented on 100% grant-in-aid basis.

Target /Beneficiaries

Rural cattle and buffalo keepers irrespective of caste, class and gender through out the country.

Components

Funds under the scheme are allocated for: a) establishment of Integrated Indigenous Cattle Centres viz. *"Gokul Gram"* b) strengthening of bull mother farms to conserve high genetic merit Indigenous Breeds c) establishment of Field Performance Recording (FPR) in the breeding tract d) assistance to Institutions/Institutes which are repositories of best germplasm e) implementation of Pedigree Selection Programme for the Indigenous Breeds with large population f) establishment of Breeders Societies: *Gopalan Sangh* g) distribution of disease free high genetic merit bulls for natural service h) incentive to farmers maintaining elite animals of indigenous breeds i) heifer rearing programme; award to farmers *"Gopal Ratna"* and Breeders Societies *"Kamadhenu"* j) organization of Milk Yield Competitions for indigenous breeds and k) organization of Training Programme for technical and non technical personnel working at the Institute/Institutions engaged in indigenous cattle development.

Procedure for Applying

State Governments are required to send the projects, duly assessed by the SIA to Government of India. Projects will be appraised and approved by Project Sanctioning Committee (PSC), Govt. of India.

Application form

General guidelines have been circulated to all the State Governments/UTs. Guidselines are available on the website www.dahd.nic.in

42.0 Advanced Technologies for Genetic Improvement

- The Reproductive technologies like Embryo Transfer (ET) and Open Nucleus Breeding System (ONBS) using MOET shall be an integrated part of cattle breed improvement programme.
- Molecular genetic studies for identification of genes of interest (Milk quality and quantity traits, fertility, draft, disease resistance, adaptive traits) and marker assisted selection (MAS) as new breeding tools need to be explored for identifying superior animals and commercial exploitation of genetic potential of indigenous cattle breeds.

43.0 Constraints in Cattle Improvement

Cattle being one of the major constituents of our livestock population is facing challenges which need to be addressed promptly and adequately to bring in rapid improvement in cattle population.

The main constrains in genetic improvement are mentioned below:

- Low heritability of the economic traits.
- Low accuracy of selection.
- Low scope/intensity of selection
- Limitations of feed resources both in qualitative and quantitative terms.
- Absence of effective field-oriented conservation strategy for indigenous breeds.
- Lack of farmers organizations and breeders societies in the country.
- Absence of effective extension network.
- Lack of unified coordinating mechanism for breeding programme with database.
- Lack of long term breeding policy and strategy with projection of requirement of breeding inputs.
- Lack of monitoring cell for certification of sperm stations and AI bulls including sourcing and use of quality bulls for breeding.
- Non-coordination in the form of fund-flow for cattle and buffalo breeding programmes available from different schemes having livestock components.
- Absence of a programme focused exclusively on draught breeds.
- Absence of an effective policy for conservation of dwindling indigenous cattle breeds.
- Lack of incentives to the farmers for rearing good quality animals.

Indigenous breeds can be made commercially viable within few generations and very few organized efforts have been made to improve the genetic potential of indigenous breeds. Usefulness of various indigenous breeds has not been fully explored. The non-renewable energy resources are bound to exhaust sooner or later. If this happens then we may have to fall back on our animal wealth for providing draught power and hence we cannot take risk of letting these breeds go extinct, as the domesticated breeds are integral part of our eco-system, culture and heritage. Thus there is imperative need to develop our indigenous breeds for milk production, draught power etc.

44.0 India Risks Losing Indigenous Native Cattle Breeds

The indigenous cattle of India not only play an important role in the economy of the country but also have some important unique characteristics for which they are well known in world. They are as much of a symbol of India as the Royal Bengal Tiger or the Taj Mahal. So it is our duty not to allow them to lose. Extensive uses of crossbreeding to enhance the milk production of country have resulted in edging out India's native breeds, and if it continues in such a way then our indigenous cattle breed may be extinct in a very short span of time. India is number one milk producer in the world and producing approximately 137.7 million tons of milk in 2013-14. With India's steady increase in population, milk production will need to continue to grow to meet demand. Hence, Government of India has spent decades promoting the cross-breeding of native dairy cattle to bulls from foreign breeds like the Holstein or Jersey cattle.

As a result of the cross-breeding program in India, Indigenous cattle are now producing milk at higher rates. But this cross-breeding program is not suitable for all Indian farmers owing to agro climatic condition and poor economic status of Indian farmers. The exotic cattle used for crossbreeding in India are well adapted at temperate region. Thus, maintenance of crossbred cattle in India is expensive that Indian farmers are unable to bear. This is important because smallholder and landless farmers own about 70 percent of India's dairy cattle. These small marginal poor farmers cannot afford to build the facilities required for crossbred cattle, and thus they need cows that thrive in India's climate. In spite of these, concept of cross breeding is now very widespread among India's cattle. Not only the exotic cattle but also best Indian cattle are also nowadays used in crossbreeding or grading up program in the country. If such practice is remain for long time then four well recognized India's dairy breeds - the Sahiwal, Red Sindhi, Gir and Tharparker may soon be extinct. This will make it harder for small farmers in India to obtain cattle they can afford to take care of. Not only this, wide diversity existed in cattle genetic resources in India will be wiped out.

Fortunately, there are some organizations working to conserve such diversity of Indian cattle. But the number of such organization in the country is not adequate as much it required. The Vechur Conservation Trust was founded in Kerala to preserve endangered livestock breeds in India. It is noteworthy that some of the retired scientist of NDRI and NBAGR formed society with their own effort to conserve indigenous germplasm. Such type of society or organization may require more in number immediately to save important native cattle germplasm.

In recent time, international actions have been oriented towards conservation of animal genetic resources. India being a signatory to many such international agreements, the country will have specific policy focus on conservation of indigenous breeds of livestock and poultry. State will take up the responsibility of conserving such threatened breeds through appropriate programmes.

45.0 Need for Conservation of Indigenous Cattle Breed

Indian cattle germplasm need to be conserved immediately for following reasons.

- India is reservoir of the cattle genetic germplasm whose genetic diversity is reflected by forty one pure cattle breed along with huge amount of non-descript cattle. Four of these-Sahiwal, Gir, Red Sindhi and Tharparkar- are well known for their milking competency. A few others, such as Hariana, Kankrej, Ongole and Rathi, belong to dual breed that have both milch and draught qualities, and the rest are pure draught breeds. Crossbreds are more productive but their tendency to wilt under Indian conditions of low input and harsh climate, susceptibility to tropical diseases warrants the conservation and development of indigenous breeds.
- The cattle populations of the country are spread out in the length and breadth of the country each having its own special features and are well adapted to their respective agro-climatic and eco-geographical conditions and plays a pivotal role in the farmer's economy as well as strong contributions in the national economy through supply of draught animal power, milk, cow dung (organic manure) and cow urine (medicinal value) for which they needs to be conserved immediately.
- Indian zebu cattle have a high degree of heat tolerance, partially resistant to ticks, many tick borne diseases and have low nutritional requirements; these make them paramount importance in the world. High degree of heat tolerance partly due to low heat production (associated with low metabolic rate

and low productivity) and partly due to a high capacity to dissipate heat; low nutritional requirements mainly due to low metabolic rate and small size and also possibly to more efficient digestion at low feeding levels; a considerable degree of resistance to ticks and also to many tick-borne diseases prevalent in tropical countries.

- It is evident that Indigenous cattle breed of India possess A2 allele of beta casein which helps to prevent some metabolic disorders like diabetes, heart diseases etc. Whole world are looking forward India as Indian cattle breed can able to produce A2 type milk which help to prevent these important diseases.
- The indigenous dairy breeds with potential for development as commercially viable milch cattle in a shorter time frame are: Sahiwal in Punjab; Rathi and Tharparkar in Rajasthan; and Gir and Kankrej in Gujarat. If these breeds are selectively crossed with genetically selected bulls through sibling and progeny testing the F_1 offsprings would be commercially viable. In this manner the entire population of the breed can be upgraded in a few generations.
- Studies of impact of climate change and effect of temperature rise on milk production of dairy animals indicate that temperature increase due to global warming will negatively impact milk production. The decline in milk production and reproductive efficiency will be highest in crossbred cattle followed by buffaloes. Indigenous cattle breeds will be least affected by climate change as they are more hardy and robust, and more heat tolerance capacity.
- In the process of inter-mating and crossbreeding, it is possible that some of the imperative breeds are continuously losing their unique features may rendering them toward the point of endangered level. It is, therefore, essential to take up necessary steps for their conservation as well as their overall improvement. The urgency for protection and conservation of indigenous breeds cannot be over emphasised. For instance breeds like Punganur, Vechur and Krishna Valley are rapidly declining, demanding immediate attention for their protection as well as conservation.

An investigation arrived at the conclusion that in ten (10) years, India will be forced to start importing milk, and that Indian cow will cease to exist. This will be happened due to several reasons. For example, India, over the past few decades, imported several exotic cow varieties to gain a boost in milk production. In Punjab, 80 percent of the state's one lakh stray cattle are exotic breeds. These breeds theoretically produce more amount of milk, but are not well-adapted to Indian conditions. It is stated that about 70 percent of Indian cows are owned by the economically poor strata of the society. They cannot afford to house these exotic breeds in regulated climate conditions.

46.0 Conservation of Indigenous Cattle Breed

At present, forty one well descript cattle breeds in addition to huge number of non-descript cattle are now available in India. Due to extensive crossbreeding throughout the country, a number of the indigenous breeds are declining due to their becoming uneconomical. Draught breed cattle those are extensively used in agriculture sector now their utility has diminished because of mechanization in agriculture. However, the Indian cattle breeds have following merits over exotic breeds as presented below:

- Indian cattle have better disease resistance capacity
- They are more suitable for low input management system
- They survive and well adapted in local environment
- Indian cattle are suitable for draught work in hot humid temperature
- Moreover, Indian cattle have some unique characteristic features

Along with these, superior indigenous cattle breeds are of valuable research inputs for developing superior breeds. It is therefore important that Indigenous breeds of cattle are to be conserved, developed and proliferated for posterity use. To protect valuable cattle germplasm of the country, appropriate conservation strategies need to be developed for which following aspects should be taken into consideration:

a) **Breeding Policy**

India is a large country having different agro climatic condition with their different needs. The vast cattle genetic resources are spread throughout the country. So each state of India needs different breeding policy for own need. The States may review their relevant breeding policy so as to highlight conservation of Indigenous breeds in their breeding tract and letting no crossbreeding of recognized indigenous cattle in their home tract.

b) **Implementation of the Breeding Programme**

The State may consider region specific and breed specific breeding programmes to implement their own conservation programme. The States may delineate and identify their respective breeding policies, the geographical boundaries of the areas where non-descript cattle should be upgraded by crossing with bulls of indigenous breeds. Once such areas are earmarked, no cross-breeding of non-descript cattle, other than with bulls of indigenous breeds, should be permitted. The areas for cross-breeding of non descript cattle with exotic breed may also be identified.

c) **Promotion of Breeders organization**

Breeding Farms: The existing States breeding farms of indigenous breeds should be declared as germplasm repositories. Only pure breeding should be practiced at these farms for getting elite pure bred bulls suppose to be used for breeding in future. ONBS can be used for further improvement as well as to avoid untoward effect of inbreeding.

Gaushala: Institute herds are maintaining small population size so conservation efforts may not be effective. There are plenty number of Gaushala available in the country. They have quite sizable populations of purebred Indigenous animals but do not have the resources for maintaining and improving these animals. Such Gaushala may be supported to maintain indigenous breeds so that they can supply improved quality of germplasm for breeding. They should be provided with scientific and technical inputs and training for genetic evaluation of animal. Larger parts of the breeding tract of the country may also be considered for their conservation.

d) **Role of voluntary organization**

Breeder Association or breed society plays a vital role in conservation programme. *In situ* conservation of cattle is more economical as animals are maintained in their own tracts and farmer can provide their support in the form of maintaining the cattle in their own house or areas. Without involvement and participation of farmer's it is not possible to conserve the breed. Improvement of Indigenous breeds can be taken up in collaboration with Breeders' association through selection of outstanding animals true to their breed types. These Breeders' association can be encouraged to form a Federation at the State/ District level to take up issues relating to conservation and development of respective indigenous breeds. States may consider having State level awards for Breeders' associations and for progressive farmers who have contributed to conservation and development of recognized indigenous breeds.

e) **Use of Science and Technology**

Technologies such as artificial insemination, frozen semen production, progeny testing, embryo transfer technology should be used for propagation, improvement and conservation of indigenous breeds. This must be used only after proper evaluation where ever required these. National gene bank should maintain the germplasm in the form of semen and embryo of our important cattle breed. Regional gene banks should meet the requirements of National gene bank. Improving economic efficiency of indigenous breeds through use of superior germplasm by selective breeding, better health coverage and providing balanced ration will be helpful for in situ conservation.

f) **Database**

Record keeping is very much essential for sustaining the conservation programme. So reliable database should be developed with regard to all the details of Indigenous breeds, including their breeding tracts, numbers, characterization, genetic makeup in the institutional farm where they are being preserved and/or conserved. The national level data base for cattle and buffalo developed by NDDB may be utilized for this purpose. A breeding network should be set up by computerizing and net working all AI outlets, semen stations, breeding farm and Gaushala. Individual farmer generally does not maintain the records. This data recording problem can be solved by covering the area of breed under Herd Registration Schemes.

g) **Creation of Public Awareness**

Available information on different breeds should be published in the form of pamphlets, books, calendar etc. This will create awareness and motivate farmers to conserve the important breeds. Some farmers are the proud owner of the popular breeds of their area. Such farmers, if encouraged through financial and veterinary facilitate will help in preservation of breeds. Breeds exhibition should be arranged for local breeds and owners should be rewarded for maintaining pure local breeds. Published success stories on local breed conservation and innovative utilization. Some incentives may be given to the farmers or cattle owners who are rearing the breeds. Government assistants are very much essential to fulfil the conservation strategies in our country.

47.0 Development and Conservation of Recognised Cattle Breed

Indigenous breeds are specially known for qualities of heat tolerance, resistance to diseases and ability to thrive under extreme nutritional stress. Considering the importance of recognized indigenous breeds in the National economy, Government has undertaken the following measures for their development and conservation.

National Project for Cattle and Buffalo Breeding has focus on development and conservation of indigenous breeds. The cattle genetic resources of India are represented by 41 indigenous breeds of cattle including Rathi, Gir, Kankrej, Tharparkar, Sahiwal, Deoni, Hallikar, Khillar, Hariana etc. Global warming is likely to increase incidences of animal diseases particularly viral and protozoan diseases in crossbred animals. Therefore, there is a need to take programmes for development and conservation of indigenous breeds.

Funds have been released to the participating states for procurement of quality bulls for natural service, initiating bull production programmes, strengthening of bull mother farms and establishment of ONBS farms for important indigenous breeds (Sahiwal, Gir, Deoni, Kankrej, Hariana, Kenkatha, Hallikar, Khillar, etc.) for their further development. During Phase-I of the project an amount of 58 crore has been released exclusively for development and conservation of indigenous breeds. An amount of Rs. 477.30 crore has been kept exclusively for development of indigenous breeds under Phase-II of NPCBB. Out of this, an expenditure of Rs. 250 crore has been made under the scheme till March 2012. In addition to this, strengthening of field AI network, semen stations, establishment of private AI workers and organization of fertility camps etc have also lead to development of indigenous breeds.

48.0 Economics of Milch Animal

Cow and buffaloes together contributes more than 97 percent of the total milk produced in the country. The best milch animals account for 25 percent of the Indian cattle population while 21 percent of the cattle population is cross-bred. Most of the indigenous breeds of cattle excel in draught capacity.

There is a paradox about the Indian livestock species 'Plenty and Poverty'. This means that the population of different species is excessive compared to land and other resources and their production potential is lower than their counterparts of American and European species. Further, it has been estimated that about 75-80 percent of native cattle and buffalo population are non-descript i.e. they do not conform to the recognized breed characteristics. It is also true, among the descript breed majority is of draught and dual purpose breeds of cattle. The average milk yield per animal in India is about 3.2 kgs, compared to a global average of 6.6 kgs. Implementation of breeding policy for cattle and buffaloes has resulted in the production of crossbred cattle and improved buffaloes of different breeds in various states of the country.

Although crossbred cattle are exceptionally rich in high milk production as compared to indigenous cattle milk but they are very much susceptible to diseases in our country. This invites a question whether crossbred cattle are more profitable for dairy production. Crossbred cattle having 50 percent or higher exotic inheritance can able to yield 15 kg milk per day or higher, while indigenous cattle usually yield much lower amount of milk. It appears that dairy farmers can earn more income from raising crossbred dairy cattle than indigenous cattle but benefit of high milk yield in crossbred cattle cannot compensate for their overall maintenance cost. However, indigenous cattle become more superior to crossbred cattle when they are considered as the multipurpose animal in integrated farming systems. Moreover, they are very much superior for disease resistance; thrive on fewer amounts of food and poor management conditions.

From the research finding, it was observed that Holstein crosses recorded higher lactation/annual yield compared to Jersey and Brown Swiss crosses as well as to non-descript cows and buffaloes in different rural areas. Consequently, net income per milch animal per annum obtained from Holstein crosses was also higher than those from other crosses and non-descript cows and buffaloes reared in different states of the country. Interestingly, non-descript cows indicated positive net income only in Kerala and Jammu and Kashmir areas. A study on the comparative performance of first and second generations of crossbred cows indicated that although second generation produced more milk presumably due to higher level of exotic inheritance than that of first generation but net income obtained from second generation was almost half than that of first generation of crossbred cows. This was due to relatively high cost of feed and veterinary medicines since second generation of crossbred cows appear to be more susceptible to various diseases. The performance of Holstein crosses was found to be the best among all other exotic breeds of dairy animals in north-western part of the country. However, Jersey crosses showed reasonably good performance in hilly regions of Jammu and Kashmir, Himachal Pradesh and West Bengal.

49.0 Central Institute for Research on Cattle (CIRC), Meerut, Uttar Pradesh

The Central Institute for Research on Cattle (CIRC) formerly known as Project Directorate on Cattle (PDC) was established on 3rd November 1987 at Military Farm School and Research Centre, Meerut, Uttar Pradesh by upgrading the status of All-India Coordinated Research Project (AICRP) on Cattle. After initial set up at Military Farm School and Research Centre, CIRC had been functional at Shastri Nagar and later on at Modipuram, Meerut, before it finally shifted to its present location occupying a 30 acres campus at Grass Farm Road, Meerut Cantt, where the Directorate's own building has come up in the year 2000. Since then the Directorate was actively collaborating with the Military Farms, Ministry of Defense to evolve a national milch breed of crossbred cattle *'Frieswal'* by crossing the Holstein Friesian with Sahiwal cattle.

Considering its sincere research and extension efforts and achievements made in cattle improvement, the Project Directorate on Cattle (PDC) was upgraded as Central Institute for Research on Cattle during 2014. The Central Institute for Research on Cattle (CIRC) is acting as a nodal institution to monitor, coordinate and support all research and development projects for cattle improvement in India.

Vision of the Institute

- The vision of CIRC is Improvement of cattle for high productivity and profitability.

Mission of the Institute

- Germplasm improvement and technology development for realizing enhanced productivity and profitability.

Mandate of the Institute

- Basic and strategic research on productivity and production enhancement of cattle including indigenous cattle.
- Dissemination of scientific information and technology for cattle production management.

Objectives

AICRP on Cattle

- To develop a national milch breed of cattle 'Frieswal' using Holstein Friesian X Sahiwal base.
- Conservation and genetic improvement of important indigenous cattle breeds.
- Production of progeny tested crossbred bulls and genetic improvement of cattle under field conditions.

ICAR-CIRC Main Scheme

- To undertake research in the field of cattle breeding, feeding, management and reproduction to enhance productivity and profitability.
- To plan, coordinate and monitor the research projects on cattle.
- To serve as national data repository and provide consultancy for cattle production and reproduction.

Future Thrust Areas

- Genetic improvement of Tharparkar, Rathi, Red Sindhi breed using conventional and modern breeding techniques.
- Studies on draught animal power of important indigenous draught breeds.
- Large scale production of quality cattle germplasm.

- Development of optimum feeding and management practices including designing of shelter to suit the local environment for enhancing cattle productivity.
- Sexing of male germplasm for production of calves of desired sex.
- Validation of therapeutic importance of cow produces like milk, punchgavaya, urine, dung etc.
- Genomic selection of bulls and use of embryo transfer technology for elite bull production.
- Biotechnological strategies including biotic and abiotic stress for understanding and improving cattle production and reproduction.
- Comparative economics of productivity of Indian cattle breeds vis-à-vis crossbred cattle.

Considering importance of the Indigenous cattle breeds for their adaptability, feed conversion efficiency and disease resistance etc., this nodal Institute has undertaken different Indigenous Breeds Development Project in collaboration with State Agricultural Universities and State Government, Non Government Organizations and sister ICAR Institutes for conservation and genetic improvement of some of the important indigenous cattle breeds (Gir, Sahiwal and Kankrej) of our country. During the 8th Five Year Plan the Field Progeny Testing programme (FPT) was also started to undertake progeny testing of crossbred bulls under the field conditions.

The Institute has undertaken research programmes related to genetic improvement of indigenous and crossbred cattle by identifying germplasm (G.P.) and data recording (D.R.) units in various government and non-government organizations. Frieswal cattle resource is available at 36 Military Farms, the bull rearing unit is located at Meerut under the administrative control of Directorate of Frieswal. Similarly, indigenous cattle genetic resources are available at different G.P. and D.R. units of respective breeds. The germplasm unit for Sahiwal is located at NDRI, Karnal (Haryana) while that of Gir, and Kankrej are located at Junagadh Agricultural University, Junagadh and SK Nagar University, Dantiwada (Gujarat), respectively. The Institute is also providing good quality germplasm to stakeholders.

It is expected that this Institute with its own strength on semen production will be developed as a nodal Institute for production and supply of superior male germplasm of different indigenous and crossbred cattle in near future. It will also act as a key player in the socio-economic upliftment of cattle owners by infusing superior germplasm in the farmer's herd for enhancing the milk and draught capacity.

50.0 Overview

- The breeds of cattle are mostly evolved out of constant inbreeding and generations of adaptability to local environment.
- The cattle population in India is so varied in structure and body conformation as to suit the different climatic conditions in which they are bred and reared.
- In general, the cattle breeds from the drier regions are well built with higher productivity, and those from the heavy rainfall areas, coastal regions and hilly regions are smaller in built and low in production performance.
- The indigenous dairy breeds of cattle with potential for development as commercially viable milch animals in a comparatively few generations are Sahiwal, Red Sindhi, Tharparkar and Gir. These dairy breeds and Hariana cattle have also been extensively used for different breed improvement programmes in different parts of India.
- A reorientation of cattle and buffalo breeding policy need to be attempted with area specific approach backed up by appropriate programs addressing our concerns for indigenous cattle breeds and draught animal power. A similar approach has been adopted in the National Project on Cattle and Buffalo Breeding.
- Keeping in view the milk production potential, draught capacity, and resistance to diseases, heat and humidity tolerance, capacity to survive on crop by-products and crude roughages, it is extremely essential to conserve these imperative Indian cattle breeds and improve their important traits in their respective home tracts.
- Considering the essence of the importance of Indian cattle genetic resources spread throughout the country following

recommendations may need to be undertaken for further genetic improvement of our indigenous cattle:

- Indigenous cattle breeds accepted by common farmers should be further developed through region specific and breed specific programs aimed at selection in the breeding tracts and supply of improved quality germplasm on demand by farmers.
- The states should be directed to specifically delineate the areas of native breeds of cattle, record their numbers breed wise and sex wise and encourage farmers to conserve them in their home tracts.
- Formation of breed associations for improvement of indigenous breeds should be encouraged. Such associations shall be involved in production of quality male stock. An effective mechanism for providing disease free quality breeding bulls and quality semen for artificial insemination will be put in place. Breeding services would be provided at the farmers' door.
- Immediate attention need to be taken to save our valuable cattle germplasm through suitable conservation strategy.
- There is an urgent need to initiate zoning exercise in the country on the basis of different cattle breeds, its density, and availability of feeds and fodders.
- Selective breeding and grading-up policy should be followed in the districts of the state wherever there is a need to introduce the milk production traits in draught or dual purpose breeds and non-descript cattle breeds.
- In order to conserve and improve the well defined indigenous breeds, crossbreeding with exotic germplasm should not be resorted to the cattle breeds belonging to well defined milch, dual purpose and draught categories. Grading up and selective breeding may serve as alternatives for these categories.
- Cross breeding through exotic cattle can be an immediate measure for improvement of non-descript cattle in different parts of India to meet up the increasing requirement of milk.
- Provision should be made to castrate the non-descript males of cattle to reduce the indiscriminate breeding through legislation and its strict implementation.

- State wise breeding policy should be framed in accordance with the production traits, economic performance and draftability of breeds along with the local requirement, agro-climatic factors, existing infra-structure and support systems.
- An integrated approach is being adopted involving creation of milch herd, improving draught power and conserving genetic diversity through a composite central project.
- The crossbreeding shall be restricted to low yielding indigenous cattle breeds.
- In view of the shortage of proven and progeny tested bulls of exotic and indigenous breeds, efforts are needed to be made to establish more number of bull farms in different states to meet the increasing requirement of quality bulls.
- In order to preserve high potential germplasm, it is essential to ban the slaughter of breedable and high genetic potential cows in different areas of the country.
- Efforts should be intensified to identify and transfer technically feasible and economically viable new technologies of livestock production systems through conducting on-farm animal research trials in different regions/zones of the country.
- It is noteworthy that all these recommendations will not be fruitful unless there is active participation of common people. Thus, extensive extention programme must be undertaken to reach out the livestock rearer who are the real beneficiaries of entire breed depevelopmental programme.
- In conclusion, the Indigenous cattle undoubtedly offer an excellent opportunity to improve the socio-economic status of our country through utilizing them in breeding programs. Hence, all-embracing lab to land efforts should be undertaken to conserve and exploit the valuable germplasm of Indian cattle breed in the future.

❑❑❑

UNIT-2

Buffalo Genetic Resources in India

1.0 Introduction

Buffalo plays a pivotal role in livestock and agriculture economy of many countries across the world. Domesticated species of buffalo are river and swamp buffalo. The habitat of these animals is tropical, subtropical, wet grasslands, marshes and swamp regions of the world. These animals cool themselves by spending a substantial part of their time in water, mud holes or rivers.

A triple purpose versatile animal, buffalo produces milk, meat and is also used as mechanical power to mankind. Due to its highly nutritious milk, leaner meat (less fat and cholesterol) and being superior draught animal in waterlogged conditions, buffalo offers immense potential for the improvement of livelihood. Buffalo is a more efficient convertor of poor quality feeds and fiber than cattle. This species have a low cost of milk production per litre which is a net outcome of physiological superiority of buffaloes over cows. Most importantly, buffalo is used as cash during needy hours thus securing the economic status of many families. Despite of immense advantages of raising buffalo, unfortunately, these animals remain underutilized. In particular, buffalo breeders and farmers are facing challenges in terms of poor reproductive efficiency, suboptimal production potential, infertility and also lower calf survival rate.

Fortunately, India is blessed with valuable livestock resources which integrated the largest population of cattle and buffalo in the world, and its breeds are admired for heat tolerance and inherent resistance to diseases and ability to thrive under different climatic condition. The buffaloes play major role in the farmer's economy and because of their strong contributions to Indian's animal husbandry sector, they are aptly termed as 'Black Goldmine'. This dairy species has been creating headlines commanding high price tags while also contributing immensely to animal protein needs of the vegetarian population of the country, as well as earning foreign exchange through surging export of buffalo meat. Buffalo, the 'Black Goldmine' of India is already shining with a glittering future. Although, buffalo is the flagship of all agricultural revolutions but unfortunately this species of animal has been neglected in the past.

2.0 History

In ancient literature, different forms of buffaloes have been described ranging from docile riding beast to furious and powerful demons in the mythology of India, China, Indo-China, Assyro-Babylonia and ancient Persia. Existence of different kinds of Indian (Asiatic) buffaloes has been recorded in all ages.

Buffalo was considered as animal of the demon group and hunted for food upto Ramayana and Mahabharata epical period. In 'Ram Charit Manas' of Tulsidas, Demon King 'Ravana' went to awake his brother 'Kumbhakarna' from his deep sleep of six months and ordered to arrange supply of thousand pitchers of wine and large number of buffaloes for the feast of Kumbhkarna. During Mahabharata period too, buffalo was listed as wild animal. However, there is mention of rearing boars, buffaloes and elephants for food and other purposes. Buffaloes were well domesticated in the Indian subcontinent by the era of medieval period and they were considered milch animals along with cow, goat and sheep (Kautilya's Arthasastra 381-186 B.C.).

Another river valley civilization, the Shang Dynasty (probably during 1766-1123 B.C.) existed along the Yangtze and Yellow rivers in China. Presence of tamed buffaloes has been mentioned in the Shang dynasty during the second millennium B.C. The importance of buffalo in the life of people during Shang dynasty, as an important animal of socio-economic and cultural significance, is evident from the depiction of buffalo in different forms on the vessels and pillars of Shang period. Studies of skeletal fossils found during breaking of land in the North-East Thailand for rice cultivation provided evidence of buffalo domestication during the second millennium B.C. around 1600 B.C. (contemprary to Shang dynasty period) in Southeast Asian countries.

Evidence is available on the seals and sculptures, mostly depicting male buffaloes crowned with typical crescentic and massive horns now prevalent among the wild Indian and Swamp buffalo. On one of the seals of the Indus valley excavation in Lahore Museum, depiction of a buffalo on feeding trough can be considered a valid evidence of domestication of buffalo during that period. Some multicoloured ceramics of Nal culture of South Baluchistan exhibit buffaloes and it is considered contemporary with the Indus valley culture.

3.0 Origin and Domestication

Most species of the present farm and pet animals were domesticated before the beginning of written history. Paleolithic man started gathering food by hunting wild animals, mostly herbivorous, because these species were grazers and browsers due to which it was easier to kill them. This process gradually changed to taming and then domestication.

The origins of the domestic water buffalo types are debated, although results of a phylogenetic study indicated that Riverine buffalo, *bubalus bubalis* may have originated from India and was domesticated nearly 5000 years ago in Iran, Iraq and Indo-Pak subcontinent, whereas Swamp buffalo, *bubalus carabensis* may have originated in China and the domestication was took place in China and other part of Southeast Asia after 1000 years.

The present domesticated buffaloes are the descendants of *Bos arni* buffaloes found in wild state even today in the North-Eastern parts of India. Indo-gangetic plain is the world's largest fertile plain where the world's first civilization was settled for food security. The large area in the Indus valley was covered with marshy grasses, dense forests and grasslands intercepted by many rivers, streams and other water resources which provided suitable environment for human settlement and buffalo domestication in the valley.

A majority of the modern historians believe that buffaloes were first tamed and then domesticated for working in various agricultural operations before 2500 B.C. in Mesopotamia during the period of Akkadian dynasty and in Indus valley civilization of Indian subcontinent extending to Harappa, Mohanjodaro and some parts of Gujarat, Rajasthan and Haryana. Till the restoration of further information on the domestication of buffaloes, it may be more appropriate to believe that wild buffaloes of the Indus valley (*Bubalus arnee*) were first tamed and domesticated in the region and then extended to Mesopotamia in the west and upto China in the east. They spread westwards from Mesopotamia.

In this way buffalo is the species which has been domesticated more recently as compared to *Bos taurus* and *Bos indicus* domesticated 10,000 years ago. Domestication of buffalo started much later than the domestication of horses, donkeys, dogs, cattle, sheep, goats and elephants. It has been suggested that buffaloes were in the service of man as early as 2500 to 2100 B.C.

The present-day river buffalo is the result of complex domestication processes involving more than one maternal lineage and a significant maternal gene flow from wild populations after the initial domestication events. Twenty-two breeds of the river type water buffalo are known, including Murrah, Nili-Ravi, Surti, Jaffarabadi, Anatolian, Mediterranean, and Egyptian buffalo in the world. China has a huge variety of buffalo genetic resources, comprising sixteen local swamp buffalo breeds in various regions.

Almost 96% of World buffalo population were found in Asia and Pacific, while they were distributed in more than 50 countries around the world, from China and India to Brazil, from USA and Europe to Australia. Most buffaloes are raised by small farmers in developing countries. During the past three decades the number of buffaloes in the world steadily and consistently increased at about 1% to 2% per year, except in some Eastern European countries, where buffalo numbers decreased during this period.

4.0 Evolution and Domestication

Buffalo belongs to family Bovidae are of two main species such as Asian buffalo (*Bubalus bubalis*) and the African buffalo (*Syncerus caffer*). Asian buffalo originated in India where its domestication occurred during the third millennium B.C. The second origin point of buffalo is China where it was domesticated earlier than in India (in fifth millennium B.C.). African buffalo originated distinctively than river buffalo and swamp buffalo that came from Asia. Furthermore, a recent study opposed to the previous mtDNA analysis results showing a distinct origin of water and swamp buffaloes.

There are two subspecies of African buffalo: the cape buffalo *(Syncerus caffer)* and the forest buffalo *(Syncerus caffer nanus)*. They have evolved independently to Asian buffalo. Furthermore, recent studies of mtDNA sequence indicated on the divergence of central Africa and cape buffalo around 130,000-100,000 years ago, during the Pleistocene period.

Evolution of large number of buffalo breeds by people in the Indian subcontinent clearly suggests the importance given to this animal as a source of food and power, which were sufficient grounds for its domestication. Deep involvement of the people of this region led to evolving several breeds of buffaloes capable of thriving and performing in the prevalent agro-climatic conditions and herbage. They are especially suitable for tilling rice fields, and their milk is richer in fat and protein than that of dairy cattle. Probably milk production formed the basis of selection and breeding which resulted in the evolution of farmers' dairy breeds of riverine buffalo like Murrah, Kundi, Nili Ravi, Jaffarabadi, Mehsana, Surti etc.

Review of the accessible ancient literature of Indian and other civilizations from the Vedic period through the Epic, Puranic and Medieval period and modern studies reveal the existence of different kinds of buffaloes in Asian, African and some European countries. However, buffaloes are considered to have originated in Asia and Africa. America and Australia were devoid of buffaloes and the Europeans introduced different types of domesticated buffaloes in these continents. The large feral population of northern Australia became established in the late 19th century, and smaller feral herds are in New Guinea, Tunisia, and northeastern Argentina. Feral herds are also present in New Britain, New Ireland, Irian Jaya, Papua New Guinea, Colombia, Guyana, Suriname, Brazil and Uruguay.

5.0 Scientific Classification of Wild Water Buffalo

Kingdom	:	Animalia
Phylum	:	Chordata
Class	:	Mammalia
Order	:	Artiodactyla
Family	:	Bovidae
Subfamily	:	Bovinae
Tribe	:	Bovini
Genus	:	*Bubalus*
Species	:	***B. Arnee***
Binomial name	:	***Bubalus arnee***
Subspecies	:	• *B.A. Arnee* (Much of India and Nepal) • *B.A. Fulvus* (Assam and neighbouring areas) • *B.A. Theerapati* (Southeast Asia)
Conservation	:	Endangered

Carl Linnaeus first described the genus *Bos* and the water buffalo under the binomial *Bubalus bubalis* in 1758; the later was known to occur in Asia and as a domestic form in Italy. Ellerman and Morrison-Scott treated the wild and domestic forms of the water buffalo as conspecifics whereas others treated them as different species. The nomenclatorial treatment of wild and domestic forms have been inconsistent and varies between authors and even within the works of single author.

In March 2003, the International Commission on Zoological Nomenclature achieved consistency in the naming of wild and domestic water buffalo by ruling that the scientific name *Bubalus arnee* is valid for the wild form. *Bubalus bubalis* continues to be valid for the domestic form and applies also to feral populations.

6.0 Water Buffalo Fact

The water buffalo or domestic Asian water buffalo (*Bubalus bubalis*) is a large bovid originating in South Asia, Southeast Asia, and China. Today, it is also found in Europe, Australia, and some American countries. The water buffalo, or Asian buffalo, as it is often called, is the largest member of the Bovini tribe, which includes yak, bison, African buffalo, various species of wild cattle, and others. Water buffalo has been domesticated for more than 5,000 years. They have buttressed humanity's survival with their meat, horns, hides, milk, butterfat, and power, plowing and transporting people and crops.

Water buffalo is a member of the bovine family. It originates from southern parts of Asia, but it has been domesticated to the rest of the world few thousand years ago. Water buffalo live in muddy waters and swamps of tropical and subtropical areas of India, Nepal, Bhutan and Thailand. Water buffalo is used as a transportation system for transfer of heavy loads and people. Because of that, it is also known as 'Tractor of the East'. Other than that, water buffalo is often killed for its horns, meat and leather. Water buffalo is an endangered species, with less than 4000 animals remaining in the wild area.

Water buffaloes spend much of their day submerged in the muddy water of Asia's tropical and subtropical forests. Their wide-splayed hoofed feet prevent them from sinking too deeply in the mud and allow them to move about in wetlands and swamps. These marshes provide good cover and rich aquatic plants to forage on, although water buffaloes actually prefer to feed in grasslands on grass and herbs.

Water buffalo milk presents physicochemical features different from that of other ruminant species, such as a higher content of fatty acids and proteins. The physical and chemical parameters of swamp and river type water buffalo milk differ. Water buffalo milk contains higher levels of total solids, crude protein, fat, calcium, and phosphorus, and slightly higher content of lactose compared with those of cow milk. The high level of total solids makes water buffalo milk ideal for processing into value-added dairy products such as cheese. The conjugated linoleic acid (CLA) content in milk ranges from 4.4 mg/g fat in September to 7.6 mg/g fat in June. Season and genetic may play a role in variation of CLA level and changes in gross composition of the water buffalo milk.

7.0 Interesting Water Buffalo Fact

- Water buffalo is a large animal. Males are three times bigger than females. They can reach 6.6 to 9.8 feet in height, and weigh between 1500 and 2650 pounds.
- Water buffalo is the second largest type of wild cattle that can be seen in the wild. Gaur is the largest species of the wild cattle.
- Water buffalo is black or white in color. It has large, backward curved horns. Males have larger horns than females.
- Horns of males are crescent-shaped with a ridge along the body of the horns. They can reach 5 feet in length.
- Water buffalo uses its horns to protect against predators such as: tigers, lions and crocodiles.
- Water buffalo is an herbivore. It eats aquatic plants, but it also grazes grass and eats different types of leaves and herbs.
- Water buffalo has large hoofed feet which prevent sinking of the animal into the mud.
- Water buffaloes live in groups composed of few/larger number of animals that provides protection for them against predators.
- Due to high outer temperature, water buffalo spends majority of its day submerged in the muddy waters. This way, animal is able to keep its body temperature stable and prevent overheating.

- Water buffalo can run very fast when it is faced with danger. Average speed of water buffalo is 30 miles per hour.
- Mating of water buffalo takes place during rainy season.
- Females give birth to a single baby every second year after pregnancy lasting between 9 and 11 months.
- Milk of water buffalo contains the greatest percentage of fat compared to other species of wild cows. This is the reason why young water buffalos grow up very fast. Humans also use milk of water buffalo to produce different types of cheese, butter, ghee etc.
- Young water buffaloes are tightly associated with their mothers in the first few years of their life. Males should leave their native herd to join bachelor herds (composed of only males) at the age of 3 years. Females usually stay with their mothers.
- Water buffalo can survive upto 9 years in the wild and up to 25 years in captivity.

8.0 Classification of Water Buffalo

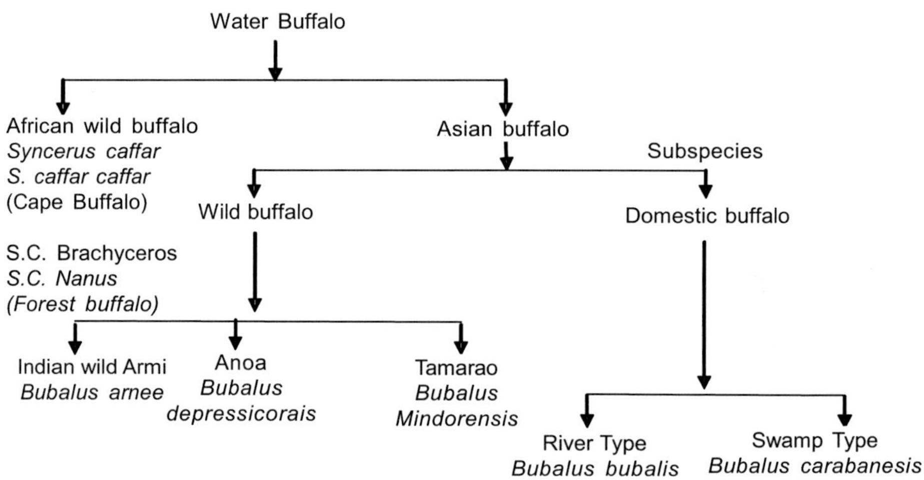

These are the general classifications of water buffalo within the United States. Throughout the world there are two general types - Swamp buffalo and River buffalo-within the River buffalo there are 18 sub-species. The sub-species are generally water buffalo-raised through centuries in a given local area. They developed their own characteristics as they adapted to their surroundings and nature.

8.1 African Buffalo

There are 26 chromosome pairs in *Syncerus caffer* and 27 chromosome pairs in *Syncerus nanus*. Likewise Asian buffalo, African buffalo can also be interbred and the progeny has 53 chromosomes. The consequences are similar to those in Asian buffalo. Chromosome arms are preserved between these two subspecies, crosses between them are fertile with 49 chromosomes in crossbreds (River x Swamp type). But, fertility and reproductive efficiency is reduced in subsequent matings. The consequences are similar to those in Asian buffalo in terms of reduced fertility resulting from unbalanced gametes and zygotes. There are four biarmed chromosomes in *Syncerus caffer* and three biarmed chromosomes in *Syncerus nanus*. All other chromosomes, including sex chromosomes, are acrocentric in both species. In *Syncerus caffer* biarmed pairs correspond to fused cattle chromosomes *viz*. 1, 13; 2, 3; 5, 20; and 11, 29.

Furthermore, *Syncerus* and *Bubalus* share no biarmed chromosome pairs. It suggests that the hybrid may be unbalanced in the karyotyping results if these genera are crossed. Thus, chromosome morphology of these animals entitles them as two separate genera.

8.2 Asian Buffalo

8.2.1. Wild Buffalo

The wild water buffalo (*Bubalus arnee*), is also called Asian buffalo and Asiatic buffalo native to Southeast Asia is considered a different species, but most likely represents the ancestor of the domestic water buffalo. Wild water buffalo are endangered and live only in a small number of protected areas stretching across India, Nepal, and Bhutan, and a wildlife reserve in Thailand, east to Vietnam, and south to Malaysia. By 1963, it had been substantially reduced numerically and eliminated from the greater part of its former range. Populations are likely to diminish also as they are interbred with domesticated water buffalo. It is even possible that no purebred wild Asian buffalo will remain. Population estimates are hampered by the difficulty in distinguishing wild buffalo from domestic, feral and hybrid buffalo. It is listed as endangered in the IUCN Red List since 1986, as the remaining population total is less than 4,000, with an estimate of fewer than 2,500 mature individuals. The population decline of at least 50% over the last three generations (24–30 years) is projected to continue. The global population has been estimated at 3,400 individuals, of which

3,100 (91%) live in India, mostly in Assam, Madhya Pradesh, although most, if not all, are believed to have interbred with domestic and/or feral buffalo.

Wild water buffalo are larger and heavier than domestic buffalo, and weigh from 700 to 1,200 kg (1,500 to 2,600 lb). Females are smaller in size and weight. Their head-to-body-length is 240 to 300 cm (94 to 118 inch) with a tail 60 to 100 cm (24 to 39 inch) long, and a shoulder height of 150 to 190 cm (59 to 75 inch). Both sexes carry horns that are heavy at the base and widely spreading upto 2 m (79 inch) along the outer edges, exceeding in size of the horns of any other living bovid. Their skin color is ash grey to black. The moderately long, coarse and sparse hair is directed forward from the haunches to the long and narrow head. There is a tuft on the forehead, and the ears are comparatively small. The tip of the tail is bushy; the hooves are large and splayed. They rank alongside the gaur as the heaviest living wild bovid species, as both attain similar average, if not maximum weights, although, with their stockier, shorter-legged frame, wild water buffalo are somewhat less in length and height than the gaur.

The wild Asian buffalo is very dependent on the availability of water. Historically, its preferred habitats were low-lying alluvial grasslands and their surroundings. Riparian forests and woodlands were also utilized. The wild Asian buffalo eats grass and leafy aquatic vegetation. It is mainly a grazer, feeding in the morning and evening and lying up in dense cover or submerging in wallows during midday. During the midday heat, the wild Asian buffalo frequently wallows in water or muddy pools, sometimes almost completely submerged, with only its nostrils showing. In addition to keeping it cool, wallowing helps to remove skin parasites, biting flies, and other pests. Where there is substantial human disturbance, the wild Asian buffalo is mainly nocturnal.

The most important threats to wild Asian buffaloes are interbreeding with feral and domestic buffalo, habitat loss/ degradation, and hunting. Diseases and parasites (transmitted by domestic livestock) and competition for food and water between wild buffalo and domestic stock are also serious threats.

The wild water buffalo represents most likely the ancestor of the domestic water buffalo. The wild Asian buffalo has been domesticated for thousands of years and bred around the world into various, mostly smaller, breeds of less than 500 kg (1100 lb). The domesticated water buffalo is now found in most tropical and subtropical regions. Archeological evidence shows that domestic buffaloes were being used in Zhejiang Province of China, just south of the mouth of the Yangtze River, 6000-7000 years ago (although some think that these may have belonged to a separate species, *Bubalus mephistopheles*, which has been reported as a wild animal from Pleistocene and early historical sites in Henan Province, China). Thailand's wild Asian buffalo is the largest water buffalo in the world.

In India, they are largely restricted to in and around Kaziranga, Manas and Dibru-Saikhowa National Parks, Laokhowa Wildlife Sanctuary and Bura Chapori Wildlife Sanctuary and in a few scattered pockets in Assam; and in and around D'Ering Memorial Wildlife Sanctuary in Arunachal Pradesh. A small population survives in Balpakram National Park in Meghalaya, and in Chhattisgarh (formerly part of Madhya Pradesh) in the Indravati National Park and the Udanti Wildlife Sanctuary. This population might extend into adjacent parts of Orissa. In the early 1990s, there may still have been about 3,300–3,500 wild buffaloes in Assam and the adjacent states of northeast India. In 1997, the number was assessed at less than 1,500 mature individuals.

Many surviving populations are believed to have interbred with feral or domestic water buffalos. In the late 1980s, fewer than 100 wild buffaloes were left in Madhya Pradesh. By 1992, only 50 animals were estimated to have survived there.

Nepal's only population lives in the Koshi Tappu Wildlife Reserve, and has grown from 63 individuals in 1976 to 219 individuals in 2009. There are two large herds comprising 87 and 99 animals, and two smaller herds of subadult males and some isolated single males. This small population is seriously threatened.

In and around Bhutan's Royal Manas National Park, a small number of wild water buffaloes live. This is a part of the subpopulation that occurs in India's Manas National Park. In Myanmar, a few wild-living animals independent of human husbandry live in the Hukaung Valley Tiger Reserve.

In Thailand, wild buffaloes have been reported to live in small herds of less than 40 individuals. A population of 25–60 individuals inhabited low land areas of the Huai Kha Khaeng Wildlife Sanctuary between December 1999 and April 2001. This population has not grown significantly in 15 years, and there may be interbreeding with domestic water buffalo.

The population in Cambodia is confined to a small area of easternmost Mondulkiri and possibly Ratanakiri Provinces. Only a few dozen individuals remain.

The origin and genetic status of the so-called wild buffalos in Sri Lanka is unclear. There is cross-breeding with domestic stock and it is believed to be unlikely that there are true wild buffalos left on the island. Wild living populations found elsewhere in Asia are feral. Water buffaloes were introduced to northern Australia, Argentina and Bolivia, where they became feral.

8.2.2 Domestic Buffalo

At least 130 million domestic water buffaloes exist, and more human beings depend on them than on any other domestic animal. They are especially suitable for tilling rice fields, and their milk is richer in fat and protein than that of dairy cattle.

The origin of the domestic water buffalo types are debated, although results of a phylogenetic study indicates that the swamp type may have originated in China and was domesticated about 4,000 years ago, while the river type may have originated from India and was domesticated about 5,000 years ago. Water buffalo were traded from the Indus Valley Civilisation to Mesopotamia, in modern Iraq, 2500 BC by the Meluhhas. The seal of a scribe employed by an Akkadian king shows the sacrifice of water buffalo. The water buffalo was known to occur in Asia and as a domestic form in Italy.

9.0 Classification of Domestic Buffalo

The domestic water buffalo *Bubalus bubalis,* belongs to the family bovidae, sub-family bovinae, genus bubalis and species arni or wild Indian buffalo. The domesticated buffaloes may be classified into two main categories: River and Swamp buffalo based on morphological, behavioral, geographical criteria and number of chromosomes. The River and Swamp buffaloes vary slightly in body structure, size and colour. They belong to the same species, *Bubalus bubalis* but have very different habitat. The river buffalo found South Asia and further west to the Balkans, Egypt, Romania and Italy, and the swamp buffalo, found from Assam in the west through Southeast Asia to theYangtze valley of China in the east. Hence, River type buffalo consist of Asian

(India and Pakistan) as well as Mediterranean breeds of buffalo. More than 70% of the total buffaloes in the world belong to the river type while almost 30% are of the swamp type. The number of chromosomes is 25 and 24 pairs in river and swamp buffalo, respectively. These subspecies differ by one chromosome because of a fusion between chromosomes 4 and 9 pair in the swamp buffalo genome. All chromosomes and chromosome arms are preserved between these two subspecies, crosses between them are fertile with 49 chromosomes in crossbreds. Male crossbred progeny have sometimes displayed fertility problems while female progeny have manifested longer calving interval only in the case of further backcross. But, fertility and reproductive efficiency is reduced in subsequent matings.

Geographical division between Riverine and Swamp buffaloes is assumed to be provided by Patkai, Barail and Arkan-Yoma mountain ranges of Burma. Buffaloes to the west of these mountains are supposed to be the River type and those distributed to the east of these mountains (Far East) are believed to be the Swamp type. All descript and nondescript South Indian buffaloes resemble Swamp buffaloes in external features with low milk yield and small body size. The karyotype of Orissa buffaloes is similar to 48 chromosomes of Swamp buffalo. All nondescript and descript north Indian buffaloes are Riverine type. Therefore, the demarcation line between distribution of River and Swamp breeds within India (North South) is yet to be established by cytotaxonominists based on karyotypes.

In India, river-type buffaloes are kept mainly for milk production and for transport, whereas swamp-type buffalo are kept mainly for work and a small amount of milk.

Examples of River Type Buffalo

1. Anatolian Water Buffalo
2. Australian Water Buffalo
3. Egyptian Water Buffalo
4. Kundi Water Buffalo
5. Water Buffalo Jafarabadi
6. Malaysian Water Buffalo
7. Murrah Water Buffalo
8. Nili-Ravi Water Buffalo
9. Pandharpuri Water Buffalo

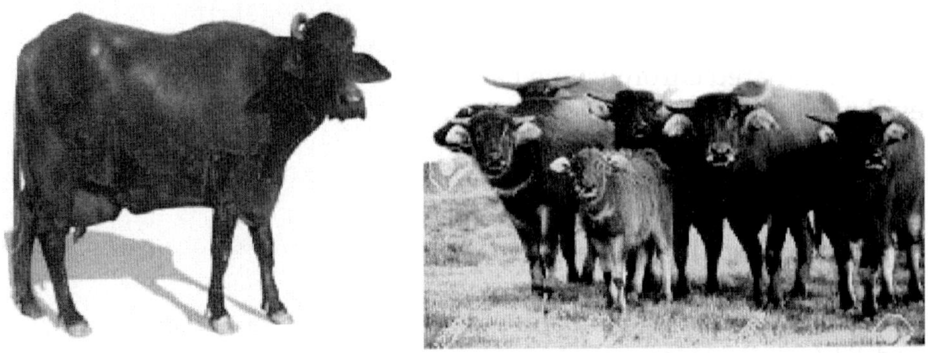

Fig. Photograph of Buffalo

9.1 River Buffalo: *Bubalus bubalis* (Chromosome, 2n=50)

- The River Buffaloes are found throughout India, Pakistan, Bangladesh, Nepal, Sri Lanka, Bulgaria, Hungary, Turkey, Italy and Egypt. They are also found in Brazil and Caucasia. As the name implies, the water buffalo, whether of the river or the swamp type, has an inherent predilection for water and loves wallowing in water or mud pools. The river buffaloes prefer to wallow in clean water and rivers, thereby the name.
- The River buffaloes have 50 chromosomes of which 5 pairs are submetacentric, while 20 pairs are acrocentric. X chromosome is large acrocentric and Y chromosome is small acrocentric.
- The River buffaloes are generally massive in size mostly with curled horns. Their horns grow downward and backward, then curve upward in a spiral. The River buffaloes have longer bodies than swamp buffaloes and weigh from 450 to 800 kilograms.
- The River buffaloes have comparatively longer faces, smaller girths, and bigger limbs than swamp buffalo. Their dorsal ridges extend further back and taper off more gradually.
- The skin of river buffaloes are usually black with occasional white markings on their head and legs, but some specimens may have dark, slate-coloured skin.
- The River buffaloes are primarily used for milk production but are also used for meat production and for draught purposes. The milk production varies between 1400 to 3000 kilograms during a 300 days lactation period. River buffaloes breeds e.g. Murrah, Nili-Ravi and others are solely used for milk production.

River buffalo has 5 pairs biarmed chromosomes and the remaining chromosome 20 pairs are acrocentric including the sex chromosomes. Based on shared chromosome banding and gene order homology, it is evident that river buffalo and domestic cattle (two members of the *Bovidae* family) are closely related. Cattle and River buffalo chromosomes are cytogenetically matched arm-for-arm. The cattle genome has 29 acrocentric chromosome pairs, with XY sex chromosome pair, while the river buffalo has 5 biarmed and 19 acrocentric chromosome pairs along with sex chromosomes XY. Each two cattle acrocentric chromosomes, *viz.* BTA1 and BTA27, BTA2 and BTA23, BTA8 and BTA19, BTA5 and BTA28, BTA16 and BTA29 fused into BBU1, BBU2, BBU3, BBU4 and BBU5 biarmed chromosome pairs of river buffalo, respectively. Thus, each of the acrocentric river buffalo chromosomes corresponds to one of the cattle chromosomes.

9.1.1 River Buffalo First Domesticated in India

The domestication history of the river buffalo has been the subject of debate for many decades, mainly due to the lack of clear archaeological evidence and scientific data, though it was believed that the animal was domesticated from the Asian wild buffalo (*Bubalus arnee*), a few thousand years ago. Scientists at the Central University of Kerala, Kasaragod, and the CSIR - Centre for Cellular and Molecular Biology, Hyderabad, have produced genetic evidence to establish that the river buffalo was first domesticated in India, from where it reached Mesopotamia and spread to other parts of the world. The scientists have now come up with evidence to prove that the river buffalo was first domesticated in the northwestern region of India, probably in the places of distribution of the present day Mehsana, Surti, and Pandharpuri breeds. Their study concluded that the domestication process involved a continuous influx of wild buffalo genes into the Indian domestic stocks after the initial domestication event. The domestication process has been traced back to the period prior to the mature phase of the Indus Valley civilisation (3300 B.C. to 1400 B.C.). Their study excluded the Mesopotamian region as the place of domestication of the river buffalo. It also reconfirms earlier findings that the river buffalo and swamp buffalo were domesticated independently.

Seals from the Indus Valley civilization dating around 2500 B.C. and those from the Akkadia era (2100 B.C. to 2500 B.C.) of the Mesopotamian civilisation have been found to depict images of the buffalo. The study indicated that the migration of the river buffalo from India to Iran, followed by genetic drift, would have contributed to the high genetic variability in the Iranian buffalo. The lack of genetic similarities between the Iranian buffalo and other buffalo populations, especially Pakistan buffalo, suggests that the migration of river buffalo from India to Iran could not have occurred through land but probably through sea.

9.2 Swamp Buffalo: *Bubalus carabanesis* (Chromosomes, 2n=48)

- The Swamp buffaloes are found principally in Malaysia, Singapore, Philippines, Thailand, Indonesia, Southern China and other countries in the fareast. Few animals are also available in north eastern states (Assam) of India. In Philippines and some other countries it is known as the Carabao, and in Malaysia as the Kerban. Various regional names are also given as Kwai Tui or Kwai Jaam, Kwai Kam etc. in Thailand.
- The Swamp Buffaloes are more or less a permanent inhabitant of marsh lands or swamp areas, where it wallows in mud, feeds on coarse marsh grass. The hottest part of the day is spent in wallows and active grazing occurs in the morning and evening hours. They have derived their name from the natural habitat which is swamp areas or marshland. Swamp buffaloes resemble the wild arni in morphological characteristics.
- Swamp buffaloes prefer to wallow in mudholes which they make with their horns. During wallowing, they acquire a thick coating of mud. Both are well adapted to a hot and humid climate with temperatures ranging from 0°C (32°F) in the winter to 30°C (86°F) and greater in the summer. Water availability is important in hot climates, since they need wallows, rivers, or splashing water to assist in thermoregulation. Some breeds are adapted to saline seaside shores and saline sandy terrain.
- The Swamp buffaloes have 48 chromosomes of which 1 pair metacentric, 4 pairs submetacentric and 18 pairs are acrocentric. The difference in number of chromosomes is due to a telomere-centromere tandem fusion between two chromosomes 4 and 9 pairs of river buffalo. X and Y chromosome are same as river buffalo

- Swamp buffaloes are recognized by their short stocky body with a pot belly, short face with wide muzzle, and short and thin legs. The forehead is flat, the eyes orbits are prominent. The tail is short, reaching only to the hocks. The udder is small and set far back in the legs. Height at withers is 129–133 cm (51–52 inch) for males, and 120–127 cm (47–50 inch) for females. The neck is comparatively long, and the withers and croup are prominent. A dorsal ridge extends backward and ends abruptly just before the end of the chest.
- Their horns grow outward, and curve in a semicircle (crescent shape), but always remain more or less on the plane of the forehead. The horns grow out laterally and horizontally in young animals and curve round in a semi-circle in older ones. In Thailand the horn shape and size varies from short horns to long straight horns.
- The Swamp buffaloes have a grey skin at birth, but with advancing age turning to slate blue.These buffaloes are usually dark grey in colour, although variations from black to albinoids are also found among the population. There are two white chevrons in neck area usually slate gray to black.
- They are primarily used for draught power in paddy fields and haulage but they do provide small quantities of milk for a farmer's family. Milk yield is very low (maximum of around 488 litres) and generally it is not used as a dairy animal. Swamp buffalo is a work animal of rice growing areas. The main use is ploughing, harrowing and puddling of rice fields. It is also used for carts and sledges and has tremendous ability for draught.
- Recently, its potential as a meat producer has been discovered. Some strains of the swamp type are larger than others, but there are no distinct breeds. The Swamp buffaloes vary in size from 300 to 550 kilograms. The weight in small types is between 300-450 kg but in larger types between 450-550 kg. They range in weight from 300–550 kg but weights of over 1,000 kg have also been observed.
- Swamp buffaloes are generally used for draft - transportation - meat - and are not used as milk producers. However, crossings between river and swamp buffaloes have been attempted in Thailand, Philippines, Vietnam, and China on a large scale. These crossbred buffaloes are powerful work animals, and produce good quality meat and more milk than the indigenous buffaloes.

In Philippines, Dr. Libertado Cruz has done extensive work in upgrading their Swamp Buffalo with River stocks.

- Swamp buffaloes generally become reproductive at an older age than river breeds. Young males in Egypt, India, and Pakistan are first mated at about 3.0–3.5 years of age, but in Italy they may be used as early as 2 years of age. Successful mating behaviour may continue until the animal is 12 years or even older.
- Although buffaloes are polyoestrous, their reproductive efficiency shows wide variation throughout the year. Buffalo cows exhibit a distinct seasonal change in displaying oestrus, conception rate, and calving rate. The age at first oestrus of heifers varies between breeds from 13–33 months, but mating at the first oestrus is often infertile and usually deferred until they are 3 years old. Gestation lasts from 281–334 days, but most reports give a range between 300 and 320 days. Swamp buffalo carry their calves for one or two weeks longer than river buffalo. It is not rare to find buffalo that continue to work well at the age of 30, and instances of a working life of 40 years have been recorded.

Chromosome Morphology of Buffalo

	Chro-mosome	Autosomes				Sex Chromosomes	
Species	**2n**	**Meta centric**	**Sub-meta Centric**	**Acro centric**	**Telo centric**	**X**	**Y**
River type	50	-	10	38	-	Large Acrocentric	Small Acrocentric
Swamp type	48	2	8	36	-	Large Acrocentric	Small Acrocentric

The Asian buffalo or the Water buffalo is classified in the genus bubalus, species bubalis. Their taming occurred at recent times (5,000 years ago) compared to taming of *Bos taurus* and *Bos indicus* (10,000 years ago). Asian buffalo includes two subspecies, the River buffalo and the Swamp buffalo are different for morphological as well as Genetical aspects.

It had been reported that the F_1 River buffalo x Swamp buffalo crosses had chromosomes numbers 2n=49. Of the chromosomes, three chromosomes included one metacentric; one submetacentric and one telocentric chromosome were not in pair. It was demonstrated that the metacentric chromosome in the three unpaired chromosomes belonged to the chromosome 1 of swamp buffalo, and the others two chromosomes were response to chromosome 1 and 9, respectively, from river buffaloes. Inter-se mating of F_1 produce the F_2 hybrid of three different karyotype categories (2n=48, 2n=49 and 2n=50).

10.0 Phylogenetics of Water Buffalo

The buffalo species originated in mainland south-east Asia and then it spread north to China and west to the Indian subcontinent where the river type buffalo evolved and was domesticated. Following domestication in China, the domesticated swamp buffalo spread through two separate routes, through Taiwan and the Philippines to the eastern islands of Borneo and Sulawesi, and south through mainland southeast Asia and then to the western islands of Indonesia. Genus *Bubalus* dispersed from Asia to Europe during the Pleistocene era. These animals became restricted to India, Indonesia, and parts of Southeast Asia when climate went dry. Water buffalo was introduced to Italy during the sixth century *via* Bay of Tunis. Moreover, buffalo was introduced in Australia, Africa and both Americas.

Water buffalo (*Bubalus bubalis*) is broadly classified into river and swamp categories, but it remains disputed whether these two types were independently domesticated, or if they are the result of a single domestication event. Based upon the existing knowledge of cytogenetic, ecological and phenotypic parameters, molecular data and present-day distribution of the river and swamp buffalo, it is suggested that these two types were domesticated independently, and that classification of the river and swamp buffalo as two related subspecies is more appropriate. River and swamp buffaloes were distinguished into two distinct clades.

The phylogenetic relationships support the evolution of domesticated swamp and river buffalo from an ancestral swamp-like animal, most likely represented today by the wild Asian buffalo (*Bubalus arnee*). On the basis of DNA (mtDNA) D-loop data analysis, the estimated time of divergence of the swamp and river types is about 28000 to 87000 years ago.

A considerable, within and between population, differences have been observed in allelic variability in 21 microsatellite *loci* in 8 swamp and 3 river buffalo populations. *Bubalus bubalis* and *Syncerus caffer* were reported as the most divergent species in the *Bos* clade when 20 bovine microsatellites among bovid species were studied based on genetic variability among Indian buffaloes using 27 microsatellite *loci*. The DNA fingerprinting analysis using amplified fragment length polymorphism (AFLP) revealed clustered African and water buffalo. This study included several phylogenetic trees with African buffalo and water buffalo. Mitochondrial D-loop DNA sequence analysis of 19 swamp buffaloes and 61 river buffaloes suggested just one domestication event of water buffalo (5,000 years ago in the subcontinent). In that study, researchers hypothesized that water buffalo was an interbred with wild buffalo or domestic buffalo from China, resulting in South-East Asian buffalo. Mitochondrial D-loop regions of Chinese swamp buffalo and other swamp and river buffaloes from Australia, India, Brazil, Italy, and Southeast posed an alternative notion of an independent domestication for river and swamp buffalo. These results indicated an independent divergence of river buffalo and swamp buffalo, before the occurrence of domestication in the subcontinent and in China.

Water buffalo interleukin-12 (IL12) sequence showed significant identity with bovine IL12. There was also a functional cross-reaction with bovine immune cells. Furthermore, Indian water buffalo interleukin-18 (IL18) showed 99% similarity in amino acid sequences with cattle IL18.

Results of mitochondrial DNA analyses indicate that the two types were domesticated independently. Sequencing of cytochrome b genes of *Bubalus* species implies that the domestic buffalo originated from at least two populations, and that the river and the swamp types have differentiated at the full species level. The genetic distance between the two types is so large that a divergence time of about 1.7 million years has been suggested. The swamp type was noticed to have the closest relationship with the Tamaraw or Mindoro dwarf buffalo (*Bubalus mindorensis*) belonging to the family Bovidae. It is endemic to the island of Mindoro in the Philippines, and is the only endemic Philippine bovine. It is believed, however, to have once also thrived on the larger island of Luzon. The Tamaraw was originally found all over Mindoro, from sea level up to the mountains (2000 meters above sea level), but because of human habitation, hunting, and logging, it is now restricted to only a few remote grassy plains and is now an endangered species. Contrary to common belief and past classification, the Tamaraw is not a subspecies of the local carabao, which is only slightly larger, or the common water buffalo. In contrast to the carabao, it has a number of distinguishing characteristics: it is slightly hairier, has light markings on its face, is not gregarious, and has shorter horns that are somewhat V-shaped. It is the largest native terrestrial mammal in the country.

11.0 Current Scenario of Indian Buffalo

- Buffalo contributes around 21.23% of the total livestock population in India as per 19th Livestock census report.
- Total number of buffalo in the country as per 2012 Census is 108.7 million.
- Buffalo population has increased from 105.3 million to 108.7 million showing a positive growth of 3.19% from 2007 to 2012.
- Female buffalo population has increased by 7.99% over the previous census and the total number of female buffalo is 92.5 million in 2012.
- The variations of animals in-milk of buffalo population during the period 2003-07 and 2007-12 is showing a decline of 56% in rural area.
- The percentage changes in - milch buffalo population during the periods has increased by 46% in rural areas.
- The percentage changes in total female buffalo population showing an increase of 10% in rural areas.
- The decline of male buffalo population is on higher side for both rural and urban areas during 2007-12.
- Milch buffaloes increased from 48.64 million to 51.05 million with an increase of 4.95% over previous census.

The world's first cloned buffalo was developed by Indian scientists at National Dairy Research Institute, Karnal, Haryana. The buffalo calf was named *Samrupa*. The calf did not survive more than a week, and died due to some genetic disorders. So, the scientists created another cloned buffalo a few months later, and named it Garima.

12.0 Buffalo Wealth and Growth Rates in India

The current buffalo population representing about 97.13% world buffalo is in Asia, with 76.92% in South Asia, 12.8% in East Asia, and only 8.4% are found in South-East Asia. Small proportions of the world population are found elsewhere: about 0.626% in America, 0.22% in Europe, and 2.90% in Africa. India has about 57% of the world buffalo population. So, in Indo-Pak region water buffalo comprise 97% of the world's buffalo population, where more people are dependent on the water buffalo than on any other domesticated species. Buffalo world population is steadily increasing at the rate of 2% *per annum* during the last two decades.

The total Buffalo contributes around 21.23% of the total livestock population of India as per report of last Livestock Census-2012. The water buffalo population in India numbered over 108.7 million head in 2012, representing 57% of the world population. As per All India Livestock Census 2012, the buffalo population in India was increased by 3.19% compared to 2007 Census. Out of the total population of Buffaloes, Recognized breeds - 17.05%, Graded buffaloes - 39.58%, Non descript - 43.37%.

Analysis of sex wise population: Male buffaloes: Calf & young stock- 13.1 million (36.5%), Used for agriculture & breeding- 3.7 million (18.9%), For bullock cart & breeding-1.2 million (6.1%), Breeding males- 0.9 million (4,6%), Female buffaloes: 85.7 million, Calf & young stock- 31.3 million (36.5%), In milk- 35.6 million (41.5%), Dry-13.0 million (15.2%), Have not calved once - 4.2 million (4.9%), Above 10 years of age- 1.7 million (2.0%). About 70% of the total buffaloes in India are non-descript and rest 30% population is descript which has been classified into 13 district breeds according to NBAGR, Karnal, Haryana, India.

The number of milch animals (in-milk and dry) cows and buffaloes has increased from 111.09 million to 118.59 million with an increase of 6.75%. The number of animals in milk cows and buffaloes has increased from 77.04 million to 80.52 million showing a growth of 4.51%. The milch buffaloes increased from 48.64 million to 51.05 million with an increase of 4.95% over previous census.

The annual growth rate during 1987-92 registered an increase of 2.08%. From 1997 to 2007, the world buffalo population increased by approximately 18 million, which is annual increase of about 1.13 per cent. This increase is due to increase in population in Asian countries. In India, percent increase was about 1.0 as compared to 1.09 in Asia and 2.58 in rest of the world. The buffaloes constituted about 22 per cent of the total livestock population in India which have increased during 1951-2012 at the rate of 2.50 per cent per annum and 3.19 percent from 2007-2012.

In addition to the fact that India has more buffaloes than any other country of the world, the Indian buffalo-breeds are some of the world's best. They are primarily of the river type and mainly used for milch purpose. Swamp buffaloes occur only in small areas in the north-eastern part of the country and are not distinguished into breeds. The Murrah, Bhadawari, Jaffarabadi, Surti, Mehsana, Nagpuri and Nili Ravi are among the important breeds.

India is gifted with rich genetic resources in terms of its buffalo breeds. The buffalo is an integral part of agriculture in India, providing a source of milk, meat, skin, hides, fertilizer, fuel, and draft power. Buffalo is the main milch producing species in our country, and cattle the main milch species to produce the draft bullocks. Hence, the contribution of buffaloes to the total milk production is larger than that of cattle. India is the home tract for some of the best buffalo breeds. India has been the centre of dispersion of reputed breeds for improvement of the species elsewhere in the world and has dominated the world trade in export of reputed breeds from the country.

The country has made a grand spectre on the World stage being top milk producer and leading meat exporter-with crucial contributing about 55 percent of the total milk produced in the country and 86 per cent of the exported meat from buffalo alone. Share of buffalo milk occupies the highest position in Indian dairy industry, contributing about more than half of the total milk produced by its varied population which is less than half that of the cattle population. Hence, Indian buffaloes are an important source of milk supply today and yield nearly three times as much milk as cows. It contributes substantially to economy of the country by producing 75 million metric tons of milk and over 1.6 million metric tons of meat. Apart from that about 7.5 million male and 0.3 million female buffaloes are also used as draught power.

Buffaloes are reared mainly for milk but some buffaloes are used as draught animals in certain parts of the country. The Indian dairy industry, of late, has come to depend more and more on the buffaloes to the neglect of the cow so much so cow milk constitutes not even 1% of the total quantity handled under the various projects, which have come up in the public, co-operative and private sectors. The private (unorganized) milk trade, which is used to supply cow milk to the urban customers until very recently in the eastern and southern States, has now started supplying buffalo milk. Buffalo has now come to occupy an important place in the dairy industry in India.

India is the first country in the world for the number of buffaloes and milk production (about 84.4 million/tons, of which 54 percent are buffalo milk). India is also the first country in Asia for scientific and technological development in the buffalo nutrition, production, reproduction, biotechnologies and genetic improvement. Moreover, India realized national programmes like as the "green revolution" (to increase crop production for animals), the "white revolution" (to increase milk productivity and satisfy the human need of proteins) and finally the "red revolution" (to increase meat production and industry), particularly depending on buffalo. The strategy of the Indian country is the genetic improvement of the local breeds through animal recording and selection. In fact India posseses the best River milch breeds of Asia, e.g. Murrah, Nili-Ravi, Surti and Jaffarabadi, which had their origin in North-Western states of India and have high potential for milk and fat production besides being used for work and surplus stock used for meat production. Indian Murrah is the most diffused animal in the world from Bulgaria to South America and all over the Asian countries.

Buffaloes are well adapted to a hot and hot humid climate and play a distinct role in the economy of the farmers, which is primarily based on agricultural production systems. They provide high quality milk, meat and source of draught power to small holders of the countries of different regions. In fact these animals are considered as an asset financially as they serve as an instrument of insurance against the risk of crop failure due to natural calamities.

13.0 Scientific Classification of Domestic Buffalo

Kingdom	:	Animal
Phylum	:	Chordata
Class	:	Mammalia
Order	:	Artiodactyla
Family	:	Bovidae
Subfamily	:	Bovinae
Tribe	:	Bovini
Genus	:	*Bubalus*
Species	:	*B. bubalis*
Binomial name	:	*Bubalus bubalis* : River buffalo
	:	*Bubalus carabanesis* : Swamp buffalo
Conservation status	:	Domesticated

14.0 Salient Feature of Buffalo

- Indian buffaloes or water buffaloes are found all over the plains and lower hills in the country. They are semi-aquatic animals, and are most abundant in humid localities. Wild buffalo is fairly abundant in India, except in the southern and western states, particularly in low-lying swampy land covered with tall grass. While the wild buffalo-cow will not breed with the tame buffalo-bull, the tame buffalo-cow readily pairs with the wild buffalo-bull, the stock being thereby improved.
- They are large, massive, and clumsy creatures, with exceptionally short, thick legs and conspicuous hoofs. The horns are thick, flat, curved or straight and marked with rings indicative of age. Light coloured brownish breeds stand in heat better than jet black ones.
- They are powerful draught animals; males are castrated for use for heavy transport as well as ploughing. They are generally not made to work during the hot parts of the day. Buffaloes are nocturnal in habit: not only do they like to wallow at night, but if left to their own devices, they will mate, suckle their calves and travel more during the hours of darkness than in day light.
- Females normally produce calves every other year after a gestation of 9 to 11 months. Young bulls typically remain with maternal herds which consist of around 30 buffaloes for three years after birth. They then go on to form small all-male herds.
- Buffalo milk is richer in butter-fat content (7%) than cow milk (4.5%). The solid not-fat (SNF) content is around 9.0 to 10.5 and is generally slight higher than that of cows milk. It is more commonly used for the manufacture of dairy products, such as butter, ghee, cheese, khoa etc.
- In general buffaloes are versatile. The buffalo breeds and their home tracts are stable, have a well-defined place in the local natural environment; consume the remnants of the crops, yet produce valuable milk and provide draft-power and dung/urine as organic manure. With excellent ability to convert poor quality feed to fodder, buffaloes provide milk that is rich in nutrition and quality, meat that is known for flavor and marbling and steady but sure-footed draft power in rural/remote areas and a host of other services, including Mozzarella cheese.

- All the recognized breeds and local populations have unique qualities for meeting local requirements of food, energy and livelihoods in an environmentally suitable manner. Buffaloes are used for all types of land cultivation and crop harvesting. They are also used as a means of transportation (by draught and pack).
- Buffaloes are less discriminating in foraging and therefore consume a large quantity of coarse fodder that is not readily eaten by cattle. This might be one of the reasons why buffaloes thrive better than do cattle on coarse fodder.

15.0 Buffalo Statistics in India

The present-day domesticated buffaloes are the descendants of *Bos arni* found in wild state even today in the north-eastern parts of India specially Assam and the surrounding areas although this species originated in India. The buffaloes are normally classified into River and Swamp types though both are called Bubalus bubalis. Most of the buffaloes in India are River type though Swamp type is also found in certain parts of the country especially in eastern parts of India.

According to the 19th Livestock Census Statistics Indian buffalo population in 2012 was 108.7 as compared to 105.3 million in 2007. Buffalo ranked on third position with regard to other livestock species in Total Livestock Population in India. Distribution of Indian buffalo population as per last Livestovk Census-2012 across different states of India is presented in following table. It is evident from the data that although buffalo population is concentrated in Uttar Pradesh but it is present in every state and region of India varying in ecology, climate, topography as well as socio economic conditions. This also showed the versatility of buffalo to be raised in all over Indian soil irrespective of geography.

Buffaloes are spread over almost all states with varying density in India. Northern and Western states comprising Haryana, Punjab, Uttar Pradesh, Rajasthan, Gujarat and Maharashtra have the majority of the population (66%). Most of the milch breeds are also found in these regions. The highest number of buffalo population present in Northen region, which is about 38% while Eastern region contributes the least number of buffalo, about only 10%. In western region 28% of buffalo head present and Southern region contributes 24% of total buffalo population.

Among different states, Uttar Pradesh has the highest buffalo population (30625334) followed by Rajasthan (12976095), Andhra

Pradesh (10622790) Gujarat (10385574) and Madhya Pradesh (8187989). Uttar Pradesh has the largest number of buffaloes, which is over 28% of the total buffaloes of India. The other major states having considerable buffaloes are Rajasthan (11.94%), Andhra Pradesh (9.77%), Gujarat (9.55%), Madhya Pradesh (7.53%), Punjab (4.75%), Bihar (6.96%), Haryana (5.6%) Maharashtra (5.15%) and Karnataka (3.19%).

The density of buffaloes is higher in the alluvial plains of North India where large quantity of fodder is available. In 1997, density of 122, 109 and 79 buffaloes per sq km in Punjab, Haryana and Uttar Pradesh were recorded respectively, which was much higher than the national average of 27 buffaloes per sq km. Population of recognized breeds constitute about 30% of the total buffalo population. About 70% of buffaloes are non-descript. Murrah is the major breed constituting about 44.39% of the population of recognized breeds.

During the last decade, there has been continuous growth of buffalo in north-western part of the country at the rate of about 2 percent per annum as against the average growth rate of approximately 1 percent of the country. Highest buffalo population growth was observed in Uttar Pradesh followed by Rajasthan and Andhra Pradesh. However, percent growth of buffalo population was recorded highest in Haryana followed by Gujarat and Rajasthan. The states which possess large population of non-descript buffaloes and have shown higher growth rate during the period are Maharashtra, Bihar and Jammu & Kashmir whereas the states which have large buffalo population and negative growth rate are Tamil Nadu, Karnataka, Orissa, West Bengal, Chhattishgarh and Assam. The high growth rate in Uttar Pradesh, Maharashtra and Andhra Pradesh has mainly been attributed to increasing trend of buffalo meat production while in Rajasthan it is primarily due to the increased demand of buffalo milk and in Haryana due to increasing demand of superior buffalo germplasm.

Recent trend indicates that the landless farmers are losing out while medium and big farmers/entrepreneurs are consolidating ownership over milch buffaloes especially high producing Murrah buffaloes. Many crossbreds like Mehsana (Gujarat), Godavari (Andhra Pradesh) and Kujang (Orissa) evolved by using Murrah breed. The performances of these crossbreds have been close to Murrah Buffalo, the pride of world.

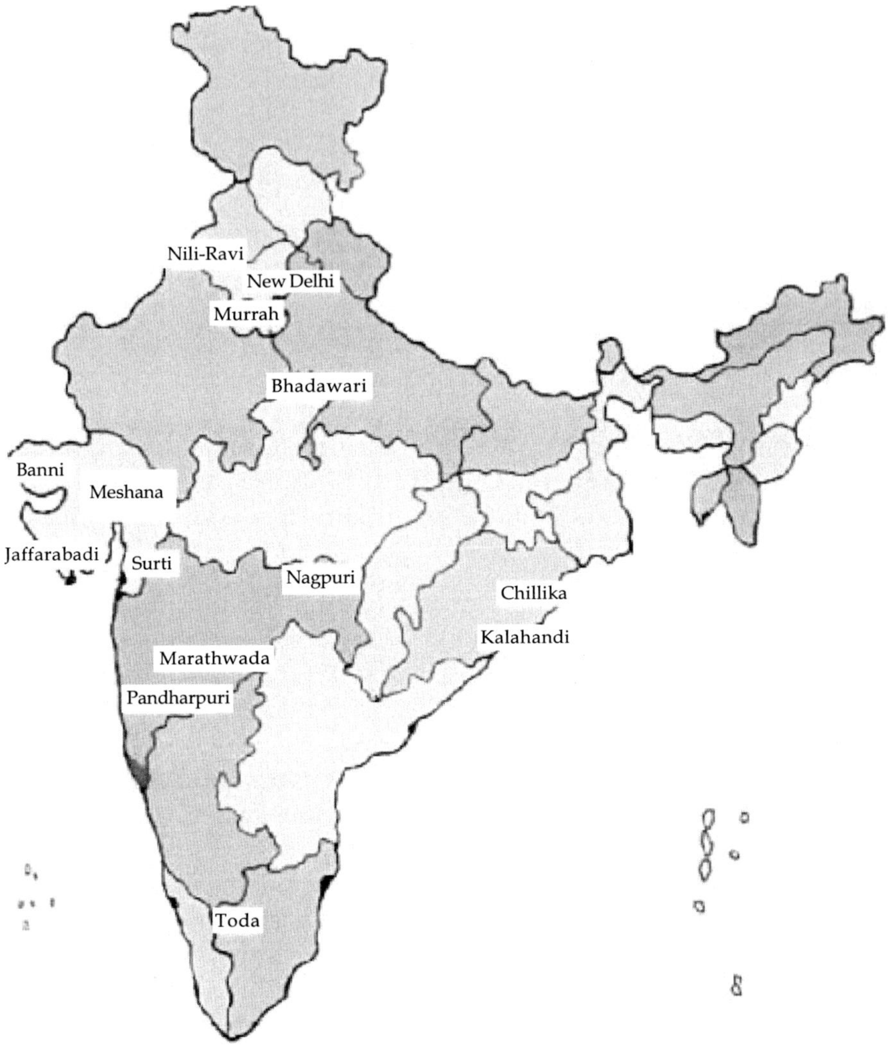

Fig. Distribution of Buffalo Breed in India

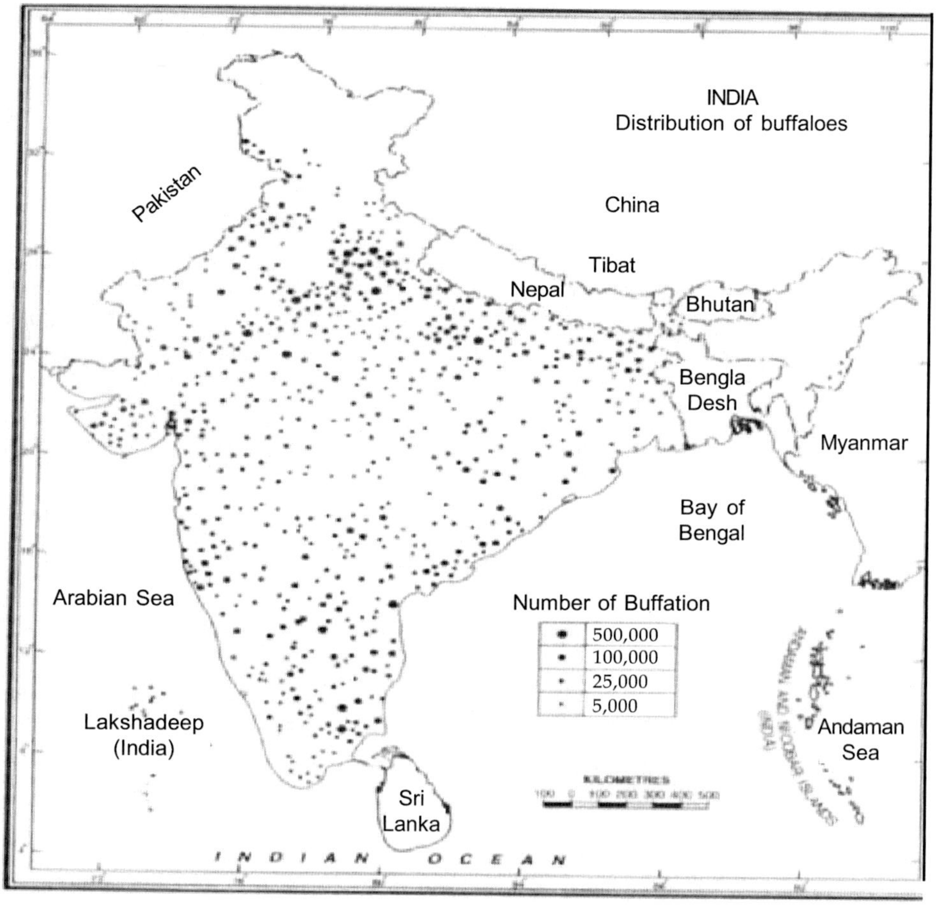

Fig. Region Wise Distribution

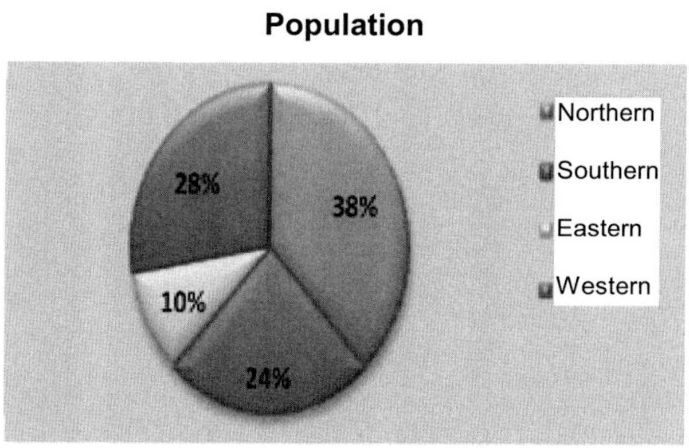

Fig. Region wise distribution In India

16.0 State Wise Buffalo Population in India as Per 19th Livestock Census-2012

Sl. No.	Name of the State	Population size	Sl. No.	Name of the State	Population size
1	Andaman & Nicobar Islands	7863	19	Madhya Pradesh	8187989
2	Andhra Pradesh	10622790	20	Maharashtra	5594392
3	Arunachal Pradesh	5970	21	Manipur	66369
4	Assam	435265	22	Meghalaya	22059
5	Bihar	7567233	23	Mizoram	5174
6	Chandigarh	14034	24	Nagaland	32720
7	Chhattisgarh	1390553	25	Delhi	162142
8	Dadra & Nagar Haveli	4062	26	Odisha	726306
9	Daman & Diu	430	27	Puducherry	2109
10	Goa	31798	28	Punjab	5159734
11	Gujarat	10385574	29	Rajasthan	12976095
12	Haryana	6085312	30	Sikkim	703
13	Himachal Pradesh	716016	31	Tamil Nadu	780431
14	Jammu & Kashmir	738989	32	Tripura	10806
15	Jharkhand	1185942	33	Uttar Pradesh	30625334
16	Karnataka	3470505	34	Uttarakhand	987775
17	Kerala	102269	35	West Bengal	597379
18	Lakshadweep	0		**Total Population**	**10 87 02 122**

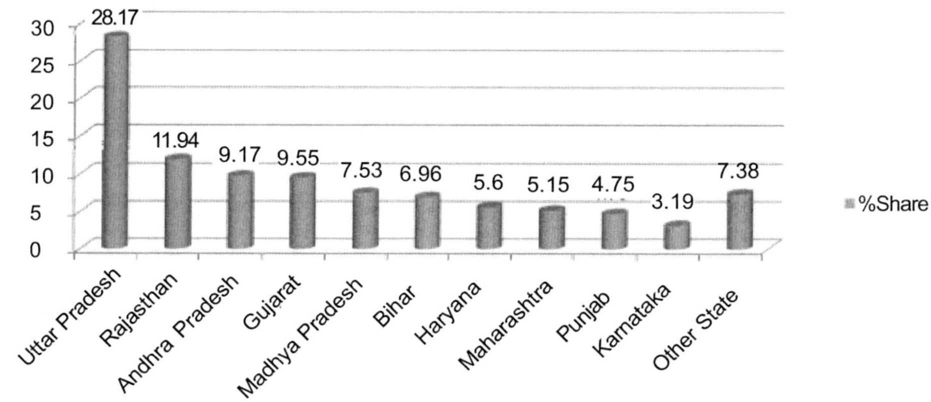

Fig. Percentage of Share of Buffalo Population In India as per 2012 Census

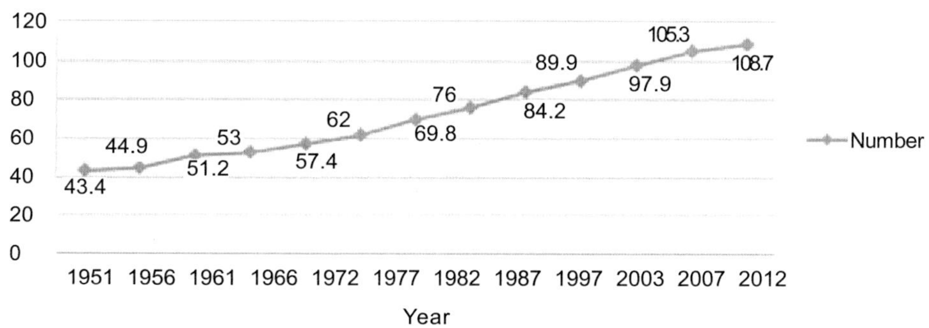

Fig. Buffalo Population in India (in million)

17.0 Breed of Indian River Buffalo

Buffaloes mainly concentrated in Asia are identified as two main types: River Buffalo and Swamp Buffalo. The buffaloes in India and Pakistan belong to the River type. They have been selected for improved milk production. They are also good meat producers and can be used for work as well. The native buffaloes in other countries belong to the Swamp type. They are used primarily for work and meat. Milk yields are very low. However, in several countries even these low yielders contribute to the income of the rural poor.

It is essential to understand the genetic architecture and relationships among different breeds, so as to design rational breeding strategies for optimum utilization and conservation of available genetic variability in India. The diversity within domestic livestock species is perceived generally in terms of differences that are referred to as breed.

Each breed is the product of mutation and genetic drift as well as separate adaptation and evolution with differing selection pressures imposed by climate, endemic parasites and diseases, available nutrition and criteria imposed by man.

About 70 percent of the total buffaloes in India are non-descriptive and rest 30 percent population is descriptive classified into Thirteen (13) recognised breeds according to NBAGR, India. Besides these descript breeds, many lesser known buffalo populations are also spread out in the length and breadth of the country each having its own special features and are well adapted to their respective agro-climatic and eco-geographical conditions. They have extremely variable composition being either non-descript or crosses among various breeds and cannot be categorized in any other well-established breed. Inter-mating among breeds located in adjoining areas is also very common. Therefore, it is very difficult to identify and ascertain the total number of animals of specified breeds. In the process of inter-mating and crossbreeding, it is possible that some of the important breeds may be at the point of extinction. It is, therefore, necessary to take urgent steps for their conservation and improvement. There is general concern that the genetic variation within the few domestic animal species is disappearing through breed substitution and inter-breed crossing. Any reduction in the diversity of genetic resource narrows the scope to respond to selective breeding.

In India there are few well defined breeds with specific physical characters that differentiate them unmistakably from other types as may be found in various states of the country. These are all milch breeds, but the number of animals belong to distinct breed is small fraction of the total buffalo population of the country. The larger section belong to a non-descript class and these vary greatly in size, weight and general features known as deshi. So, it is therefore necessary to characterize these large amount of deshi buffalo for strengthening the whole buffalo genetic resources in our country. The well defined Indian buffalo breeds distributed in different regions of the country are now classified into distinct group and are presented in the folloing table:

17.1 Indian Buffaloes grouped under the following Heads

On the Basis of Milk Production		
Superior Milch Breed	:	Average milk production more than 1500 kg/Lactation Example: Murrah, Nili-Ravi, Surti and Mehsana
Average Milch Breed	:	Average milk production 500-1000 kg/ Lactation Example: Jaffarabadi, Nagpuri and Bhadawari
Draught Purpose Breed	:	Average milk production less than 500 kg/Lactation Example: Toda
On the Basis of Body Size		
Large sized	:	Murrah, Nili-Ravi and Jaffarabadi
Medium sized	:	Mehsana, Nagpuri, Bhadawari, Surti, Toda, Banni, Chilika, Kalahandi, Marathwada and Pandharpuri
Other Populations	:	Manda, Paralakhemundi, Sambalpuri, Jerangi, Godavari, Ganjam, Dharwadi/ Gowli, South Kanara and Swamp
On the Basis of Region		
North and North-Western Breed	:	Murrah, Nili-Ravi, Kundi, Bhadawari, Tarai
Central Indian Breed	:	Nagpuri, Pandharpuri, Manda, Jerangi, Kalahandi, Sambalpur
South Indian Breed	:	Toda, South Kanara
Western Indian Breed	:	Surti, Jaffarabadi, Mehsana
On the Basis of Phenotypic similarity and the Breeding tracts		
Murrah Group	:	Murrah, Nili-Ravi, Kundi
Gujarat Group	:	Jaffarabadi, Surti, Mehsana, Banni
Uttar Pradesh Group	:	Bhadawari, Tarai
Central India Group	:	Nagpuri, Pandharpuri, Kalahandi, Sambalpuri, Manda, Jerangi
South India Group	:	Toda, South Kanara

Out of all, Six breeds viz., Murrah, Nili-Ravi, Jaffarabadi, Bhadawari, Surti and Mehsana are high quality milch breeds of the country and they all come from Northern and Western parts comprising Punjab, Rajasthan and Gujarat states. The breeds of Central and Southern parts are noted as draught purpose due to the fact that they have swamp as well as river characteristics.

18.0 Registred Breed of Buffalo in India

S.No.	Breed	State/Home Tract	Accession Number
1	Murrah	Haryana	INDIA_BUFFALO_0500_MURRAH_01001
2	Nili Ravi	Punjab	INDIA_BUFFALO_1600_NILIRAVI_01002
3	Bhadawari	Uttar Pradesh and Madhya Pradesh	INDIA_BUFFALO_2010_BHADAWARI_01003
4	Mehsana	Gujarat	INDIA_BUFFALO_0400_MEHSANA_01004
5	Surti	Gujarat	INDIA_BUFFALO_0400_SURTI_01005
6	Jaffarabadi	Gujarat	INDIA_BUFFALO_0400_JAFFARABADI_01006
7	Nagpuri	Maharashtra	INDIA_BUFFALO_1100_NAGPURI_01007
8	Pandharpuri	Maharashtra	INDIA_BUFFALO_1100_PANDHARPURI_01008
9	Marathwadi	Maharashtra	INDIA_BUFFALO_1100 MARATHWADI _01009
10	Toda	Tamilnadu	INDIA_BUFFALO_0018_ TODA _01010
11	Banni	Gujarat	INDIA_BUFFALO_0400_BANNI_01011
12	Chilika	Odisha	INDIA_BUFFALO_1500_CHILIKA_01012
13	Kalahandi*	Odisha	INDIA_BUFFALO_1500_KALAHANDI_01013

* Breed Registration Committee of NBAGR in its meeting on 14th May, 2012 at New Delhi approved registration of **'Kalahandi'** as one newly identified breed of buffalo germplasm in India. Hence, the total number of Indian buffalo breed is Thirteen (13).

19.0 Breed Wise Buffalo Population in India

Buffaloes in the country are third major contributors in the total livestock population but largest contributors in the production of milk. According to the 19th Livestock census, buffaloes have 21.23% share to the total livestock population in 2012. NBAGR recognized a total of 13 descript buffalo breeds in the country besides a large population remains as non-descript buffaloes. Breed Survey conducted in 2013 consider these thirteen descript buffalo breeds. The following table shows the number of animals in various breeds of buffaloes.

20.0 Estimated Number of Animals Under Indigenous Buffalo Breed

S. No.	Name of the Breed	Pure (number)	Graded (number)	Total No. of Animals	Percentage share
1	Murrah	1,16,86,198	3,65,68,676	4,82,54,874	44.39
2	Surti	18,86,280	20,06,614	38,92,894	3.58
3	Mehsana	26,76,699	9,48,426	36,25,125	3.33
4	Jaffarabadi	5,71,077	12,00,421	17,71,498	1.63
5	Bhadawari	5,83,599	11,70,188	17,53,787	1.61
6	Nili Ravi	1,29,411	5,47,834	6,77,245	0.62
7	Pandharpuri	2,87,751	1,95,987	4,83,738	0.45
8	Banni	2,39,572	1,42,550	3,82,122	0.35
9	Marathwadi	2,78,502	98,093	3,76,595	0.35
10	Nagpuri	73,584	1,17,410	1,90,994	0.18
11	Kalahandi	1,15,213	26,802	1,42,015	0.13
12	Toda	3,003	2,533	5,536	0.01
13	Chilika	2,599	787	3,386	0.00
	Descript Buffalo	**1,85,33,488**	**4,30,26,321**	**6,15,59,809**	**56.63**
	Non-descript Buffalo	-	-	4,71,42,313	43.37
	Total Buffaloes			**10,87,02,122**	

20.1 Breed group of Buffalo

The following diagram shows the distribution of indigenous buffaloes under three major categories i.e. pure, graded and non-descript. Out of total buffaloes, 17.05% are pure breeds, 39.58% are graded and remaining 43.37% are in non-descript category.

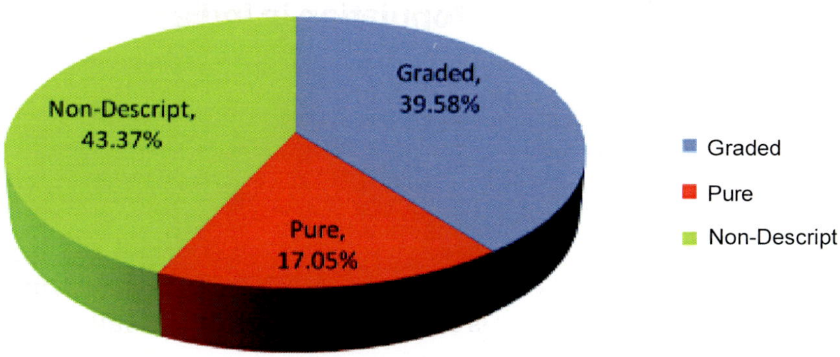

Fig. Distribution of Total Buffaloes Population

The Following Graph shows the distribution of various major indigenous breeds of buffalo in the country. The Murrah breed of buffalo contributes 44.39% of the total buffalo population followed by Non-Descript category which contributes 43.37%. Among the other breeds, Surti and Mehsana have percentage contribution of 3.58% and 3.33% respectively whereas the Jaffarabadi and Bhadawari breeds, contribute 1.63% and 1.61% respectively. All other recognized breed individually has less than 1% contribution in their breed spectrum.

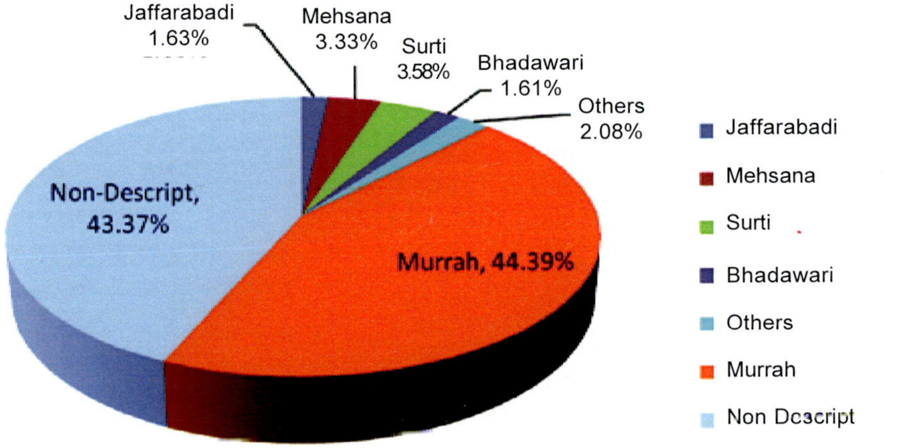

Fig. Percentage Contribution of Various Breeds of Buffalo Including Non-Descript

20.2 Buffalo: Indigenous and Graded breeds

The Following Graph gives a picture on the percentage share of pure and graded breeds excluding non-descript category. Among the individual breeds it shows that only 5 breeds namely Mehsana, Banni, Marathwadi, Kalahandi and Chilika are having their pure breeds more than 60% in number. In all other breeds major contributions is from graded breeds.

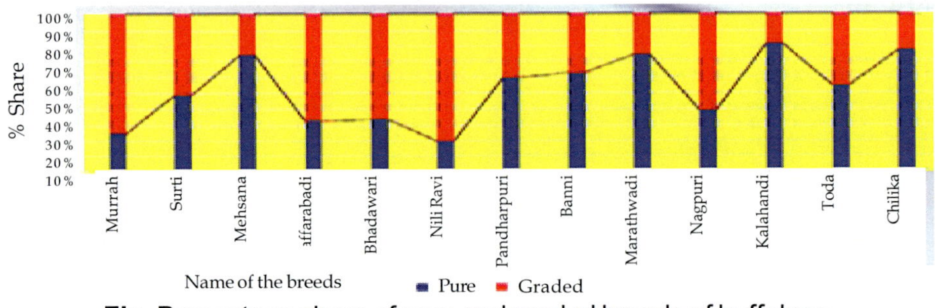

Fig. Percentage share of pure and graded breeds of buffaloes

21.0 Characterization of Indian Buffalo

The buffaloes of India have evolved within their ecosystem over several centuries and have thus acquired adaptive characteristics and still remain useful in food production. However, they have been subjected to genetic manipulation such as selection and crossbreeding only during recent past decades. By virtue of the fact that it is often considered a neglected species, much of its genetic variation may not have been lost except through natural selection in the domestic environment. However, the main areas of concern are that a complete documentation and evaluation of the variability and characterization of the various breeds and strains are lacking. Such information is vital in agricultural planning strategies and allocation of animals and breeding programs to various farmers and farming systems.

Gene technologies are being promoted and utilized in many fields of livestock production. For instance, higher productivity is being realized through manipulating the genetic variation within and between breeds that multiplies genetic gain in traditional breeding value. Therefore, gene technologies have application in distinguishing molecular phenotypes for their accurate characterization which in turn improving the use of genetic resources of domestic buffalo.

Hence, phenotypic and molecular characterization of the recognized and lesser known buffalo breeds have been taken up and the breed descriptors have been in the recent past prepared. The breed descriptors contain detailed information on the geographic distribution, population status, morphological characters, physical traits and production and reproduction performances. At present, most of the breeds have been identified on the basis of morphological characters; information on genetic architecture is available for few breeds. The molecular characterization of buffalo for establishing genetic distances among various breeds has been undertaken using microsatellite based DNA markers.

22.0 Breed Description of Indian Buffalo

The main evolutionary forces of mutation, selection, and genetic drift have created a vast diversity which ended in the formation of many well-defined breeds used for a variety of purposes with differing levels of performance. The knowledge of the genetic variability and process that underlie its origin and maintenance is vital to provide critical insights into the structure and dynamics of populations. Genetic variability also provides the opportunity for tracing the history of populations, species, and their ancestors through DNA based markers. For the overall breed improvement and to meet future challenges there is an urgent need to characterize buffalo breeds. Moreover, the future improvement is dependent on genetic variation present within breeds and between breeds variation. Detailed knowledge of genetic variation within and among different breeds is very much important for understanding and improving traits of economic importance. Keeping this aspect in view, a brief description of each of the buffalo breed available in India is delineated here.

1. Murrah

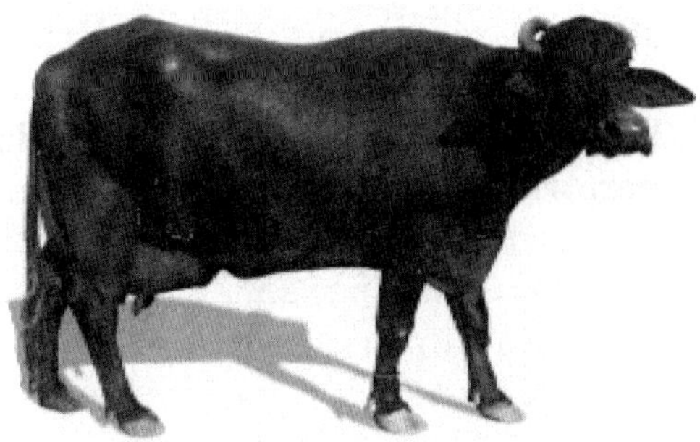

Synonym: Kundi, Kali, Delhi buffalo

Origin and Distribution: Murrah is the most important milch breed of buffalo whose breeding tract is Rohtak, Hisar and Jind districts of Haryana state, and Nabha and Patiala districts of Punjab state and Delhi. Rohtak in Haryana is a well-known market from where thousands of high yielders are exported. The name Murrah was given to the buffalo for their tightly curled short horns.

Morphological Characteristics

- Colour is usually jet black with white markings on tail face and extremities.
- Tightly curled short horn is an important character of this breed.
- Deep massive frame body, neck and head are comparatively long.
- Hips are broad and fore and hind quarters are drooping.

- Skin is soft, smooth with scanty hair.
- Short massive limbs with good bones.
- Eyes should not be walled i.e. the cornea should not have whiteness.
- Long tail reaching upto fetlock joint with black or white switch.

Performances: The average milk yield per lactation is 1500 to 2500 kg with 270 to 305 days lactation length. On an average the daily milk yield is found to be 8-10 kg, whereas a cross breed Murrah buffalo gives 6-8 kg per day. Butter-fat content of milk is 7 percent. The age at first calving is 45 to 50 months in villages but in good herds it is 36 to 40 months. The intercalving period is 450 to 500 days. The bullocks are good draft animals though slow and powerful. The body weight on average is 550 kg for male and 450 kg for female.

Remarks: Murrah buffaloes are highest milk producers among the buffalo breeds not only in India but probably in the World. The bulls of this breed are extensively used to upgrade the non-descript buffalo stock in India and also used extensively for upgrading inferior stock of many countries of abroad. This breed has even formed an important place in the livestock industry of many developing countries like Bulgaria, Philipines, Malaysia, Vietnam, Brazil and Sri Lanka. It performs well in coastal and slightly cold climatic areas. The Indian Council of Agricultural Research is maintaining a Herd Book for Murrah buffalo breed.

2. Nili-Ravi

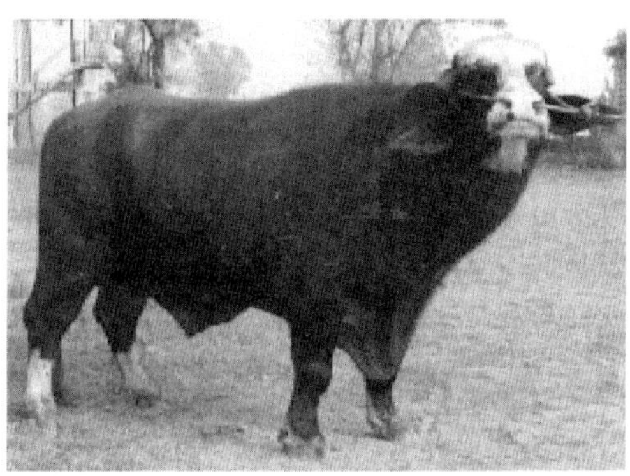

Synonym: Panch Kalyani

Origin and Distribution: The native breeding tract of Nili-Ravi is spread in Sutlej River in Ferozpur district of Punjab and in the Sahiwal district of Pakistan (bred around Ravi River). They are found mainly in Lahore, Sheikhupura, Faisalabad, Sahiwal, Multan and Bahawal Nagar districts in Punjab Province. The best animals are found in the riverine tract along the Sutlej River, south-west of Pakpattan tehsil, Mailsi tehsil of the Multan district and Bahawalpur State. The name of this breed is supposed to be derived from the deep blue colour (Nili means blue) water of the river Sutlej.

Nili and Ravi are two types of buffaloes being similar to Murrah were originally two distinct breeds as they belonged to geographically isolated areas. Previously these were described as two breeds - Nili was found in the Sutlej valley and particularly in Multan and Montgomery districts (both in Pakistan) and in Ferozepur district (Punjab, India) and Ravi was found in the Sandal Bar area of Ravi river valley (also called as Sandal bar Breed) particularly in Lyallpur, Montgomery, Gujarat and Thang districts (all in Pakistan) and in Frozepur and Amritsar district (India). Both areas are in the central Punjab of Pakistan. Frequent movement of animals with improvement in communication has resulted in their blending into a single identity.

Nili and Ravi breeds were almost similar in appearance except in the facial conformation. Nili had a more convex profile, more coarse hairs on head and face, and a more conspicuous double chin. The horns were finer, more tightly coiled and circular in cross section. In Ravi, horns were oval in cross section and the transverse rings or pits were more conspicuous. Ravi breed is heavier than Nili buffalo, but their yields are hardly to be distinguished from each other. In spite of the distinct features between these two types, due to free movement and admixture of animals, the body features had been mixed and it became difficult to differentiate them on the basis of phenotypic characters. There is no essential difference between the two types although for a long time they were treated as different breeds, but close study indicated that it was a distinction without a difference. Today therefore, they are not regarded to be different breeds and now they are officially teated as one breed. Hence these animals were officially declared as single breed i.e. Nili-Ravi, during All India Cattle Show (ICAR, 1960). In Pakistan too, Nili and Ravi are no longer regarded as separate breeds.

In early 1930s, Nili and Ravi were referred as varieties of Murrah, which differed little except in geographical location. However, Nili was shown as a breed for the first time at the first All India Cattle Show held in 1938. After the second and third cattle shows, Nili and Ravi were described separately in ICAR bulletins (1941).

Morphological Characteristics

- Usually the colour is black with white marking on forehead, face, muzzle, legs, and switch and around bright eyes.
- The most desired character of the buffaloes with such white markings is highly desired and popularly called 'Panj Kalian'.
- They have wedge shape and massive frame body.
- The head is elongated, bulging at top and depressed between eyes.
- The head is long and convex and the double chin is conspicuous.
- The horns are small and tightly curved and circular in cross section.
- The neck is long, thin and fine.
- It is the face and forehead distinguish this breed mainly from the Murrah.
- The peculiarity of the breed is the wall eyes.
- The tail is long, almost touching the ground.
- Pink marking are sometimes seen on the udder and brisket.
- The udder is well developed with squarely placed long teats.
- The milk veins are very prominent.
- The hooves and switch of tail are white in colour.

Performances: The average lactation yield is 1945 kg in Nili-Ravi buffaloes which ranges between 1688 to 2317 kg in 250-300 days of lactation. Average fat of Nili-Ravi buffalo milk is 6.9% and is less in comparison to various reports on milk of Murrah buffaloes. The intercalving period is 500 to 550 days. The age at first calving is 45 to 50 months. Average age at maturity is 30 months in male and 36 months in female. Longevity of production is good. The average weight of male and female is 600 and 450 kg respectively. The bullocks are good for heavy trotting work and draught work.

Remarks: The Nili-Ravi buffalo is a milch type buffalo breed. This is considered to be one of the best dairy breed of buffalo in India, next only to the Murrah. Nili-Ravi buffaloes are very similar to Murrah and have got many characteristics in common except for some white markings on extremities, and walled eyes. They closely resemble each other in appearance as well as in milk production. Along with Murrah, this breed is extensively used for Urban milk production.

3. Jaffarabadi

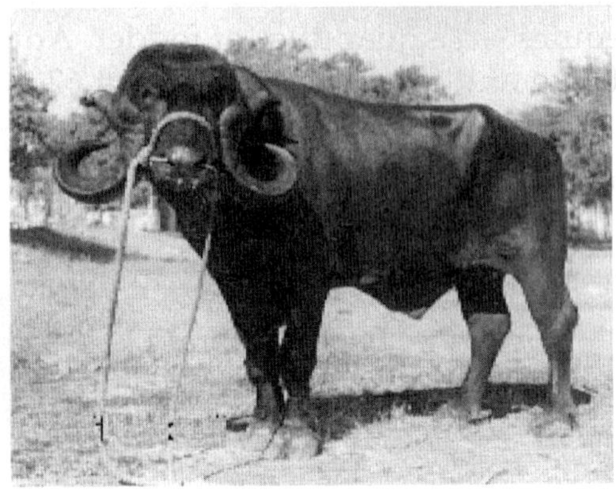

Synonym: Bhavnagri, Gir, Jaffari

Origin and Distribution: The breeding tract of this breed is Kutch, Junagarh, Rajkot and Jamnagar districts of Gujarat state. These animals are mostly maintained by traditional breeders called Maldharis, who are nomads. The animals are found in their purest form in the Gir forest of Kathiawar where they are bred in large numbers. The breed is named after the town of Jaffarabad of Gujarat State. This breed is known for its ability to fight with lions in Gir forest.

Morphological Characteristics

- The body is massive but not much compact, head and neck are massive.
- The forehead is very prominent and wide, with a slight depression in the middle.
- Their noticeable feature is heavy horns which are inclined to droop on each side of the neck and then turning up at point but not in such a tight curl as in Murrah buffaloes (drooping horns).
- Shape of horns make their eyes to look small termed as study eye, especially in males.
- The dewlap in females somewhat loose and udder well developed.
- Black in colour with white patches on face and legs.

Performances: The average milk yield is 2150 to 2340 kg with 8-9% fat. Animals are heavy milkers ranging from 15 to 18 kg per day. They yield appreciable quantity of milk, with an exceptionally high butter-fat content. These buffaloes characteristically differ from other breeds mainly in terms of kilo fat. Age at first calving is 45 months. Calving interval is about 15 months. They are very efficient in the conversion of roughages into milk with a high butter fat content. Males are good draught animals for hauling heavy loads as well. The bullocks are heavy and are used for ploughing and carting. These animals require large quantities of fodder. Adult body weight of male is about 700 kg and for female it is about 620 kg.

Remarks: Jaffarabadi is the **heaviest** of all the Indian breeds of buffaloes. This breed is reared almost solely for ghee production.

4. Nagpuri

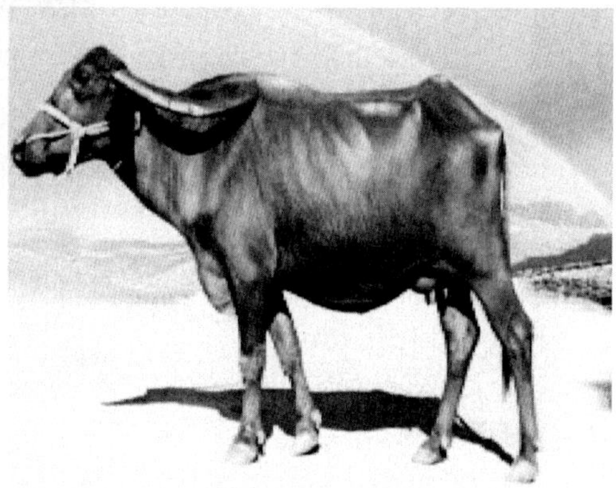

Synonym: Berari, Gaorani, Puranthadi, Varhadi, Ellichpuri, Gaolavi, Arvi, Gaolaogan, Gangauri, Shahi, Chanda.

Origin and Distribution: The breeding tract of this breed is Nagpur, Akola and Amarawati districts of Maharashtra. As the name applies, these animals are mostly found in Nagpur including Wardha, Yeotmal, Akola, Buldana, Amrawati and Achalpur in Maharasta. This breed derives its name from the place of its origin. All popular names are based on the names of respective regions.

Morphological Characteristics

- The face is long and thin with a straight profile. The neck is also somewhat longer with heavy brisket. The limbs are light.
- These are black coloured animal occasionally white markings are observed on the face, legs and switch.
- This breed has got several strains differing in colour and other superficial traits. Puranthadi strain is slightly brownish.
- The tail is comparatively short reaching a little below hocks. Naval flap is short or almost absent.
- The horns are long, flat and curved, bending backward on each side of the back almost to shoulder (like a pair of swards).
- The average height at withers in male 142 cm and that of cows 132 cm; heart girth is 210 and 205 cm for male and female respectively.

Performances: The females are moderately good yielders, producing on an average 1,000 kg milk per lactation of 300 days with butter fat content between 7.0-8.5 percent. The milk yield is ranged from 700 to 1200 kg per lactation. The age at first calving is 45 to 50 months and inter calving period is 450 to 550 days. The bullocks are good for heavy trotting work but slow in movement. Buffaloes need cooling facility e.g. wallowing tank or showers / foggers with fan. Male body weight averages 525 kg while female attains about 425 kg. These buffaloes are used for heavy draught purpose.

Remarks: This breed is known as lighter than the Murrah or other breeds of northern or western India. Farmers of this region prefer to maintain this breed mainly due to its very low maintenance cost, high fat in milk and regularity in breeding, efficiency of feed conversion, moderate production and better adaptation to local climatic conditions.

5. Marathwada

Synonym: Ellichpuri and Dudhana Thadi.

Origin and Distribution: Breeding tract includes Parbhani, Nanded, Jalna, Latur district of Marathwada Region of Maharashtra. This breed named after place of its origin.

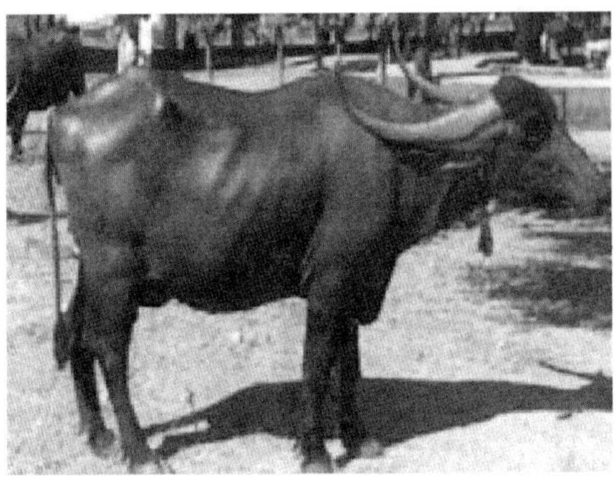

Morphological Characteristics

- They are greyish black to jet black-colour some animals have white markings on forehead and lower parts or limbs.
- Horns are medium in length and parallel to the neck, reaching upto shoulder but never beyond shoulder blade for this buffalo but in pondharpuri, horns reach upto pin bones.
- They are medium in size.

Performances: This buffalo produces on an average 1118 kg milk yield per lactation Fat% varies from 6 to 10%. The average age at first calving and calving interval are 52 and 17 months, respectively.

These animals are medium sized with an large body weight of 480 to 500 kg.

Remarks: They are used for milk, draught and transport purposes.

6. Pandharpuri

Synonym: Nil

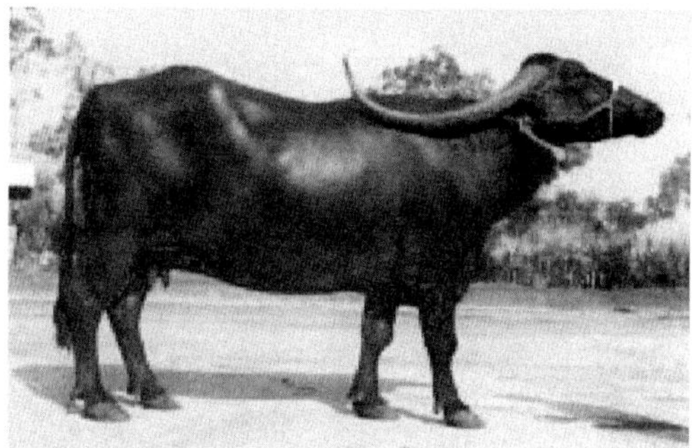

Origin and Distribution: The main breeding tract of Pandharpuri buffalo is Solapur, Sangli and Kolhapur districts of Maharastra state which is mostly drought prone. The name Pandharpuri is from the town Pandharpur in Solapur district which is the home range of this buffalo breed.

Morphological Characteristics

- Body colour varies from light black to deep black. White markings are found on forehead, legs and tail in few animals.
- Medium sized compact body animal having long narrow face, very prominent and straight nasal bone.
- Typical characteristic of this breed is its horns which are very long, curved backward, upward and usually twisted outwards.
- The breed can be easily identified by its long, sword shaped, sometimes twisted horns, which measure from 45-50 cm upto 1-1.5 m in length.
- Horns are very long extending beyond shoulder blade up to pin bones.
- Head is long, narrow with prominent nasal bone and the horizontal ears.
- Udder is compact, trough shaped with cylindrical teats.

Performances: On an average, they produce 1790 kg milk / lactation. Average age at first calving and calving interval is 44 and 14 months, respectively. Under average management conditions and hot-dry climate, these buffaloes yield 6-7 kg of milk per day. However under good management they are reported to yield upto 15 kg of milk in a day. The breed is famous for its high reproductive ability, producing a calf every 12 months. The Pandharpuri are medium sized with average body weight of 450-470 kg.

Remarks: It is an important breed in south east Maharashtra. They are hardy and suited to dry condition.

7. Bhadawari

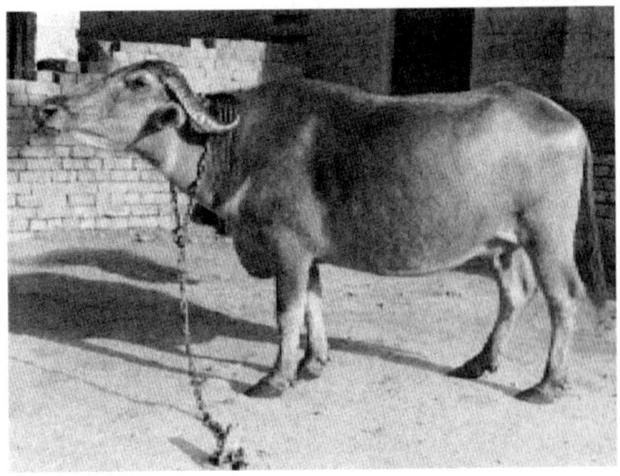

Synonym: Etawah

Origin and Distribution: This breed is found in the Bhadawari estate and Bhadawari Tehsil in Agra district and Etawah district of Uttar Pradesh state and Gwalior district of Madhya Pradesh state. Animals are found scattered in the surroundings of Yamuna and Chambal rivers. These buffaloes were the proud possession of Bhadauria clan of the former Bhadawer State before independance and has possibly derived its name from that state.

Morphological Characteristics

- The body is medium sized and wedge shaped. Barrel is short but well developed. Face is comparatively narrow with slightly marked nose. Forehead is slightly broad and deep in the middle. The ears are small. Eyes are prominent, active and bright.
- Comparatively small head bulging towards horns. Horns are black, curling slightly outward, downward before running backward parallel and close to neck, and finally turning upward.
- The legs are short and stout and the hooves are black. The hind quarters are uniform and higher than the forequarter.
- The body is usually of light copper colour with short hair of black or brown colour which is peculiar to this breed. Eye lids are generally copper or light brown colour.
- Two white lines 'Chevron' locally called as Kanthy are present at the lower side of the neck similar to that of Surti buffaloes.

- The tail is long, thin and flexible with black and white or pure white markings reaching up to fetlock.

Performances: Average milk yield ranges from 2000 to 2070 kg in a lactation period of 305 days with a high fat percentage. They are recognized for high fat content [14%] in their milk. The fat content varies from 6 to 12.5 per cent. Average age at first calving is 45 months and calving interval is about 16 monhs varies from 13 to 21 months. This breed is an efficient converter of coarse feed into butterfat. The bullocks are reputed as good draft animals with better heat tolerance than darker breeds. Adult body weight of male is about 475 kg while female weight is about 410 kg. Because of its small size these animals can be reared even by marginal and landless farmers. The male animals of this breed are considered to be one among the best for ploughing the marshy paddy fields and the mortality rate in the calves is quite low as compared to other breeds. The animals can easily tolerate the extreme weather conditions in the ravines where maximum temperature goes up to 48°C.

Remarks: Bhadawari buffaloes are recognized for high fat content in their milk, which goes as high as 14%. This breed is an efficient converter of coarse feed into butterfat and is known for it high butter fat content. They are said to be resistance to many tropical bovine diseases.

8. Surti

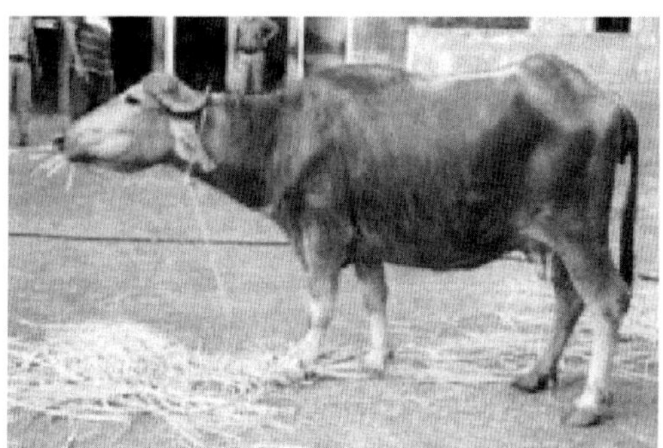

Synonym: Charotari, Deccani, Gujarati, Talabda and Nadiadi

Origin and Distribution: The home tract of Surti breed is mainly Kaira, Surat and Baroda districts in the south-western part of Gujarat state in India. The best animals of this breed are found in Anand, Nadiad and Baroda districts. The animals are also commonly found in South Rajasthan extending over to Udaipur, Bhilwara, Rajsamand, Chittorgarh and Dungarpur districts. This breed is named after place of its origin.

Morphological Characteristic

- The body of Surti breed is well shaped and medium sized; the barrel is wedge shaped.
- The animals have a very straight back. The neck is long and thin in female but massive in male and there is no dewlap.
- The skin colour is black or brown and the colour of the hair varies from rusty-brown to silver-grey.
- The head is long and fairly broad with prominent eyes. The breed has got a fairly broad and long head with a convex shape at the top in between the horns.
- The horns are sickle-shaped, moderately long and flat which grow in a downward and backward direction and then upwards at the tip, forming a hook.
- The peculiarity of the breed is two white collars, one round the jaw and the other at the brisket.
- The tail is long, thin and flexible usually with a white switch.
- The udder is well developed and well shaped and the teats are medium sized and squarely placed between the hind legs. The skin of the udder is pinkish in colour.

Performances: The average lactation yield of well-bred animals is around 1,500-1,700 kg with a fat content of 7.5 percent having record of yielding upto 2,500 kg. The peculiarity of this breed is very high fat percentage in milk (8 to 12 percent). The age at first calving is 40 to 50 months with an intercalving period of 400 to 500 days. The female has an average weight of 600 kg and the male about 700 kg. The bullocks are good for light work. Animal consumes less feed, thrives well both on limited and without green, and produce milk with higher fat and SNF content.

Remarks: The Surti buffalo is lighter in body size as compared to heavy breeds. Surti is an economical producer of milk and butter-fat. It is maintained easily by landless, small and marginal farmers. These animals are preferred by city milk producers, due to its body size and regularity in calving.

9. Mehsana

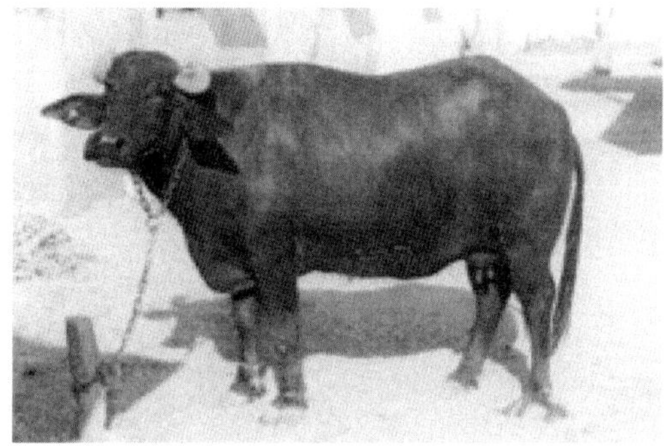

Synonym: Mehesani, Mehsani

Origin and Distribution: The breeding tract of this breed is in and around Mehsana, Sabarkantha and Banaskanta districts of the northern part of Gujarat state. Animals of this breed are also found in Palanpur in Banaskantha district and Radhanpur and Tharad in Sabarkantha district. This is supposed to have been evolved out of crossbreeding between the Surti and the Murrah. It derives its name from its home tract of the town Mehsana district located in the northern region of Gujrat state.

Morphological Characteristics

- The breed is a medium sized animal with a low-set deep body. As compared to Murrah breed the body is longer and tighter. The animals have a long body, higher limbs and a longer and heavier head. The neck is long and fine.
- The horns resemble the Surti or Murrah breed, i.e., they may vary from long sickle type of the former to a curved knot of the latter. The horns usually are less curved at the end compared to Murrah breed but are longer and could be of irregular shape.
- Eyes are very prominents black and bright bulging from their sockets with folds of skin on upper lids.
- The skin colour is mostly jet black and occasionally brown grey with some white markings on the face, legs or tips of the tail.
- It has well developed udder carried well behind, generally hind quarters are more developed than the fore-quarters with uniformly placed teats. The teats are fairly thick, long and pliable.

Performances: Milk production ranges between 598 to 3597 kg in a lactation of 300 days. Average Lactation Milk Yield: 1988 kg. Daily milk yield (kg): 11.53 (range 5.00 to 26.00). Milk Fat%: 7 to 7.5% (range 4.00 to 12.10). Lactation length averages: 305 days. Age at first calving: Average 42-48 months. The intercalving period ranges between 450 and 550 days. Average calving interval: 372 days. On an average, adult body weight of male is about 565 kg and female it is about 484 kg. The bullocks are good for heavy work but rather slow. Mehsana females are reputed for regular breeding and persistent milking.

Remarks: Mehsana buffaloes are good dairy type milch buffaloes which mature early and bred regularly yielding milk over prolonged periods. This breed is an economical producer of milk and butter-fat among the dairy buffalo breeds of India. It is docile and can stand stall feeding, and be reared under grazing conditions. Mehsana is very popular for city milk production. It is also highly valued for ghee production.

10. Banni

Synonym:

Kutchi or Kundi

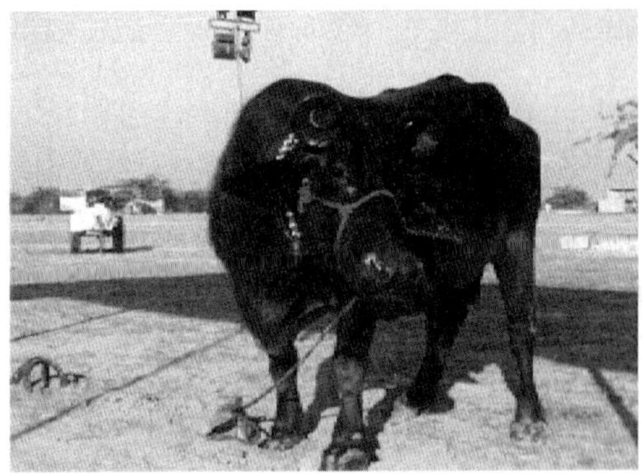

Origin and Distribution: The breeding tract includes the Banni area of Kutchchh District, Gujarat. Banni was evolved over centuries by 'Maldharis', the traditional livestock keepers of the region. They have good adaptability to harse climatic conditions and drought resistance.

Morphological Characteristics: Banni buffalo is black or copper or brown in colour. Horns are tightly coiled vertically with single or double coiling. No slope towards base of horns. Brisket is highly prominent and loose.

Performances: Average age at first calving is 40 months and calving interval is about 13 months. Milk yield on average is 1857 kg with 6.65% fat.

Remarks: This is considered as milch buffalo breed. Banni buffalo in Gujarat state, now recognized as a breed, entirely follows organic practices (Biocultural Community Protocol-BCP on Banni Buffalo). There is a need to earmark their respective breeding tracts and save this buffalo breed for organic production of milk and meat, the by-products like dung and urine under the suitable breeding strategies.

11. Chilika

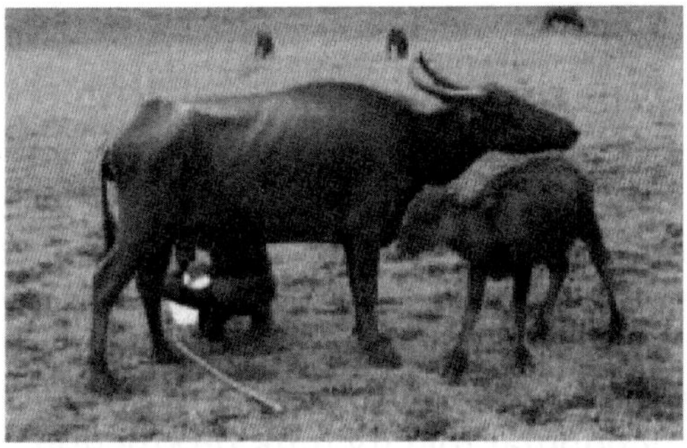

Synonym: Deshi

Origin and Distribution: Actually this breed is originated in and around Chilka lake in Odisha. This breed gets its name from the name of its native tract which is surrounding the Chilika lake in the state of Odisha.

Morphological Characteristics: The colour of the breed is brownish black or black. The buffalo is of medium size body, short legs. Horns-Typical sickle shaped, grow upward. Tail extends just below the hock.

Performances: Average age at first calving is 45 months and calving interval is 14 months. This buffalo can able to poduce only 500 kg milk per lactation which ranges from 440 to 514 kg Fat% is about 8.7%. The milk and curd of these buffaloes have been better taste and preservaton quality, and is prefered by local people. The curd from milk of Chilika buffalo can be preserved for 5-7 days at room temperature. Male are used for ploughing, threshing and power purposes. Adult body weight is about 352 kg for male and 342 kg for female.

Remarks: Mainly uses for agricultural operations as they are having good heat tolerance capacity.

12. Kalahandi

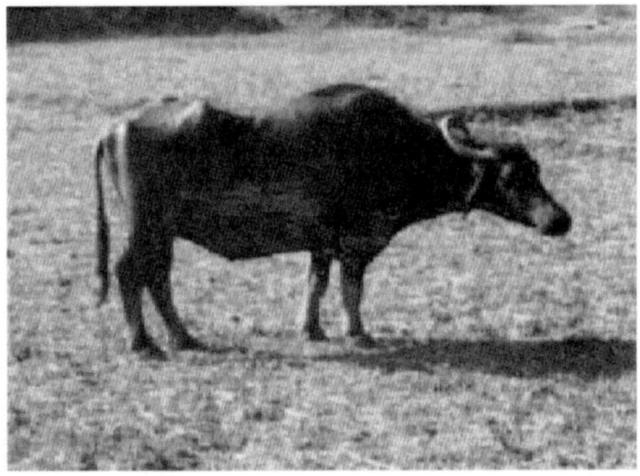

Synonym: Nil

Origin and Distribution: It is found in Kalahandi and Rayagada districts of Odisha and eastern part of Andra Pradesh. This breed gets its name from Kalahandi.

Morphological Characteristics

- Medium sized animal with well developed chest. Head convex, hump small, udder round.
- Tail is medium length and extends below hock with coarse hairs on Switch.
- Slghtly protuberant forehead covered with golden hairs is its special character.
- Body colour is between grey and ash grey. Muzzle eyelids, tail and hooks are black.
- Long, strong and half circled horns with broad base and half curved horn running backward at the tip.

Performances: Milk yield ranges from 680 to 912 kg per lactation. Fat% varies from 7.8 to 8.2%. Age at first calving is 50 months and calving interval is 18 months. Adult body weight of male is 377 kg and female is about 350 kg. Kalahandi buffaloes are dual type; used for milk and draught purpose in Kalahandi and Rayagada districts of Odisha.

Remarks: Animals are excellent in heat and drought tolerance. Kalahandi buffalo of Odisha state entirely and naturally follow organic practices. There is a need to earmark their respective breeding tracts and take appropriate breeding strategies for organic production of milk and meat. The by-products like dung and urine are superior as organic bio-fertilizer and bio-pesticide for the soil to produce organic forage and feeds.

13. Toda

Synonym: Nil

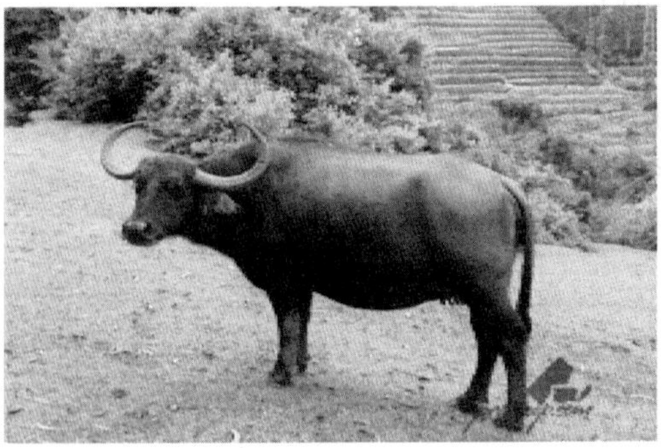

Origin and Distribution: Among Indian breeds of buffaloes, the Toda buffalo breed is a quite distinct from other breeds and a genetically isolated population, confined to the Nilgiri hills of Tamil Nadu. Toda breed of buffalo is named after an ancient tribe,

Toda of Nilgiri hills of Tamil Nadu State who rear this breed. It is a semi-wild buffalo breed.

Morphological Characteristics

- The animals have long strongly build body, deep and broad chest, and short and strong legs.
- Coat colour of the calf is generally fawn at birth, changes to ash grey at about 2 months of age. In adult the predominate coat colours are fawn and ash-grey.
- Horns are usually set wide apart run outward, upward and then inward at the top. Horns are quite large, semi circular and wide apart or cresent shape.
- Along the crest of the neck, hump area and back, there is a thick growth of hair like a mane which imparts a bison like appearance.
- There are two chevron markings - One just around the jowl and the other anterior to the brisket.
- Udder- small, not so prominent.
- They are gregarious in nature. The animals are not always docile. All of a sudden they may become furious and dangerous particularly to unknown persons. When necessary, they fight against even tigers and other wild animals in an organised team.

Performances: The average daily milk yield in Toda buffaloes was reported to be 2.53 kg with the maximum yield of upto 6.65 kg. Besides, Toda buffaloes are known for high milk fat content of 8.27 per cent with the range of 4.8 to 14 per cent, possesses typical well-flavoured taste. Milk Yield: 800 kg per lactation. Adult body weight is about 380 kg for both male and female.

Remarks: This is one of the important breed of buffalo other than Kaziranga buffaloes of Assam which thrives well in the high rainfall and high humid area.

Other Buffalo Populations

There are a number of other less well-known breeds such as Manda in Orissa, Godavari in Godavari and Krishna deltaic area, Tarai in Tarai area of Uttar Pradesh. Kujang buffalo breed evolved by using murrah buffalo in Orissa and Their performance is very close to murrah buffalo. But the population of these is very small, and they are only found in isolated pockets but are distinct because of their morphological traits.

The large number of buffaloes found in Northern Districts of Karnataka state is called as Dharwari. South Kanara buffaloes found in Dakshina Kannada and Udupi districts of Karnataka state now have been used in the local buffalo races called Kambala. So, characterization of these buffaloes need to be done for improving milk production or draft power or meat production capability.

14. Manda

Synonym: Parlakimedi, Ganjam.

Origin and Distribution: The animals are bred in the hills above Parlakimedi and Mandasa on the boarders of Orissa and Andhra Pradesh. Basically this breed is reared in areas of thick forest usually on natural herbage and brought down to the plains for sale.

Morphological Characteristics

- The breed is a medium sized animal.
- The forehead is flat with short muzzle. Neck and forelegs are also short but stout with well developed chest.
- The eyes are sharp with a broad red margin around the lids.
- The horns are broad and semi-circular extending backward and inward.
- The general colour is brown or grey with yellowish tufts of hair on the knees and fetlocks, and switch is yellowish white.

Performances: Milk yield is satisfactory. Males are hardy and like a bullock can work in the hot sun. It can draw a load of about a ton but at a slow pace.

Remarks: This is drought type buffalo breed.

15. Godavari

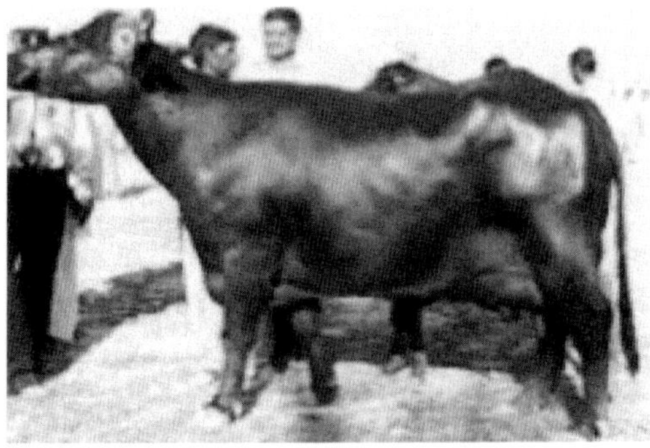

Synonym: Nil

Origin and Distribution: The home tract is Godavari and Krishna deltaic area. Godavari is a result of crossing of native buffaloes with Murrah bulls.

Morphological Characteristics

- The animals are of medium stature with compact body.
- The colour is predominantly black with a sparse coat of coarse brown hair.
- Its horns are short, flat, curved slightly downward, backward and then forward with a loose ring at the tip.

Performances: Godavari buffaloes are reputed for high fat with daily average milk yield of 5-8 kg and lactation yield of 1200-1500 kg. The animals breed regularly and have a short calving interval compared to Murrah.

Remarks: This is breed is developed through cross breeding.

16. Tarai

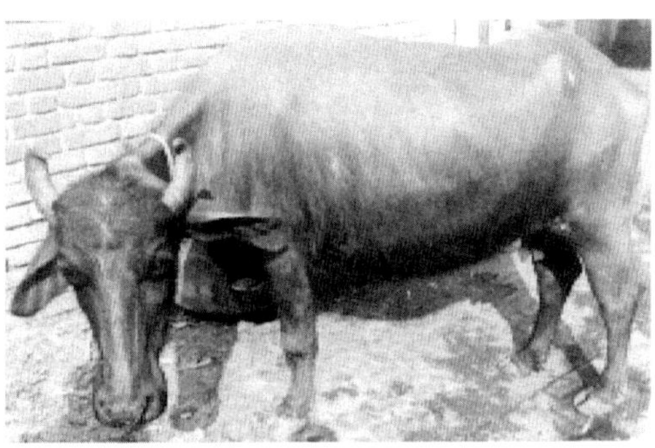

Synonym: Nil

Origin and Distribution: The breed gets the name from the Tarai area of Uttar Pradesh, where it is mostly found between Tanakpur and Ramnagar. The breed is native to hilly area, They are frequently crossed with Murrah bulls.

Morphological Characteristics

- It has moderate body, slightly convex head with prominent nasal bones.

- The eyes are rather small but ears are long and coarse.
- Legs are short but strong.
- The tail is long, reaching below the hocks. The switch of the tail is white.
- Horns are long and flat with coils, bending backwards and upwards having pointed tips.
- The colour of the skin varies from black to brown. Sometimes there is a white blaze on the forehead.

Performances: The breed is poor regarding milk production, which may be as low as 2-3 kg daily. Males are efficient draught animals used for agricultureal operations as powers including transport. Tarai breed is well adapted to the difficult environmental situations and nutritional conditions of the Tarai region.

Remark: This is draught buffalo breed.

23.0 Morphological Features of Indian Buffalo for Identification

S.No.	Breed	Unique Feature
1	Murrah	• Colour usually Jet Black • Short tightly curled horn • White markings on tail and face and extremities • Long tail with white switch reaching to the fetlock
2	Nili-Ravi	• Peculiarity of the breed is the wall eyes • White marking on forehead, face, legs switch • Tail long, almost touching the ground • Face and forehead distinguish from Murrah • Pink marking seen on udder and brisket
3	Jaffarabadi	• Heavy horns inclined to droop on the neck • Prominent forehead with depression in middle • Massive body • Usually black in colour • Black with white patches on face and legs
4	Nagpuri	• Sword shaped horns • Naval flap short or almost absent • Tail short reaching a little below hocks

		• Small-sized buffalo, entirely different from Murrah • Usually black in colour
5	Marathwada	• Greyish Black or Jet Black colour • Horns medium in length and parallel to neck
6	Pandharpuri	• Horns very long and extend beyond shoulder blade. • Black colour but vary from light to deep black
7	Bhadawari	• Light copper brownish coloured scanty short hair • Two white lines at the lower side of the neck • Tail long reaching up to fetlock • Medium size and wedge-shaped body • Face comparatively narrow with slightly marked nose
8	Surti	• Horns sickle-shaped • Skin colour brown • Colour varies from rusty-brown to silver-grey • Two white collars at the jaw and brisket
9	Mehsana	• Body longer than in Murrah and the limbs lighter • Horn resembles the Surti or Murrah breed • Skin colour Jet black occasionally brown grey
10	Banni	• Horns tightly coiled with single or double coiling • No slope towards base of horns • Brisket–highly prominent and loose • Black/copper/brown in colour
11	Chilika	• Horns-Typical sickle shape • Colour brownish black or black • Tail extends just below the hock
12	Kalahandi	• Half circled horns with broad base • Forehead with golden hairs slightly protuberant • Broad horns and half curved running backward • Colour between grey and ash grey
13	Toda	• Grey skin • Hair like a mane which imparts a bison like appearance • Hump and dewlap are absent • Horn-quite large and semi circular • Horns out-ward, upward inward at the top

24.0 Characteristic Feature of Phenotypic Trait

Breed		Phenotypic Trait
1. Murrah	Horns	Tightly curled short horn
	Colour	Jet Black
	Size	Long body with Massive frame
	Forehead	Light neck and head
	Tail	Long white switch
2. Nili-Ravi	Horns	Small and curled
	Colour	Black, White spots on forehead, muzzle, feet
	Size	Medium to large
	Forehead	Heavy head convex at center
	Tail	Long
3. Jaffarbadi	Horn	Curved downward, compressing head
	Colour	Black, Dark tan
	Size	Massive with long and tender neck
	Forehead	Heavy and wide head
	Tail	Medium
4. Nagpuri	Horn	Long, flat, curved backwards on sides of neck
	Colour	Black
	Size	Medium with slightly deep back
	Forehead	Long, Cone shaped, straight nasal bone
	Tail	Short, White switch common
5. Marathwada	Horn	Medium length and parallel to neck
	Colour	Grayish Black or Jet Black.
	Size	Light to medium compact stature
	Forehead	Long narrow face, white mark on head common
	Tail	Short, white switch common
6. Pandharpuri	Horns	Long, sword shaped
	Colour	light black to deep black
	Size	Medium
	Forehead	Long narrow face, Prominant thick neck
	Tail	Short, white switch common

7. Bhadawari	Horns	Curling downward, backward then upward
	Colour	Copper coloured hair, Gray skin, White ring under neck
	Size	Medium with wedge shaped body
	Forehead	Small and bulging between horns
	Tail	Thick and long with brown switch
8. Surti	Horns	Sickle shaped
	Colour	Black as well as brown
	Size	Medium
	Forehead	Broad, long and convex between horns
	Tail	Long thin flexible, White switch common
9. Mehsana	Horns	Slightly curved upward, inward
	Colour	Black, Dark tan
	Size	Medium
	Forehead	Wide and slight depression in middle
	Tail	Long, Switch black, Brown/white also common
10. Banni	Horns	Tightly coiled
	Colour	Black/copper/brown
	Size	Medium
	Forehead	Medium
	Tail	Thin
11. Chilika	Horns	Typical sickle shape
	Colour	Brownish black
	Size	Medium
	Forehead	Medium
	Tail	Tail extends just below the hock
12. Kalahandi	Horns	Long, strong, half circled
	Colour	Grey and ash grey
	Size	Medium
	Forehead	Golden hairs on forehead
	Tail	Medium
13. Toda	Horns	Large, semi circular, wide
	Colour	Fawn and ash-grey
	Size	Medium long with broad and deep chest
	Forehead	Broad and concave
	Tail	Long and slim with black switch

25.0 Average Performance of Buffalo Breed

	Breed	Milk Yield in kg (305day)	Age at First Calving (months)	Lactation Length (in days)	Calving Interval (in days)
1.	Murrah	2000	44.0	300	453
2.	Nili Ravi	1950	45.3	300	487
3.	Jaffarabadi	1850	50.7	300	440
4.	Nagpuri	1200	55.8	270	430
5.	Marathwadi	1000	55.7	300	435
6.	Pandharpuri	1400	44.8	350	465
7.	Bhadawari	1100	50.0	270	478
8.	Surti	1400	56.4	290	535
9.	Mehsana	1700	42.2	310	476
10.	Banni	1857	40.0	315	459
11.	Chilika	500	45.0	280	423
12.	Kalahandi	700	50.0	265	535
13.	Toda	700	47.0	250	480

26.0 Present Status of Indian Buffalo Breed

These breeds have been developed mainly as a result of farmers' wisdom over the past thousands of years. Buffalo breeds with distinctive inheritable traits have adapted to local environmental conditions over thousands of years. In this period, genes for many fitness traits have been tested. Each breed of buffalo thus consists of a unique pool of genes. Approximately 70 percent buffaloes in India are nondescript as these animals do not resemble any of the thirteen well characterized breeds. India is losing its wealth of genetic resources in domesticated animals. Native buffalo breeds which are well-adapted to adverse climatic conditions are being lost due to misdirected crossbreeding, indiscriminate crossing of native stocks, and slaughter of animals for export. The semen (or germplasm) of these 'elite' breeds was used extensively for crossing with non descript indigenous breeds, some of which are now truly endangered.

In case of cattle and poultry, it was realized many years ago that populations of native breeds are declining alarmingly, but the people capable of reversing or halting this trend stood by silently. On the other hand, realising the potential of genes of domestic animals found in India, developed countries took samples of their tissues and patented them. These countries are selling germplasm from Indian breeds to India for a profit, even as they are on the verge of extinction in their home country.

The present status of the well recognized breeds in India are as follows:

Breed	Status
Murrah	Stable
Nagpuri	Stable
Jaffarabadi	Stable
Surti	Stable
Mehsana	Stable
Marathwada	Stable
Pandharpuri	Stable
Banni	Stable
Nili-Ravi	Declining
Bhadawari	Threatened
Toda	Endangered
Chilika	Endangered

Toda (raised by the Toda tribe in the Nilgiri hills) breed is heading towards extinction. Unless the Toda buffalo can be put to some economic use, conservation efforts will not serve any purpose. For conservation, the breed has to be utilised, for which its genetic traits need to be investigated and mapped. Chilika of Odisha is another endangered buffalo breed in India.

Bhadawari buffaloes have a high milk yield and are good draught animals, are now threatened. A preliminary survey of 40 villages in its native tract in Uttar Pradesh and Madhya Pradesh some years ago revealed that just one village had 20 buffaloes, while the rest had only two or three.

The fate of the Murrah buffalo in its home tract Rohtak, Jind and Sonepat districts in Haryana is no better. A survey revealed that though there was an increase in milk production in Haryana, average milk yield had declined. This is an alarming trend, since India is supposed to have the best buffalo germplasm in the world. The decline has been attributed to mismanagement. Superior animals have been ignored by breeders and artificial insemination facilities are inadequate. Farmers favour natural breeding of their buffaloes, and select bulls on the basis of body weight rather than their dairy merit. Successive generations just do not have the genetic potential for high milk yield.

Another disturbing trend is increase in the number of high-yielding buffaloes exported from rural areas. The cost of maintaining buffaloes when not in milk and declining yields over the years induces affluent farmers to sell them off to slaughter houses in cities, from where the beef is exported. When buffaloes which have the genetic potential for high milk yield are slaughtered, the number of fertile generations is reduced to one or two, affecting the number of breeding females. There is no replacement of these animals in the breeding tract; the movement is one-way, from rural to urban areas.

27.0 Reasons for Loss of Buffalo Genetic Resources

There are a number of factors which can cause loss to buffalo genetic resources. However, the common reasons for loss are as follows:

- Cross breeding of buffaloes
- Not adequate buffalo breeding policy
- Changing market requirements
- Natural disasters
- Deterioration of ecosystems
- Unrestricted inbreeding among different breeds
- Reorganization of geographical area
- Indiscriminate breeding
- Modern agricultural practices
- Inadequate inputs of feeding, healthcare etc.

Movement of high producing buffaloes to metropolitan cities from the breeding tract to meet the milk requirement of city dwellers further leads to genetic erosion of valuable germplasm due to slaughter of these animals after completion of lactation.

Lack of genetic diversity in a population/breed affects its performance by:

- Reducing the fitness of the population
- Affecting the achievement of breeding objectives
- Decling the number or even extinction of breed
- Spreading the infections diseases more easily
- Reducing the sustainability of rare domestic breed
- Restricting the options available to meet unpredictable future requirements.

Loss of variation within breeds is continuously countered by the introduction of new variation through mutation, but the variation among breeds cannot be readily regenerated. So by using genomic techniques, genetic variation can be assessed and accordingly remedial measures should be taken to preserve genetic diversity for the future. The genetic diversity of low-production breeds is likely to contribute to current or future traits of interest, they are considered essential for maintaining future breeding options.

28.0 Buffalo Breeding in India: Present and Future

India has basically been an agricultural country and it is likely to continue to be so far a long time to come. At present 70 percent of Indians are dependent for their livelihood on agriculture. Thirty percent of the total land holdings are held by 70 percent of small and marginal farmers who held 80 percent of the total livestock in the country. Crop agriculture in India depends mainly on bullocks which contribute ample amount of power to agricultural operations.

In spite of highest number of buffalo in India the country has been unable to be assured of needed supplies of animal products including milk till today. During the period of last few decades, it has been possible to achieve substantial progress and build up a buffer stock of few graded buffaloes and some new breed of buffaloes are identified. More than fifty percent of country's milk production is supplied by this species. A number of Indian buffalo breed has been used for upgrading or genetic improvement of local buffaloes all over the country. The current yield levels for crossbred and indigenous cows and buffaloes are 1800, 900 and 1200 kg per year, respectively. It could safely be increased to the targeted levels through increased availability of feeds, culling of low producers, strengthening of field programmes of selection and progeny testing of bulls for milk and providing breeding and other input services at the farmers' door.

The indepth analysis carried out about the progress and prospects of Indian buffalo breeding has shown the existence of potentialities. It is necessary to make everyone in the country aware of these potentials, as also the tasks to be performed, to realize these potentials for milk comsumption as well as animal meat food of the country in particular and the world in general.

The production and use of animal products in the human diet is receiving tremendous attention. With this objective in view, the need for developing buffalo breeding has been recognized very well. The other objectives are to provide animal power for farmings, adaptation of better land use pattern- the land which is not suited for arable cropping should be put under grass or trees - so much needed for protection to soil. Among other objectives of Animal Husbandry, the utilization of agro-industrial by-products for converting those into valuable animal products is so much needed by all of us. The creation of thousands of employment opportunities throughout the year by adopting animal industry on large scale, shall also be a part of the objectives of Buffalo breeding in India.

29.0 Buffalo Development Programmes in India

- The important schemes initiated by the government for the development of buffaloes are Key Village Scheme (KVS) and Intensive Cattle Development Projects (ICDPs). These schemes aimed at all round development of indegineous cattle and buffalo in their breeding tract. Over 35,000 artificial insemination (AI) centres was set up for this purpose.
- Central Herd Registration Scheme was started in the year 1949 for improvement of buffalo genetic resource in India. During Third Five Year Plan the breeding tracts of important breeds were covered to organize breeder's societies for taking up this work.
- The All India Coordinated Research Project (AICRP) on buffaloes was started in 1970-71 for two buffalo breeds viz. Murrah and Surti at two centres for each breed. The centres for Murrah were

NDRI Karnal and PAU Ludhiana whereas for Surti the centres were university of Udaipur at Vallabhnagar of Rajasthan and UAS Dharwar of Karnataka.

- Seven central cattle breeding farms at Suratgarh (Rajasthan), Dhamrod (Gujarat), Alamadhi (Tamil Nadu), Chiplima and Suncheda (Orissa), Andeshnagar (U.P.) and Hessarghatta (Karnataka) are engaged in scientific cattle breeding programme and progeny testing of selected breeds of indigenous as well as exotic cattle and buffaloes.
- The embryo transfer technique is the latest technology which was also adopted successfully in buffalo for increasing their productivity. The first buffalo calf through embryo transfer technique was produced at Sabarmati Ashram Gaushala, Bidaj, Gujarat in December 1987. Buffalo Breeding Centre, Salon (Rai Bareli, UP) work exclusively on buffaloes through embryo transfer technique.

30.0 All India Coordinated Research Project on Buffalo

For systematic breeding studies, All India Coordinated Research Project (AICRP) on buffaloes was started in 1970-71 by ICAR for two buffalo breeds viz Murrah and Surti at two centres for each breed. The centres for Murrah were NDRI Karnal and PAU Ludhiana whereas for Surti the centres were University of Udaipur at Vallabhnagar (Rajasthan) and UAS Dharwad. The two northern centres maintained Murrah breed of buffaloes and the two southern centres medium-sized Surti/Mehsana breed of buffaloes. Facilities for semen freezing and exchange of breeding doses between the two northern centres and similarly in the case of medium-sized breeds between the two southern centres were also established. A centre for study on endocrinological problems; especially those associated with summer sterility in buffaloes, was added since 1977 at Gujarat Agricultural University, Anand. A Central Institute for Buffalo Research was established in 1984 at Hisar in Haryana State. The objective was the progeny testing to identify the bulls of high genetic merit and to distribute the young bulls produced from mating of elite buffaloes with proven sires at different farms in the country. Later on the field units were attached to each of the centres for testing of sires under transfer to technology.

The breeding plan for all the four centres was to maintain 220 breedable females and a separate elite herd of 70 buffaloes. It was decided to evaluate 8 bulls at each centre and finally selecting only 2 bulls out of these 8 bulls for mating with elite buffaloes. But in 1980 the technical programme was changed to test 12 sires in testing herd every 2 years in the two herds of Murrah as well as Surti breed and finally selecting 2 bulls for mating in elite herds of both centres as one unit for both the breeds. Coverage of 3000-4000 breedable females in field units attached to each centre was also recommendaded. The semen of each bull had to be used in testing herds and 2 field units. Further, it was recommendaded to freeze a minimum of 2000 doses of semen of each bull and to distribute 700 dosses from each bull to the 2 herds and other associated herd. In 1985, the technical programme was changed as:

- To Keep Surti breed at Dharwad and Vallabnagar
- To Keep Murrah at NDRI Karnal and to associate CIRB Hisar
- To change over to Nili Ravi buffaloes at PAU Ludhiana and its associate herd of Nabha (Punjab) centre of CIRB. Under progeny testing programme 68 bulls in 9 sets at CIRB Hisar, 53 bulls in 8 sets at PAU and 47 bulls in 8 sets at NDRI were evaluated till 1993. Three sets of Surti buffalo bulls at Vallabhnagar and 5 sets at Dharwad were progeny tested.

31.0 Network Project on Buffalo

An effort was made to collaborate the various institutional and organized buffalo farms under the Network Project on Buffaloes for their improvement. For Murrah Buffaloes - the participating units were CIRB Hisar with its substation Nabha - PAU Ludhiana - NDRI Karnal - HAU Hisar - IVRI Izatnagar and CBBF Alamadi (Tamilnadu). The participating units for Surti buffaloes were RAU Vallabhnagar - GAU Navsari and Anand - CCBF Dhamrod and UAS Dharwad. Elite dams each from Murrah and Surti buffalo breed were selected from different units participated in this improvement project. All male calves born from elite mating to be saved for breeding and were kept at their respective units till 12 months of age. The bull rearing and semen producing units for Murrah were taken at CIRB, PAU and NDRI. In 1998 new centres added for Murrah buffaloes were GLF Hastinapur and Majhra in Meerut (UP) - Banvasi and Mamnoor (AP).

Subsequently - the Network Project was involved to improve the buffaloes at Institutional Farms as well as field conditions. The Institutional Farm for improvement of Murrah buffalo included were PAU, HAU, NDRI, IVRI, CIRB and CCBF Alamadi (TN) and Murrah buffaloes under field conditions were around CIRB, PAU and NDRI. Institutional centres including field testing for different breeds were for Jaffarabadi buffaloes at GAU Junagarh - Nili Ravi buffaloes at CIRB substation Nabha - Bhadawari at IGFRI Jhansi - Pandharpuri at MPKV Kohlapur - Godavari buffaloes at BRS, ANGRAU - Surti at LRS Vallabhnagar - Murrah at NDUAT Faizabad - Swamp at AAU Khanapara.

32.0 Current Priorities of Government of India

The Government of India has given major thrust on the following activities for improvement of our buffalo genetic resources.

- Genetic upgradation of buffaloes and improvement in delivery mechanism of breeding inputs and services to farmers including promotion of clean milk production.
- Extension of dairy development activities in non-operational flood, hilly and backward areas.
- Provision of nutritious feed and fodder through promotion of fodder crops and fodder trees.
- Provision of adequate animal health coverage services including creation of disease free zones and control of foot and mouth disease.
- Provision of credit facilities to farmers.

To achieve the above goals, the Government adopted the following strategy:

- Expand and strengthen infrastructure for artificial insemination, improve efficiency and effectiveness of AI by using frozen semen technology for cross breeding.
- Create a germplasm bank of superior bulls and bull mothers to serve as nucleus germplasm pool.
- Facilitate genetic improvement of important native breeds through selective breeding and crossbreeding of low productive non-descript stock for both milk and drought purposes.

- Improve productivity of pasture lands, through introduction of improved fodder varieties and development of wastelands for forage production.
- Provide animal health services with special emphasis on control of foot and mouth disease.
- Promote technological inventions for adding value to livestock products.
- Improve the database of livestock performance and products.

33.0 Buffalo Breeding Policy

The improvement in the descript breeds of buffaloes is being brought about through selection and up-grading in non-descript and low milk producing animals through breeding with superior indigenous breeds. However, the breeding policy has not been properly defined area-wise within each state. Besides, it is well known that the adoption of artificial insemination in buffaloes has been very poor due to poor conception rate and availability of uncastrated buffalo males used for transport and farm operations with the medium and large farmers, are also used for natural service. Crossbreeding in buffaloes has been undertaken both within riverine breeds and riverine type with swamp type. Available results of crossbred buffaloes have been reported to be encouraging in respect of certain production traits and reproduction performance. Hence, the Present Buffalo Breeding Policy of India is as follows:

- Improving buffaloes by selective breeding in breeding tracts.
- Grading-up of non-descript buffalo with pure-bred bulls of superior breeds in other areas.
- Improving milk yields in the well defined breeds.
- Introducing more milk in dual purpose and draught breeds without impairing their draught capacity to any appreciable extent.

34.0 Breeding Strategies for Buffalo in India

The Indian buffaloes comprised of about 70 percent non descriptive and rest 30 percent descriptive. The descriptive buffalo population of India classified into 13 distinct buffalo breed according to nodal Institute NBAGR, Karnal, Haryana, India. There are mainly two breeding strategies are recommended for improvement of our indigenous buffaloes genetic resources: one is for the non-descript population and second is for the recognized breeds.

S.No.	Type of animal	Breeding strategy	Purpose
1	Indigenous dairy breeds of buffaloes	Selective breeding	Milk production
2	Indigenous draught breeds of buffaloes	Selective breeding	Draught power
3	Non-descript buffaloes	Grading up	Milk production / draught power

34.1 Grading up for non-descript buffaloes

This vast number of non descriptive buffaloes in different parts of the country may be upgraded by mating them with superior bulls of high genetic merit those are belonging to Murrah, Nili Ravi, Mehsana and Surti breeds available in the country. Upgradation of this low yielding indigenous buffaloes can enhance the milk production about 2 to 3 times from 500 kg milk of non-descriptive buffaloes to about 1200 kg of first generation upgrade buffaloes. With continuous grading up of upgraded buffaloes in 4 to 5 generations will convert the non descript low producing buffaloes into comparatively high producing upgraded buffaloes which may be very nearer in conformation to that well defined breeds used in upgradation. It may be explored to collect semen from 50 percent graded breed bull and distribute for field insemination in the places with inadequate management and feed / fodder resources for sustaining the improvement achieved in the first generation of grading up programme.

It has been recommended that Murrah breed of choice for upgradation of non descriptive buffaloes available in the states of Assam, Bihar, West Bengal, Uttar Pradesh, Orissa, Andhra Pradesh, Tamil Nadu, Maharashtra, Rajasthan, Haryana, Goa and Delhi. The grading up of non descript buffaloes with Surti have been recommended for the Karnataka, Kerala and some parts of Gujarat and Rajasthan. Murrah and Surti bulls can be used in Karnataka. The use of bulls of Murrah and Nili Ravi breeds has been recommended for Punjab. The upgrading programme is expected to make an improvement in milk yield by more than 5 percent annually.

34.2 Selective breeding for well-defined breeds

The selective breeding under progeny testing programme for buffaloes on large scale prerequisites to strengthen the existing organized farms of well known breeds like Murrah, Nili Ravi, Mehsana, Surti, Nagpuri, Bhadawari and Jaffarabadi and some more farms should be developed for the production of breeding bulls. Murrah breed is considered as a breed of choice in the states of Haryana, Punjab, Delhi and some part of Uttar Pradesh. The Surti breed is preferred in the states of Gujarat, Rajasthan and Karnataka. The Mehsana and Jaffarabadi are the breeds of Gujarat state whereas Nagpuri and Pandharpuri are the breeds of Maharashtra state. The Nili Ravi has good population in Punjab where Bhadawari are abundant present in Uttar Pradseh. The progeny testing programme should run in associating different herds as well as the farmer's herds when the population size of the organized herds is small. The methodology of progeny testing programme for buffalo is almost similar to that of cattle. It is expected that genetic improvement of 1 to 1.5 percent per annum in milk production will be achieved organized farms by selective breeding, through networking of multi-herds of a particular breed and 8 to 10 percent per annum in farmers' herds through introducing germplasm of high yielding buffalo bulls.

35.0 Schemes for Development of Buffalo in India

To develop indigenous buffaloes available in the country, Government of India had initiated three schemes namely:

35.1 National Project for Cattle and Buffalo Breeding

35.2 Central Herd Registration Scheme

35.3 Central Cattle Breeding Farms

Now, the above mentioned three schemes are presented in details as below.

35.1 National Project for Cattle and Buffalo Breeding

Genetic improvement in bovine is a long term activity and Government of India had initiated a major programme 'National Project for Cattle and Buffalo Breeding' (NPCBB) on October 2000. This was a 10 years project in two phases each of five years. The allocation for Phase I was 442 crore. In order to consolidate gains made during Phase-I, Phase-II of NPCBB was formulated taking into account recommendations of the evaluating agency (NABARD) and was initiated on December 2006 and valid up to December 2010 with an allocation of Rs 775.9 crore. The NPCBB envisaged genetic upgradation on priority basis with a focus on development and conservation of important indigenous breeds. The project envisaged 100% grant-in-aid to the State Implementing Agencies (SIAs).

A major new component of Phase-II was bull production programme. India is well known for world famous Murrah buffaloes. Murrah buffaloes are high milk producers with high fat content in addition to being efficient feed converters even when fed poor quality roughages. Murrah is the breed of choice in various parts of the country in order to upgrade non-descript population in different states of India. In spite of having best genetic resources, the productivity of Murrah buffaloes has not increased, as expected, mainly because of negative selection pressure due to poor acceptability of artificial insemination among buffalo population, availability of poor quality of sires at semen stations and use of bulls with unknown genetic potential under natural service. This situation has left the Murrah population in a state of genetic stagnation. In order to develop buffalo population, Murrah bull production programme with an allocation of Rs 128.28 crore was taken up in Phase-II.

The National Project for Cattle and Buffalo Breeding (NPCBB) was merged in the National Programme for Bovine Breeding and Dairy Development (NPBBDD) on February 2014. This scheme is no more in operation now.

Objectives

1. To arrange for delivery of vastly improved artificial insemination service at the farmer's door-step.
2. To bring progressively all breedable females among cattle and buffalo under organized breeding through artificial insemination

or natural service by high quality bulls within a period of 10 years.

3. To undertake breed improvement programme for indigenous cattle and buffaloes so as to improve the genetic makeup as well as their availability.

4. To provide quality breeding inputs in breeding tracts of important indigenous breeds so as to prevent the breeds from deterioration and extinction.

Components

The project components specially designed to address the existing inadequacies will focus on the hitherto neglected natural mating system as well as the Artificial Insemination network with particular attention to:

- Streamlining storage and supply of Liquid Nitrogen by ensuring supply from industrial gas manufacturers and setting up bulk transport and storage systems for the same.
- Introduction of quality bulls with high genetic merit.
- Promotion of private mobile AI service for doorstep delivery of AI.
- Conversion of existing stationary government A.I. centres into mobiles centres.
- Quality control and certification of bulls and services at sperm stations, semen banks and training institutions.
- Study of breeding systems in areas out of reach of A.I.
- Induction of breeding bulls for natural service in the areas not under AI coverage.
- Institutional restructuring by way of entrusting the job of managing production and supply of genetic inputs as well as Liquid Nitrogen to a specialized autonomous and professional State Implementing Agency.

State Implementing Agencies (SIAs)

At the Central Government level, a Central Project Management Unit (CPMU) with a core group of professional staff implemented the project. There was a broad based Steering Committee for the project to provide guidance to the CPMU. In a total 28 States and one UT were participated under the project. Financial assistance to the tune of Rs 398.36 crore was released to these States upto 2007-08. During next financial year Rs 89.70 crore was made available under the scheme. Since inception of the project in October, 2000, 27 SIAs were constituted under the project in 28 States. These agencies had professional approach in implementing the project. In case of small States, which were unable to constitute viable SIAs, funds were released to the State Governments for implementation of the project.

Achievements

- Semen production in the country was increased from 22 million straws (1999-2000) to 44 million straws (2007-2008) and the number of inseminations was increased from 20 million to 41 million.
- Semen production was increased from 50.5 million to 62 million and AI number from 50 million to 52 million between 2009-10 and 2010-11. Conception rate was increased from 20% to 35%.
- 36000 Government Stationary Artificial Insemination (AI) centres were converted into mobile AI centres.
- 21000 Private AI centres were established or under establishment. 4000 private AI workers were utilized between 2009-10 and 2010-11.
- 21700 breeding bulls with high genetic merit were inducted or under induction. 3000 quality breeding bulls were inducted for natural service between 2009-10 and 2010-11.
- 50,000 existing AI workers were trained in all the aspects of frozen semen technology including funds released for training of existing AI workers.
- 1800 professionals were trained outside the State at reputed training centres.
- 49 frozen semen bull station were strengthened as per Minimum Standard Protocol (MSP) for semen production; in order to improve quality of semen production in the country. MSP for semen production were formulated and implemented at all semen station in the country.

- Central Monitoring Unit (CMU) were constituted for evaluation of semen stations one in two years and implementation of MSP for semen production in the country.
- 22 semen stations were graded as 'A', 17 as 'B' and 3 as 'C' during 2010-11 against 11 as 'A', 16 as 'B' and 7 as 'C' during 2007-08. A and B graded semen station were increased to 39 against 27 in earlier evaluation.
- 34 semen stations in the country were acquired ISO certification.
- Number of animals in milk was increased from 62 million during 2000 to 77 million during 2008 i.e. about 14 million improved milch animals was added to milch herd of the country.
- Crossbred cattle population was increased from 20 million (1997) to 33 million (2007)
- MSP for progeny testing and standard operating procedures for AI technicians were formulated and circulated among all the States.

35.2 Central Cattle Breeding Farms (CCBF)

Government of India has started Central Cattle Breeding Farms scheme for propagation of superior indigenous cattle and buffalo germplasm throughout the country. Seven Cattle Breeding Farm of recognized breed were established in the country for maintenance / propagation and distribution of pure bred cattle and buffalo bull calves.

Objectives

- Progressive genetic improvement of milk production of cattle and buffalo by scientific selection and mating system.
- Production and distribution of superior bulls for cattle and buffalo breeding programme in the states/country.
- Conservation of threatened indigenous cattle and buffalo breed of national importance.
- Production of upgraded crossbred animals suitable for specified breeding tracts.

Implementing Agency

These seven Cattle Breeding Farms in the Department are implementing the above stated objectives. The Farms are subordinate offices of the Department implementing the assigned technical programme. Out of them only one is established at Alamadhi (Tamil Nadu) for Murrah buffalo.

S.No.	Name & location of the farm	Breed maintained
1	Suratgarh (Rajasthan)	Tharparkar
2	Dhamrod (Gujarat)	Surti Buffalo
3	Chiplima (Orissa)	Red Sindhi (RS) and RS X Jersey
4	Hessaraghatta (Karnataka)	Holstein Friesian
5	Semiligud/Sunabeda (Orissa)	Jersey
6	Alamadhi (Tamil Nadu)	Murrah Buffalo
7	Andesh Nagar (U.P.)	Holstein Friesian X Tharparkar

This centre was engaged for producing high pedigree bull calves of important buffalo breeds for distribution to States for use in the buffalo development programmes. The bull calves are produced from Surti and Murrah buffalo breeds. The bulls and bull calves are for sale and distribution to the State Governments.

Target Group / Beneficiaries

Various cattle and buffalo development agencies are benefited from the scheme by way of using high quality bulls produced at the farms. These bulls are used for semen production and natural breeding to help upgrade the animals in the country.

35.3 Central Herd Registration Scheme

Government of India has initiated Central Herd Registration Scheme for identification and location of superior germplasms of cattle and buffaloes, propagation of superior genetic stock, regulating sale and purchase, help in formation of breeder's societies and to meet requirement of indigenous bulls in the different parts of the country. Four CHRS units were established in different breeding tracts of the country. For milk recording, 103 milk recording centers were set up. Indigenous buffalo breeds covered under the scheme are Murrah, Jaffrabadi, Surti and Mehsana. During 2001-2002 final registration for 1795 animals were completed. The criteria for registration are laid down in the scheme. Funding Pattern of this scheme is 100 percent Central Grant in aids.

Objectives

- Identification and location of superior germplasm.
- Using data for producing superior germplasm.
- Preservation of indigenous germplasm.
- Development of Milk Recording System for indigenous germplasm.

Implementing Agencies

- CHRS Unit Rohtak in Haryana
- CHRS Unit Ahmedabad in Gujarat
- CHRS Unit Ajmer in Rajasthan
- CHRS Unit Ongole in Andhra Pradesh

Target Group / Beneficiaries

The primary aim is to identify elite germplasm for further improvement in milk production. Indigenous breeds covered at present are Murrah, Jaffrabadi, Surti and Mehsani of buffaloes. Under the scheme incentives for rearing of elite buffaloes and their male calves is given to the owners of the elite animals.

36.0 Interventions Towards Genetic Improvement of Buffalo

Genetic improvement for milk production of indigenous buffaloes is not an easy task and it will take much time owing to low heritability estimate of milk yield. For genetic improvement of buffalo population in India, it is observed that Selective breeding is the main strategy for recognized breeds of buffaloes while the non-descript buffaloes are improved through grading up program with Murrah and Surti breeds to augment the milk production potential. In the recent past, Indian Council of Agricultural Research and State Agricultural Universities had started several schemes for improvement of defined breeds as well as other inferior quality buffalo available in the country. Progeny-testing scheme was taken up in the Third Five-Year Plan to ensure identification of superior Murrah bulls tested on the basis of performance of their progeny rather than only the dam's yield. The tested bulls were used through Artificial Insemination for achieving higher genetic gain. Subsequently, field progeny testing programs for Murrah and other indigenous breeds of buffaloes supported by the Government, Cooperatives Dairies, Research Institutes and NGOs have also been made to select the superior bulls for the production and supply of semen throughout country. Under the AICRP/Network Project approach, genetic improvement and conservation of indigenous buffalo is being undertaken at a number of ICAR Institutes and in collaboration with the SAUs. Such activities have also been taken up by State and Central Government Farms, NDDB and some NGOs including Gaushalas.

State sponsored scheme 'National Project on Cattle and Buffalo Breeding' envisaged raising AI facilities for buffalo breeding in the country was started in 2000. A field oriented approach 'Central Herd Registration Scheme' implemented at some of the locations undertook earmarking of elite buffaloes at the farmers level with regular recording and genetic selection.

37.0 Buffalo Breeding for Milk Production

- Imperative dairy breeds of buffaloes found in India are being selectively bred for enhancing their milk production.
- Breeding programs for improving the production potentiality of country's Swamp buffalo through crossbreeding with Riverine buffaloes are being undertaken.
- Crossbred offspring performed better than either parent breed or intermediate performance between the two parent breeds are more common under similar conditions.
- Nucleus herds of dairy buffalo breeds can be conveniently established in our country (unlike the case of dairy cattle breeds). The bulls from the nucleus herds can then be used to breed the inferior buffaloes even where A.I. is not feasible.
- Choice of selection strategy within sire versus dam breeds may depend on the accuracy of estimates of polygenic breeding values within each breed, population size, inbreeding, etc.
- Current breeding policy recommended by the National Commission on Agriculture (NCA) and adopted by the Central

and State Governments was based on the important considerations which were similar to those of the scientific panel on Animal Husbandry.

- Major features of present buffalo breeding policy in organized and rural herds are to improve the buffaloes by selective breeding in organized herds or in breeding tracts and grading up with recognized breeds in other areas.

38.0 Constraints to Buffalo Production and Future Outlook

- Delayed puberty, seasonal breeding, long calving interval, and poor estrus detection hampered the reproductive efficiency in the female buffalo and have been identified as the major problems and constraints in buffalo development. Artificial Insemination (AI) is also limited in buffaloes due to the weakness of oestrus symptoms and variability of oestrus length. Improvement in veterinary services, especially in breed improvement, would definitely enhance buffalo production considerably.
- Lack of genetic selection programs for the propagation of superior germplasm is the primary factor affecting productivity. Although, progeny testing program of indigenous buffalo breeds are implemented in country. However, consistent and systematic long term programs aimed at improving genetic potential of local buffalo breeds is required.
- Feed resources consist of green fodder, crop residues and concentrates. These resources are not enough to meet the requirement of existing livestock in general. Buffalo, being larger in size than cattle, have more nutrient requirements and suffer greatly with the shortage of feed resources. Thus the full genetic potential has not been achieved. Use of improved fodder varieties, utilization of non-conventional feed resources, scientific feeding methods and preservation of fodders may be some of the useful strategies to overcome nutrient deficiencies.
- Lack of access to loans for expansion in the herd is a critical problem for small farmers. Unfortunately, there is little access to formal credit through the cooperatives. Informal credit is available from private traders and agents of private companies, but the interest rate is very high. Government intervention to extend loan facility to small and landless farmers on interest free basis may solve this issue.

- Collaborative public-private partnership efforts to conduct applied research for improvement in different aspects of buffalo productivity, consistent Government policies and establishing a permanent vocational and outreach training program for capacity building are some of the key factors which will undoubtedly enhance buffalo production.
- Unfortunately, the production potential of buffalo has not been exploited in the past. Buffalo has some claim to be regarded as the World's most neglected animal but having promising potential and thus may be called as the animal of future. Although, India has large buffalo population well adapted to the local environment condition and production systems, but productivity per unit of this versatile animals is very low.

39.0 Genetic Aspects of Some Characteristics of Buffalo

The degree of genetic inheritance of trait of a population is expressed in terms of heritability (h^2). The estimate of heritability can theoretically ranges from zero to one or zero to hundred percent. The value of heritability estimate of a trait indicates the effectiveness of its improvement by genetic approaches as the character is controlled by genetic as well as environmental factors. It is very important to have information on the heritability estimates of traits of buffaloes before implementing a long-term genetic improvement progamme. Hence, the heritability estimate of some characteristics in the buffaloes is appended here.

39.1 Milk production trait

In general, it can be said that heritabilities of the most milk yield characteristics in the river buffaloes ranged from low to moderate. Genetic selection to improve milk production in buffaloes should be able to achieve a medium rate of success. So, along with genetic improvement for milk production attention needs to pay also for improvement of non-genetic factors. There has been no research report on the genetics of milk production in swamp buffalo since milk yield is not important in such type of buffalo.

39.2 Meat production trait

Genetics studies concerning traits related to meat production in buffaloes have been very limited, especially in swamp buffalo, since there have been very long-term genetic studies. The estimates of heritabilities of various body weights of the river buffaloes generally ranged from medium to high. This estimate indicates that genetic selection for body weights in buffaloes can be successful at medium to high rates. In general, it is believed that animal's draught ability is related to its body weight. Hence, selection for larger or heavier buffaloes will automatically improve working capacity as well as meat production of the animals.

39.3 Reproductive trait

The heritability estimates obtained by researchers revealed that it is in general low except for age at first calving. So, genetic improvement for these traits is not significant direction as compared to time and money spent for it. It is therefore recommended that most reproductive traits should be improved through feeding and herd management, as well as culling of animals with low reproductive efficiencies.

40.0 Cattle vs. Buffalo Crossbreds for Dairy Production

Although buffalo milk is exceptionally rich in high percent butterfat (7-8%) as compared to cattle milk but buffalo milk product is not traditional food for local people of our country. This invites a question whether cattle crossbreds such as Holstein crosses or buffaloes are more suitable for dairy production. Crossbred cattle having 50 percent or higher exotic inheritance can able to yield 15 kg milk per day or higher, while crossbred riverine buffaloes usually yield lower (6-8 kg) amount of milk i.e. almost half amount. It appears that dairy farmers can earn more income from raising crossbred dairy cattle than crossbred buffaloes where the benefit of high butterfat in buffalo milk cannot compensate for their lower milk yield. However, crossbred buffaloes become more superior to crossbred cattle when they are considered as the multipurpose animal in integrated farming systems. Moreover, they are very much superior to utilize farm wastes and by-products, natural grasses and tree leaves, as well as marginal lands such as highway shoulders and scrub forest. Hence, crossbred buffaloes are able to produce moderate milk yield under poor management and feeding conditions.

41.0 Need for Conservation of Buffalo Breed

Indian buffalo breeds need to be conserved because of their following importance.

Genetic diversity: The genetic diversity existed in buffaloes of the country is represented by thirteen distinct recognized breeds besides several lesser-known breeds/strains comprising about 21 percent of the total livestock population in India. Rest of the buffaloes are non-descript in type and have extremely variable composition being either non-descript or crosses among various breeds and cannot be categorized in any other well-established breed. Altogether, India is definitely rich reservoir of all breeds of the riverine buffalo genetic resources in world. Indian buffalo breeds with distinctive inheritable traits-have adapted to local conditions over thousands of years. In this period, genes for many fitness traits have been tested. Each breed of buffalo thus consists of a unique gene pool. There is general concern that the genetic variation within the few domestic animal species is disappearing through breed substitution and inter-breed crossing. Any reduction in the diversity of genetic resource narrows the scope to respond to selective breeding.

Leading dairy animal: The buffalo is the most important dairy animal and occupy an important place in the agricultural economy of India because of their adaptability to harsh climatic conditions, tolerance to tropical diseases and survival under poor feeding and management practices. Although, total number of buffaloes are almost one-half in number as compared to cattle but buffaloes alone contribute more than fifty per cent of the total milk production in the country. It is well known fact that the organized dairy sector in India is principally dependent on buffalo milk because of their contribution to total milk production with rich fat and total solid content. Their contribution in terms of meat is also noteworthy.

Multipurpose use: The versatile buffalo produces milk, meat and also used as draught purpose animal. Buffaloes in India have a place of pride in all respects: production – productivity - population in the world - diversity/breeds - service to the underprivileged - clean draft power - footed transport - rich food/nutrition - support to a host of industries and livelihoods. For the purpose of a continued and sustained use of this important species - it is necessary to pay more attention for their conservation as well as improvement of these diverse breeds as a global resource. Already, the world is looking at this Black Gold as a hope for food in the near future - especially in the face of imminent global warming.

Unplanned breeding: Well-defined breed of buffalo constitute a valuable genetic resource which needs to be conserved on priority basis. The rich biological diversity of this species is progressively being eroded due to unplanned breeding. Except in few organized farms which maintain small herds of pure breed - there is almost unrestricted interbreeding among different breeds and there is a marked decline in the availability of unique animals conforming to the attributes of defined breeds - particularly in their native breeding tracts. This situation is further complicated by the fact that there exists no breed societies or breed registration/improvement societies to register animals of specific breeds - maintain herd books and ensure the purity of the breeds. Hence - proper conservation measures have to make to preserve the valuable buffalo genetic resources of India for their sustainable utilization.

Non-judicious utilization: There has been a non-judicious utilization of buffalo genetic resources in the country. The males are only partially utilized in the form of bulls and bullocks. There is always a scarcity of breeding bulls of superior genetic merit. Above all - the high producing milk buffaloes from the breeding tract - representing the best germplams - are taken to metropolitan cities in large numbers for milk production. After completion of lactation - these buffaloes are slaughtered - causing a serious erosion of elite germplasm.

Adaptability: There also exist a number of buffalo populations - known for their adaptability to harsh climatic conditions - tolerance to tropical diseases and survival under meager feeding and poor management practices. These local varieties have not been defined as breeds and hence they have to be assessed - defined and recognized. The buffalo breeds habituated in different agroclimatic zones of India have evolved themselves more through genetic isolation and natural selection than through deliberate intervention by man. They have been distributed in extremes of climates i.e., from saline condition (i.e., Chilka buffalo of Orissa) to high altitude mountain areas up to 2,000 m.s.l (i.e., Toda buffaloes).

Feeding custom: The buffalo breeds and their home tracts are stable - have a well-defined place in the local natural cycles - consume the remnants of the crops - yet produce valuable milk and provide draft-power and dung/urine as organic manure. With excellent ability to convert poor quality feed to fodder - buffaloes provide milk that is rich in nutrition and quality - meat that is known for flavor and marbling and steady but draft power in rural/remote areas and a host of other services - including Mozzarella cheese. All the recognized breeds and local populations have unique qualities for meeting local requirements of food - energy and livelihoods in an environmentally suitable manner. Besides the cultural and religious considerations - buffaloes are contributing significantly to food and agriculture in terms of milk-meat-manure-fuel and draft power. Variations in regional demand for animal products have influenced the use of different buffalo genetic resources.

Keeping in mind the above facts, the valuable germplasm of buffalo needs to be conserved without elapsing further more time for the following reasons in brief:

- They possess adaptive characteristics to thrive in the stressful environment which could be lost through dilution and intensive selection for production traits.
- They also possess the ability of converting poor quality feed resources into meat, milk and working capacity in the field.
- The genetic variability should be maintained which is the basis for genetic improvement for the future.

42.0 Strategies for Conservation of Buffalo

Conservation of animal genetic resources usually refers to strategies, plans, policies and actions undertaken to ensure that the diversity of animal genetic resources being maintained to contribute to food and agricultural production and productivity, or to maintain ecological, cultural values of these resources to present generation and further use for future generation. Thus, the conservation covers both continued maintenance of genetic variability through pure breeding or upgrading and their sustainable utilization for mankind. For conservation of live specimens of buffaloes - besides demanding proper planning skills- substantial manpower, valuable space and costs are also required. The most critical steps for conservation are to monitor the population of breeds over a time interval, identify breed(s) at risk, prioritize the breeds for conservation, preferably for in situ and apply proper conservation strategies. There is no single method of conservation/preservation which is optimal for all situations. During taking the decision for optimal conservation strategy, the available resources and capacities, risk of failure and costs of conservation methods should be considered. The proper guide line for conservation cattle and buffalo genetic resources as described by ICAR-National Bureau of Animal Genetic Resources (Indian Council of Agricultural Research), Karnal-132 001 (Haryana) India are now presented below:

There are three major strategies are normally recommended for conservation of cattle and buffalo farm animal genetic resources namely a) *in situ* conservation b) *ex situ* in vivo conservation c) *ex situ* in vitro conservation. The first two involves conservation of living population while last one encompasses conservation of living ova, embryo, semen, somatic cell or other animal tissue, DNA etc. stored cryogenically in liquid nitrogen. *Ex situ* in vitro (cryopreservation) should complement *in situ* conservation. *In situ* conservation of livestock through involving livestock keepers in the production system is very much essential to maintain a breed in a dynamic state. Now details about these are given below.

42.1 In situ Conservation

- This involves the maintenance of live cattle and buffalo in their original and natural environment where animal continues to evolve and be developed for sustainable use. The active in situ conservation is equivalent to breed development through animal breeding programme whereas the passive in situ conservation is the maintenance of live animal populations within their environments for the breeds which are at risk of loss.
- Information on present status of the population, communities maintaining the breed and their socio economic status, breed management and improvement programme, specific measure to conserve breeds at risk and expenditures on their maintenance are very much essential for this conservation.
- Selection of animal should be carried out for its traditionally valued characteristics and in the environment to which it is adapted. The herds must be maintained within the natural environment for that breed and need to be exposed to conditions prevalent in the field. Nucleus herd should be established in respective native tract of particular breed.
- Farmers maintaining the breed should be given incentives for encouraging more rearing of animals and breed society need to be established for them. The owners of animals of the breed may

be given incentives in form of husbandry inputs to compensate low production level for replacement of breed under same management system.

- The existing farms of indigenous breeds should be used for production of quality breeding males and only pure breeding should be practiced at these farms. Adequate facilities of frozen semen technology may help to disseminate the pure breed semen at the entire area of breeding tract. Respective Gaushalas can be used for maintaining the purebred animals of different indigenous breeds.
- There should be linkage between state owned breeding farms with local breeders association/groups so that breeding males could be make available to the communities. Suitable laws and regulations should be formulated to protect livestock keeper's rights as well as grazing lands to strengthen the conservation efforts further.

42.1.1 In situ Conservation Involving Farmers

- The area comprising of two villages belong to each of 5 blocks from the core zone of native tract of the breed should be identified first. At the commencement around 150 females should be recorded for identified parameters. 100 elite unrelated females based on production performance should be identified and inseminated/mated with the semen of superior males of the same breed. The owners should be provided incentive from government so that the animals are retained and kept in good health. 40-50 unrelated males should be selected at the farmers' premises and financial incentive should also be provided them. The farmers should maintain these males and provide breeding services with certain charge to the animals in that area through natural mating. The external support from the government should be gradually withdrawn while allowing the breed society to take over and continue the efforts in this direction. Breeding services like artificial insemination at farmers' doorstep, animal health services and feed supplements may be provided either free of cost or at subsidized rates.
- A nucleus herd comprising of about 200 breeding females with at least 20 breedable males (10:1 ratio) should be established in the native tract of the breed with the help of government support.

An open nucleus breeding system should be followed with bi-directional flow of germplasm from farm to field and *vice versa.* For a nucleus herd of 200 breeding females, the best 20 females may be selected from the villages each year as replacements for the animals to be culled from the nucleus herd. The same should be followed for breedable males also by replacing breeding males in the herd with young males from the field. An efficient field recording system should be in place to identify the elite animals as well as to monitor the genetic improvement.

42.1.2 In situ Conservation Involving Institutes

- Some of the important indigenous breeds are kept by ICAR institutes, SAU's animal breeding farms, central and state Government livestock farms. Such Institute should be identified in respective native tract of the breed to maintain the animals. The young animals should be identified and procured from the farmers' households, at least 100 females and 20 males (5:1 ratio) on the basis of true to type breed characteristics. These animals should be reared at the institutional farms. About 5 females should be mated with each bull of the same breed. Regular performance recording should be followed. Among the progeny best 10 young males should be selected through multistage selection in each generation. Selected young males should be trained for semen production. At maturity a total of 5 males should be selected on the basis of growth, semen quality and freezability. Mating should be planned to avoid the relationship in form of circular mating after developing sire lines. After each five generations, 5 young males may be incorporated in institutional herd procuring from farmers of native tract. A minimum of 2000 semen doses from each male should be collected, cryopreserved and used in for breed improvement and conservation. The surplus breeding males are distributed to the farmers for natural mating in the breeding tract.
- Associated herd progeny testing program may also be initiated if there are more such farms available for an indigenous breed so as to couple the conservation program with systematic genetic improvement.

42.1.3 Breeding Policy for in situ Conservation

- Each state should consider region specific and breed specific breeding strategies and programmes in view of conservation of Indigenous breeds in their breeding tract.
- Breeding tracts should be marked for each of the breed. Selective breeding should be followed within the breeding tracts and cross breeding is strictly prohibited in this area. In case of cattle, the states should identify the geographical boundaries of the areas for non-descript cattle. These should be upgraded by crossing with bulls of indigenous breeds.
- Animal Husbandry Departments and Livestock Development Boards of concerned State should implement the breeding programmes for conservation. The existing State Breeding Farms and Central Breeding Farms of indigenous distinct breeds should be declared as germplasm repositories and used for production of breeding males. Only pure breeding should be practiced at these farms. Improvement of Indigenous breeds can be taken up in collaboration with Breeders' associations and Gaushalas.
- Data base with regard to all the details of Indigenous breeds, including their breeding tracts, population, phenotype and performance characterization, genetic makeup, the institutional farm where they are being preserved and/conserved should be developed and updated routinely. The national level database for indigenous breeds developed by ICAR-NBAGR and NDDB should be updated routinely for this purpose. An information network related to germplasm should be set up by linking various agencies and institutions working for livestock improvement and conservation. Available information on different breeds should be published in regional languages in the form of any extension material to create awareness among the farmers to conserve the important indigenous breeds.

42.2 *Ex situ in-vivo* Conservation

- The *in situ* conservation may not be feasible for the breeds which are economically not viable and hence they may be lost due to economic pressure. The *ex situ* conservation can be an alternative in this situation. The *ex situ* conservation can be classified as in vivo and in vitro. In *ex situ in vivo* conservation, small numbers of live animals keep away from the main breeding tract of the breed. This type of conservation has the limitation of adverse effect of inbreeding. It is not possible to keep the large herds of breeds which are economically not viable. The live animal reservoir or breed safari or park or institute may help to conserve the precious germplasm of breeds of domestic animal as a self-sustaining unit.

- For ex situ in vivo, a very limited number of animals may be kept outside their natural habitat. During reconstruction of a population with frozen semen, we can use the few purebred *ex situ in vivo* conserved females as founders. As an alternate, the young males from elite females should be selected and procured. The males should be reared to maturity under intensive management. The semen can be utilized in the breeding tract through SAHD/NGO network for up-gradation and improvement of the breed.
- For cattle and buffalo, at least 20 unrelated young male progeny of elite animals from the breeding tract should be procured and maintained at the organized farm for one year. These males should be trained to donate semen. A total of 2000 semen doses per male should be procured from 15 males making the total number of doses as 30,000. The semen from these males after evaluation should be frozen and stored. The males progeny of elite cows can be extensively used for breed improvement in the tract. Embryos from different breeds can also be stored for posterity by raising females at farm. The breeding males can either be supplied to breeders or breeding services are provided at central place. The target should be to produce the desired number of progeny in the tract either by AI or through natural service depending upon the species, demand and facilities. The progeny thus produced should be followed for data recording. Such scheme should be sponsored for 10 years and transferred to any developmental agency in locality.

The general approach to be followed for conservation of cattle and buffalo genetic resources is live animals. Actively breeding population should be maintained- perhaps - each line or variety in a different farm to reduce costs. The major advantages of live animal conservation are: they are always available for immediate utilization in the event of any setbacks in the upgraded population. They are constantly exposed to new strains of diseases and their resistance evaluated. Such live animals would also contribute to education and to community awareness of the indigenous fauna. A major problem that needs to be defined is the type of selection to be practiced without altering the genetic variability. It is suggested here that both random selection as well as overall merit should be practiced with minimum intensity.

Cryogenic storage of germplasm is convenient and cheap and further work needs to be done. Another advantage is that the genotype will not be subjected to genetic drift. A disadvantage is that the animals - especially in the case of females - have a time lag when live adults are urgently required. DNA genetic material storage is a useful tool but certainly not an immediate task.

43.0 Development and Conservation of Recognized Buffalo Breed

- Based on the population the major breeds are classified into two groups and the *group-1* comprises of stable breeds viz. Murrah, Mehsana, Jaffarabadi, Nagpuri and Pandharpuri - since they do not face reduction in their numbers over the decades. The *group-2* comprises of the breeds facing dilution and reduction in numbers - the breeds are Nili-Ravi, Bhadawari, Surti, Marathwadi and Toda.
- Both in-situ and ex-situ conservation efforts have been made under different schemes at the institutional level to conserve these breeds for sustainable utilization. Conserving the live animals that exist in nature is in-situ conservation. The animals are maintained in their original habitats under native conditions with no interference in their mode of management- feeding and other conditions. The main problem of in situ conservation is inbreeding and genetic drift typical of small populations. The ex- situ conservation is used when the endangered population is miserably low in numbers - as this process has its own innate problems. It may suffer from spread of disease or neglect during periods of institutional weakness - besides being costly in long term preservations and losing the relatedness of current genotype with environment - when one of these is preserved for long time.
- Under the in-situ conservation scheme - a set of 150 buffaloes have been identified on the basis of their peak yield and then the

milk production is recorded at monthly interval. The owners are provided an incentive for two years so that the animals are retained and kept in good health. The tagged females are inseminated with the semen/bull of the same breed of higher genetic merit. The farmers' rear the male progeny from these females up to six months- incentives are provided to retain the calf. As these calves grown up - a total of 50 unrelated males are selected as future bulls. Under the ex-situ conservation program - live animals are maintained at the different government institutional farms and semen samples of the superior bulls (3000 doses/animal) are collected and stored in the liquid nitrogen container for future revival.

- Buffalo plays an integral part of farming system and its numbers have been maintained or increased in some breeds and erosion is observed in some breeds. As a part of conservation measures - various river breeds have been documented and evaluated. Strains of swamp buffalo have been observed but attempts to characterize them genetically have yet to be made. Conservation measures should begin with a proper sampling technique to represent the existing variability and in sufficient numbers. In these populations for conservation- selection should be minimal and to maintain population size constant- either random culling or culling based on total merit should be practiced. However - for the national herds - genetic improvement could be achieved through selection and grading up with Murrah and Surti breeds. For both - germplasm collection and national herd - data banks are essential to monitor their genetic progress.

- Considering the importance of recognized indigenous breeds in the national economy, Government has undertaken some measures for their development and conservation. National Project for Cattle and Buffalo Breeding has focus on development and conservation of indigenous breeds. The buffalo genetic resources in India are represented by 13 distinct breeds of buffaloes including Murrah, Jaffarabadi, Mehsani, Surti etc. Indigenous animals are sturdy, endowed with quality of heat tolerance, resistance to diseases and have ability to thrive under extreme nutritional stress. Global warming is likely to increase incidences of animal diseases particularly viral and protozoan diseases in crossbred animals. Therefore, there is a need to take programmes for development and conservation of indigenous breeds.

- Funds have been released to the participating states for procurement of quality bulls for natural service, initiating bull production programmes, strengthening of bull mother farms and establishment of ONBS farms for important indigenous breeds for their further development from Government of India. During Phase-I of the NPCBB project an amount of 58 crore has been released exclusively for development and conservation of indigenous breeds. An amount of Rs. 477.30 crore has been kept exclusively for development of indigenous breeds under Phase-II of NPCBB. In addition to this, strengthening of field AI network, semen stations, establishment of private AI workers and organization of fertility camps etc have also lead to development of indigenous breeds.

44.0 Steps for Protection and Conservation of Native Breeds of Cattle and Buffalo

In order to complement and supplement the efforts made by the States for protection and conservation of indigenous breeds of cattle Government of India has undertaken following measures:

- Rashtriya Gokul Mission a new initiative initiated as a part of National Programme for Bovine Breeding and Dairy Development exclusively for development and conservation of indigenous bovine breeds including indigenous breeds of cattle.
- National Dairy Plan-I a World Bank assisted project being implemented in 18 major dairy States covering development and conservation of 12 indigenous breeds of cattle and buffaloes namely (i) Gir; (ii) Kankrej; (iii) Tharparkar; (iv) Sahiwal; (v) Rathi; and (vi) Hariana cattle breeds and (i) Marrah; (ii) Mehsana; (iii) Pandharpuri; (iv) Jaffarabadi; (v) Banni and (vi) Nili Ravi buffalo breeds.
- Government has also established three subordinate organizations namely (i) Central Cattle Breeding Farms (CCBFs) (ii) Central Herd Registration Scheme and (iii) Central Frozen Semen Production & Training Institute. These organization are also undertaking development and conservation of indigenous breeds namely (i) Tharparkar; (ii) Red Sindhi; (iii) Gir; (iv) Kankrej; (v) Ongole; (vi) Hariana and (vii) Rathi breed of cattle and (i) Surti; (ii) Murrah; (iii) Meshsana and (iv) Jaffarabadi breeds of buffaloes.

45.0 Observation on Buffalo Traits For Future Improvement

The cattle and buffaloes are phylogenetically very close to each other. The following characteristic features which are usually observed in buffaloes but uncommon in cattle. This may raise a question whether these are controlled by genetic or environmental factors. So, research investigation need to be carried out to confirm these.

45.1 Tick Resistance

Cattle and buffaloes are raised together in small farms by small farmers in tropical Asia. But it is observed that buffaloes generally are not suffered with tick infestation while cattle either *Bos indicus* or *Bos taurus* breeds have problem with ticks and some tick-borne diseases such as anaplasmosis. Some may argue that swamp buffaloes are free of ticks because they like to lie down in mud hole and as a result prevent themselves from ticks. So research investigation needs to be carried out on this observation in order to prove whether tick resistance in buffaloes is due to genetic or environmental factors. If buffaloes' resistance to tick is due to genetic influence then with the help of available Genetic engineering techniques, buffaloes can be a very valuable genetic resource for future animal improvement.

45.2 Ability to use low-quality roughages

There are acute shortage of roughages for cattle and buffaloes during dry hot seasons. At this time, cattle would lose much body weight and become rather thin because of limited sources of roughages on small holder farms while the buffaloes on the same farm maintain their body conditions at rather satisfactory level. This could be partly owing to their less selective grazing behavior, but nowadays many researchers believe that buffaloes may have different kinds of rumen microbes as compared with cattle. These microbes enable buffaloes to utilize low quality roughages such as rice stubbles or high-fibrous residues more efficiently. Moreover, some research reports indicated that swamp buffaloes have a total nitrogen balance either equal to or higher than that of zebu cattle due to a reduced nitrogen output in the urine. It will be very useful to study in further details concerning these superior traits of buffaloes, especially on their genetic information.

45.3 Milk and Meat

It is well recognized that Buffaloes produce milk with high butterfat percentage (7-8%). Buffalo milk has 58% more calcium, 40% more protein but 43% less cholesterol than cow milk. Buffalo milk is richer source of phosphorus, vitamin A, protein and contains high levels of the natural antioxidant. It is reported that Buffalo meat contains cholesterol half as much compared to that in cattle beef. These special characteristics in buffaloes deserve further investigation in order to utilize this superior genetic resource for human use in the long term. Genetic studies utilizing modern biotechnological tools available at molecular or DNA level will be very useful in the future.

46.0 Some Considerations for Certain Breeding Strategies for Buffalo

Indian riverine buffaloes are well reputed in the world for unique characteristic features and also for production performances while Swamp buffaloes found in some regions of India are not well performed in yield. But they are also important in some aspects. Hence, the some of the following considerations should keep in mind while formulating any breeding strategies of buffaloes in the country.

46.1 Breeding buffaloes for draught purpose

Improvement of buffaloes for draught purpose through genetic selection within population is not only expensive but also slow as compared to improvement by other methods such as feeding and management, health care, and use of improved farm tools and harness systems. From breeding aspects, it appeared to be generally agreed that the draught ability of buffaloes could be improved as a secondary purpose within the improvement programs for meat or milk production by simultaneously selecting for animal body weight and height.

Crossbreeding of swamp buffalo with Murrah and Nili-Ravi in order to improve draught ability as well as milk and meat has been conducted in some countries such as the Philippines and China. Some crossbreds were found to have higher body weights than the swamp (local) buffalo at the same age, while the working ability of crossbreds having the same body weight and heat resistance were comparable to the local. It was reported the crossbred buffaloes in China were superior to local swamp buffalo in working ability, i.e. draught power, area ploughed per unit time, ploughing speed, and duration of work. This could be attributed to the higher body weight of the crossbreds. Therefore, it is very important to provide superior buffalo bulls for breeding at village level. Artificial insemination of buffalo cows with semen from superior bulls has had limited impact at farm level as far as draught buffaloes on small farms are concerned. This is due to various socio-economic, technical as well as institutional constraints facing village farmers.

46.2 Breeding buffaloes for meat or meat-and-draught purpose

Meat production from buffalo has provided an important part of total national beef supply in many Asian countries. Hence, breeding strategies to improve buffalo for meat or meat-and-draught can be quite useful for India like other Asian countries.

The traits related to meat production in buffaloes such as weights at different ages and growth rates are expected to be medium to highly heritable. There has been scanty genetic study on buffalo carcass traits so far but judging from experiences in beef cattle breeding they can be expected to be highly heritable, which means that breeding improvement can be effective.

Crossbreeding for beef and draught, crossbreeding of swamp buffalo with river breeds such as Murrah has been carried out in various countries in Asia in order to improve meat production and draught ability. F_1 crossbred of Swamp buffalo and Murrah are fertile and perform well under rural conditions. Their working ability is comparable to the swamp parent, while body size and growth rates in some cases equal or are slightly better.

One major concern relating to crossbreeding of the swamp buffalo (diploid chromosome number or 2n=48) with river buffalo (2n=50) is the unequal number of chromosomes, which result in unbalanced chromosome numbers (2n=49) in the F_1 crossbreds. So far no breeding work in the field has been reported to indicate that the fertility of F_1 crossbreds is negatively affected by this cytogenetical phenomenon. However, some recent investigations showed the occurrence of meiotic impairment which affected the semen quality in the crossbred buffalo male carrying unbalanced karyotype of 49 chromosomes. No report on the effect of unbalanced chromosomes on the fertility of crossbred buffalo cows is available so far. F_2 and F_1 upgraded backcross to river breeds buffaloes have been produced in different countries but the long-term ultimate breeding goal is often unclear while sufficient and good data are lacking to carry out comparison of production and reproductive performance of crossbreds and their parental breeds.

46.3 Breeding buffaloes for meat-milk-and-draught purpose

Crossbreeding between the swamp buffalo and the riverine breeds is often aimed at producing milk in addition to meat and draught in the crossbreds, as reported in China and the Philippines. Crossbred buffaloes can produce 3 to 5 kg of milk per day which can be used for household consumption, where only 1 or 2 buffalo cows are kept. Hence, buffalo crossbreeding in this case is aimed at improving nutritional status and human health as well, especially for children and the elder.

Only moderate levels of milk and meat production is expected from crossbred buffaloes since most dairy and beef characteristics in bovine animals are genetically negatively correlated. Under village conditions where feed resources and feed quality are commonly limited, milk production by an animal could mean that less nutritional supply available for meat production. Similarly, to use crossbred buffaloes for farm works resulted in decrease of milk production by 12 to 17 percent. However, with appropriate feeding levels dairy cows could be used for draught purpose without any detrimental effects on fertility, except for extended calving interval and small reduction in milk. Further feed supplementation to dairy cows used for work could result in a satisfactory level of milk production, but socio-economic considerations at small farm level may render feed supplementation of the multi-purpose animals impractical and uneconomical. Improved milk production of buffalo cows will definitely increase growth rate and body weight of offspring at weaning age.

46.4 Breeding buffaloes for milk production

The use of buffaloes as dairy animals by rural farmers has been well known in many countries such as India and Pakistan. River buffaloes of at least 15 breeds had been described by various authors. Some of the river breeds such as Murrah and Nili-Ravi have been introduced to some other countries such as China and the Philippines to cross with local buffaloes in order to use the crossbreds as dairy or multi-purpose buffaloes. Different types of crosses are commonly carried out in various countries, especially in SEA and China where only swamp buffaloes exist only.

Only the Murrah and the Nili-Ravi have been used more extensively so far in crossbreeding programs with the swamp buffalo in Asia. The milk yield and lactation period of dairy buffaloes of different genotypes appeared to be at satisfactory levels.

Some crossebreeding schemes of Swamp X River buffaloes

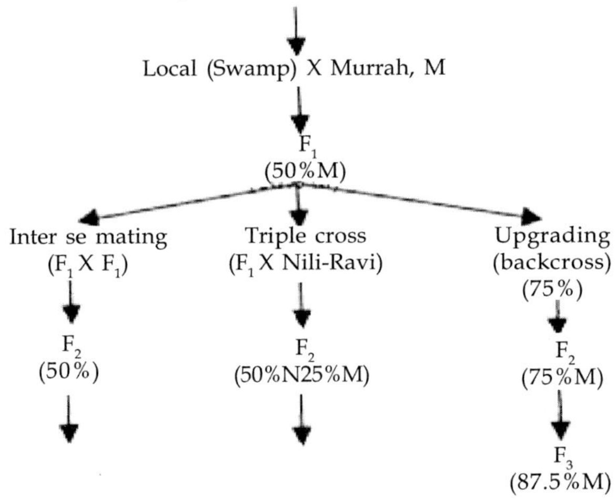

47.0 Central Institute for Research on Buffaloes (CIRB), Hissar, Haryana

Central Institute for Research on Buffaloes, Hisar, Haryana - the world's largest premier institute for buffalo research - is located 170 km from Delhi, at Hisar in the north Indian state of Haryana. It came into existence on 1st February 1985 when the *Progeny Testing Bull Farm Hisar-* which was earlier part of the Government Livestock Farm, Hisar - was transferred from the Government of Haryana state to the Indian Council of Agricultural Research for research on Buffaloes (CIRB). On 11 December 1987 - a sub-campus near the *Bir Dosanjh Wildlife Sanctuary* at Nabha in Patiala District was opened to undertake research on Nili-Ravi breed found in Punjab. This Institute has the main campus at Hisar - with satellite campus at Nabha in Punjab - and two regional stations in Andhra Pradesh and Gujarat respectively. The institute was set up with the aim to create a core breeding population of important buffalo breeds - conducts comprehensive research on buffalo breeding and production and transfer technology to the farmers, institutes, NGOs, etc, - collate and disseminate comprehensive information on buffalo.

Soon after its establishment - the institute came to lime-light in the 'buffalo world' by successfully hosting the II World Buffalo Congress during 1988. The institute embarked upon active research programmes to unravel the physiological, nutritional and genetic virtues and distinctiveness of this species through numerous research projects including some outside funded projects and others with international cooperation as well. In 2016 - it became world's second center to produce cloned buffalo. The first ever successful cloning of buffalo was done by the National Dairy Research Institute, Karnal in 2010.

Vision of the Institute

To develop and propagate high yielding elite buffalo germplasm for quality milk and meat production while retaining inherent draughtability across different regions of the country.

Mission of the Institute

To improve the buffalo through identification, conservation and propagation of elite germplasm; having high efficiency of reproduction and nutrient utilization for sustainable production and commercialization.

Mandate of the Institute

- To undertake research and transfer of technology on all aspects of buffalo production.
- To establish nucleus breeding herds of important buffalo breeds.
- To act as repository of information on all aspects of buffalo production and development

CIRB operates a nation-wide network of 10 research centres to undertake breed improvement on more than 7 native and several other breeds. The main local breed at CIRB is Murrah buffalo and Nili-Ravi at Bir Dosanjh sub-station. It also networks with other institutes to undertake research, and collate and disseminate information on the 10 recognised breeds of the Indian river buffalo [Murrah, Nili-Ravi, Jafarabadi, Mehasana, Marathwada, Nagpuri, Pandharpuri, Bhadawari, Surti Toda and Banni] and Swamp buffalo found in Assam. CIRB carries out research on various aspects of buffalo improvement including conservation of germplasm, development of optimum diets and feeding systems, enhancement of reproductive efficiency and health management practices for augmenting milk, meat and draught performance of the species.

This Institute created world's first and most comprehensive online Buffalopedia in several languages. Annual Buffalo festival is held every year at Hisar main campus on CIRB foundation day of 1st February, as an extension and awareness day where usually large number of farmers and breeders attend. Another annual Buffalo mela is also organsied at Bir Dosanjh subcampus every year on 11th December.

48.0 Cloned Buffalo in India

National Dairy Research Institute, Karnal, Haryana, India has privileged reputation for production the first in vitro fertilized buffalo named as *'Pratham'* in the world. Later on a series of hand guided cloning techniques has been used to develop cloned buffaloes in India.

Name		Place
Samrupa	:	The world's first cloned buffalo calf was born on February 6, 2009 at NDRI, Karnal. It survived for only six days and died on February 11, 2009 due to lung infection.
Garima	:	The world's second cloned buffalo calf through the Advanced Hand-Guided Cloning Technique was born at NDRI, Karnal on June 6, 2009. It survived for more than two years but she died of heart failure on August 18, 2011.
Gamini	:	On August 22, 2010, a cloned calf of female buffalo *'Garima-2'* nicknamed *'Gamini'* was born from embryonic stem cell; she is the mother of a calf named *'Mahima'*.
Shrestha	:	On Aug 26, 2010, a cloned calf of male buffalo *'Shrestha'* was born from the somatic cell from the ear of an elite bull; it has been producing a good-quality of fertile semen.
Mahima	:	On 25 January 2013 at 1.51 PM by normal parturition first female calf was born from cloned buffalo Garima-2 through hand-guided cloning technique in the world. NDRI has named the newborn female calf *'Mahima'*.

Swarn	:	On March 18, 2013, a clone of male buffalo *'Swarn'* born from the somatic cell of semen and it is alive and healthy.
Purnima	:	On September 6, 2013, a clone of female buffalo *'Purnima'* born from a high milk-yielding animal; it survived for 21 days before dying.
Lalima	:	On May 2, 2014 *'Lalima'* was born through the NDRI's 'hand-guided cloning technique'.
Rajat	:	On July 23, 2014, a male cloned calf named *'Rajat'* was produced through the 'Hand-guided Cloning Technique'.
Karishma	:	On December 27, 2014, Garima-2 gives birth for the second time to female calf *'Karishma'*
CIRB Gaurav	:	CIRB becomes second centre to clone buffalo calf produced from cells of ventral side of tail of superior bull buffalo. This part is least exposed to sunlight and may have less mutation rate.
Deepasha	:	India's first cloning of Chhattisgarh's endangered wild buffalo met success with birth of healthy female calf born on December 12, 2015 through the 'hand-guided cloning technique' at NDRI at Karnal in Haryana.

49.0 Buffalo Breeding Farm in India

Name of the Breed	Name of the Farm
1. Murrah	**Haryana** • Central Institute for Research on Buffaloes, Sirsa Road, Hisar • National Dairy Research Institute, Karnal • Government Livestock Farm, Hisar **Punjab** • Punjab Agricultural University, Ludhiana **Uttar Pradesh** • Cattle Breeding Farm, Bahugarh, Ghaziabad • Cattle Breeding Farm, Bharari-Jhansi • Cattle Breeding Farm, Chak Ganjaria, Lucknow • Cattle Breeding Farm, Hastinapur, Meerut

- Cattle Breeding Farm, Lakhimpur, Kheri
- Indian Veterinary Research Institute, Izatnagar

Andhra Pradesh

- Cattle Breeding Farm, Ashwaraopet, Khammam
- Government Livestock Farm, Banavasi, Kurnool
- Government Livestock Farm, Kakinada, East Godavari
- Government Livestock Farm, Mamnoor, Warangal
- Government Livestock Farm, Reddipalli, Anantpur
- Government Dairy Farm, Visakhapatanam
- Cattle Breeding Farm, Kareemnagar
- Cattle Breeding Farm, Horesikullu

Tamil Nadu

- Central cattle Breeding Farm, Alamadhi
- Central cattle Breeding Farm, Avadi, Madras
- Central Breeding Farm, Chettinad, Madurai
- Cattle Breeding Farm, Orthanad, Thanjavur
- Cattle Breeding Farm, Pudukkottai
- Cattle Breeding Farm, Tirunelveli

Madhya Pradesh

- Cattle Breeding Farm, Kiratput, Itarsi
- Cattle Breeding Farm, Ratona, PB-2, Sagar

Karnataka

- Cattle Breeding Farm, Bankapura, Dharwad
- Cattle Breeding Farm, Kurikuppi, Bellari
- Livestock Farm, Hessarghatta, Bangalore

Assam

- Livestock Farm, Barpeta, Kamrup
- Livestock Farm, Berhampur, Nowgong
- Livestock Farm, Guwahati
- Livestock Farm, Khanikar, Dibrugarh
- Government Livestock Farm, Khanapara
- Government Livestock Farm, kaliapani

Bihar

- Cattle Breeding Farm, Sariakala, Ranchi, Jharkhand
- Cattle Breeding Farm, Sepaya, Ranchi, Jharkhand
- Cattle Breeding Farm, Dumraon

	Chhatisgarh • Cattle Breeding Farm, Anjora, Durg **West Bengal** • Cattle Breeding Farm, Haringhata **Jammu and Kashmir** • Cattle Breeding Farm, Beli Charana, Jammu Cantt.
2. Bhadawari	**Uttar Pradesh** • Cattle Breeding Farm, Babugarh, Meerut • Cattle Breeding Farm, Saidpur, Lalitpur • Agricultural College Dairy Farm, Kanpur
3. Jaffarabadi	**Gujarat** • Cattle and Buffalo Breeding Farm, Junagadh Agricultural University, Junagarh • Livestock Research Station, Anand Agricultural University, Anand • Central Cattle Breeding Farm, Dhamrod, Surat
4. Surti	**Gujarat** • Livestock Research Station, Navsari Agricultural University, Navsari. **Goa** • Composite Livestock Farm, Dhat, Sangeum **Karnataka** • NDRI(SRS), Bangalore Dairy Farm, Dharwad campus, Krishinagar, UAS, Dharwad
5. Nili-Ravi	**Punjab** • Military Dairy Farm, Ferozpur • Bull Mother Farm and Exotic Cattle Farm, Bhattian, Khanna, Ludhana · Buffalo Breeding Station, Nabha
6. Mehsana	**Gujarat** • Livestock Research Station, S.D. Agricultural University, Sardarkrushinagar. Banaskantha.
7. Banni	**Gujarat** • Livestock Research Station, S.D. Agricultural University, Sardarkrushinagar. Banaskantha.

50.0 Overview

- About 70 percent of Indian buffalo are of non-descriptive type and remaining percentage is descriptive type which could be classified into 13 distinct breeds. The breeds of buffalo are mostly evolved out of generations of adaptability to local environment. They are either adapted to the prevalent conditions and climatic factors in different parts of the country or thrive only on the particular environments in which they are bred and reared. Often many of them resemble each other with slight morphological changes but because of constant inbreeding in the locality where they are now found these have been evolved as independent breeds.
- Most of these buffalo breeds have enormous potential to become high producing commercial milch animals, and there is a need for the development of these breeds. Pre-requisite for the development of a breed are large enough population size, a wide selection differential for economic traits.
- Buffalo production has undergone a major transformation resulting into a substantial increase in milk production thus helping our country to achieve top position in milk production in the world. Even though various animal breeding and management programmes have contributed to this improvement, there are constraints hampering the growth which require proper attention by initiating realistic breeding policies for genetic improvement of buffaloes.
- Although India ranks at the top in bovine inventory, the inventory of buffalo has been found to be declining in a few states. This indicates a growing shortage of buffalo meat. However, such a decline cannot be related to the export of buffalo meat from the country as there are no registered export units in these states. Secondly, slowdown in increase of population is not only due to slaughter but can also be due to urbanization and conversion of agricultural areas into housing/commercial/industrial land.
- Buffalo is an important species as well as valuable assets of the country contributing significantly to Indian economy. Present buffalo breeds have gene pools of wide representation and valuable combination of genes. There is urgent need to study genetic diversity between and within breeds using appropriate

set of microsatellite markers which can be further supplemented by using genome sequencing data, phonemics and high density arrays. It is our responsibility to conserve, preserve and maintain this genetic diversity.

- It is evident that the buffalo plays an integral part of our farming system and its numbers have been maintained or increased in some breeds and erosion is observed in some breeds. As a part of conservation measures, various river breeds have been documented and evaluated. Strains of swamp buffalo have been observed but attempts to characterize them genetically have yet to be made. Conservation measures should begin with a proper sampling technique to represent the existing variability and in sufficient numbers. In these populations for conservation, selection should be minimal and to maintain population size constant, either random culling or culling based on total merit should be practiced. However, for the national herds, genetic improvement could be achieved through selection and grading up with Murrah and Surti breeds. For both, germplasm collection and national herd, data banks are essential to monitor their genetic progress.

- The indigenous breeds of buffalo are essentially the products of long term natural selection and are better adopted to withstand tropical diseases and perform under low and medium input. Many of these breeds may have useful genes for high yielding of milk production and other economic traits also. Such utility genes and breeds shall be identified, conserved and utilized. In recent time, international actions have been oriented towards conservation of animal genetic resources. India being a signatory to many such international agreements, the country will have specific policy focus on conservation of indigenous valuable breeds of buffalo. State will take up the responsibility of conserving such threatened breeds through appropriate programmes.

- Keeping in view the milk production potential, draught capacity, and resistance to diseases, heat and humidity tolerance, capacity to survive on crop by-products and crude roughages, it is extremely essential to conserve these imperative Indian breeds of buffalo and improve their important traits in their respective home tracts.

- Considering the essence of the importance of Indian buffalo genetic resources spread throughout the country following recommendations may need to be undertaken for further genetic improvement of our indigenous buffaloes.
- Buffalo Breeding Policy should be framed keeping in view the production traits, economic performance and draftability of breeds of animals along with the local requirement, agro-climatic factors, existing infra-structure and support systems.
- In order to conserve and improve the well defined indigenous breeds of buffalo, crossbreeding with well defined germplasm should not be resorted to in the buffalo breeds belonging to well defined milch categories found in the centres of origin and other selected pockets. In these well defined indigenous breeds, selective breeding through superior, preferably progeny tested bulls should be done.
- Selective breeding and grading-up policy should be followed in their own native tract wherever there is a need to introduce the milk production traits in draught or dual purpose breeds and non-descript buffalo.
- In view of the shortage of proven and progeny tested bulls of high yielding breeds, efforts are needed to be made to establish more number of bull mother farms in different states to meet the increasing requirement of quality bulls.
- In order to preserve high potential germplasm, it is essential to ban the slaughter of breedable and high genetic potential cows and buffaloes and make an arrangement to buy back dry milch animals from private dairy farms established in urban areas of the country.
- In the areas where grading-up, selective breeding and crossbreeding are being done through artificial insemination and where adequate infra-structure for buffalo development exists, provision should be made to castrate the non-descript males of buffaloes through legislation and its strict implementation.
- The newer breeding and reproductive technologies like Embryo Transfer (ET) and Open Nucleus Breeding System (ONBS) shall be an integrated part of breed improvement. Efforts should be intensified to identify and transfer technically feasible and economically viable new technologies of livestock production

systems through conducting on-farm animal research trials in different regions/zones of the country.

- Molecular genetic studies for identification of genes of interest (milk quality and quantity traits, fertility, draft, disease resistance, adaptive traits) and marker assisted selection (MAS) as new breeding tools need to be explored for identifying superior animals and commercial exploitation of genetic potential of indigenous breeds.
- There is need for a sustainable buffalo production system in the country to meet the future demand of buffalo meat. Therefore, priority should be given to implementation of a male buffalo calf rearing programme for the long-term benefit of the farmers, country and the trade.
- Policy intervention for culling and slaughtering of unproductive, infertile, old and disabled and stray animals is badly needed and should be implemented. It will go a long way in reducing the burden on the national economy on the one hand and in increasing income of the farmers as well as of the nation through meat export on the other. The breeding of buffaloes for development of meat breeds should also be taken up.
- There is a need to initiate zoning exercise by all the agricultural universities in the country on the basis of different bovine breeds and density, and availability of feeds and fodders.
- Top-down approach is being followed to design breeding policy in different areas. However, it is essential to ascertain the farmers and farmer organisation's perspective about the existing breeds and breeding policy. Therefore, focused Rapid Rural Appraisal (RRA) Participatory Rural Appraisal (PRA) should be conducted by a multi-disciplinary team of scientists and technicians in all the states to study livestock production systems and farmers' perception about production traits and breeding problems of different breeds of bovines. This bottom-up approach would help in designing suitable breeding policy in the country.
- A reorientation of cattle and buffalo breeding policy would be attempted with area specific approach backed up by appropriate programs addressing our concerns for indigenous buffalo breeds and demand of milk as well as draught animal power. A similar approach has been adopted in the National Project on Cattle and Buffalo Breeding.

- State wise breeding policy should be framed in accordance with the production traits, economic performance and draftability of breeds along with the local requirement, agro-climatic factors, existing infra-structure and support systems.
- In view of this, optimum breeding policies for various classes of buffaloes are presented with their strengths and shortcomings. Technologies for selection of superior genotypes and multiplication of their germplasm are also being required. Finally, some breeding policy strategies for proper implementation of these programmes are recommended for adoption.
- The vast amount of genetic/genomic resources for cattle research will serve as shortcuts for the water buffalo community to study functional genomics. Buffalo genome resources are going to contribute to develop genome technologies for researchers and policy makers and may serve to improve reproductive performance and production potential of buffalo.
- All these recommendations will not be fruitful unless there is an active participation of common people. Thus, extensive extention programme must be undertaken to reach out the livestock rearer who are the real beneficiaries of entire buffalo breed depevelopmental programme.
- Indian Buffaloes obviously provide an excellent opportunity to improve the economic status of our country. Hence, sort of efforts should be considered to conserve and exploit this valuable germplasm for posterity use.

❑❑❑

UNIT-3

Documentation of Cattle and Buffalo Genetic Resources

Cattle and Buffalo constitute important genetic resources in country that provide strength to the livelihood security in agriculture based system. Besides, their significant contribution to the national economy, they play important role in ensuring rural employment as well as women's empowerment in India. Each animal population is specific combinations of alleles forming specific gene pool, which serves a particular purpose for mankind in their natural habitat. Despite contribution to the society, a large part of Cattle and Buffalo Genetic Resources distributed all over the country is yet to be characterized, documented and evaluated scientifically. Documentation of cattle and buffalo diversity is the key to ensure sustainable development of agriculture not only in the present context but also in future. However, with the change in utility and socioeconomic conditions of the people as well as increasing globalization, Animal Genetic Diversity is becoming highly vulnerable. Even some of the unique germplasm may become extinct if no proper corrective measures are taken. Therefore, search for new germplasm, its characterization and evaluation and documentation should be undertaken on priority as breed is generally taken as reference point for the animal genetic diversity.

1.0 National Bureau of Animal Genetic Resources (NBAGR), Karnal, Haryana

As early as in 1926 - the then Royal Commission on Agriculture recommended that livestock production in India required research efforts in a planned and systematic manner. The commission had critically analysed the situation prevailing at that time and had stressed the need for the establishment of an Institution on Animal Genetics and Breeding. Its beginning was made when a Genetic Research Unit was established at Imperial Veterinary Research Institute, Izatnagar,

Uttar Pradesh in the early forties which gradually developed into a full-fledged division soon after independence. This acted as a stimulus and later genetic research on milk animals was started at National Dairy Research Institute, Karnal, Haryana in the late fifties. In the early sixties - several agricultural universities and colleges too started research and training programmes in this important discipline of Animal Genetics and Breeding.

With the realization of unique significance of tropical animal and poultry genetic resources and their potential utilization at global level - a need was felt for an organization which could undertake the responsibility of evaluating - certifying and conserving the rich and varied germplasm resources available in the country and whose genetic base is shrinking fast. Thus - the establishment of National Bureau of Animal Genetic Resources/National Institute of Animal Genetics in 1984 was culmination of sustained efforts made by the leading geneticists in the country over the years.

The establishment of National Bureau of Animal Genetic Resources/Institute of Animal Genetics was approved in principal during IV Five Year Plan. In this regard - effective follow-up steps were taken in this V and VI Five Year Plan. Finally - the Institute was set up on 21st September, 1984 at the campus at National Dairy Research Institute (Southern Regional Station), Bangalore in the form of twin institutes namely National Bureau of Animal Genetic Resources and National Institute of Animal Genetics. These two Institutes then shifted to Karnal in 1985. The National Bureau of Animal Genetic Resources and National Institute of Animal Genetics were merged in 1995 to function as a single unit in the form of National Bureau of Animal Genetic Resources. The new office cum lab building of NBAGR was inaugurated on 28th November 1998. Now National Bureau of Animal Genetic Resources of Indian Council of Agricultural Research is the main nodal authority for breed registration of different livestock species and poultry of the country.

Vision of the Institute

- Striving for excellence in innovative research to identify genetic potential of indigenous livestock for improvement and conservation.

Mandate of the Institute

- Identification, evaluation, characterization, conservation and sustainable utilization of Livestock and Poultry Genetic Resources.
- Coordination and capacity building in animal genetic resources management and policy issues.

Objectives of the Institute

- To conduct systematic surveys to characterise, evaluate and catalogue farm livestock and poultry genetic resources and to establish their National Data Base.
- To design methodologies for ex situ conservation and in situ management and optimal utilization of farm animal genetic resources.
- To undertake studies on genetic characterisation using modern biological techniques such as molecular cytogenetics, immunology, DNA Fingerprinting, RFLP analysis etc.
- To conduct training programmes as related to evaluation, characterisation and utilisation of animal genetic resources.

The Bureau has traveled a long journey in endeavoring for excellence in innovative research to identify the uniqueness and genetic potential of country's vastly distributed livestock biodiversity and its sustainable development. Among the major achievements to its credit are the phenotypic and genetic characterization of majority (> 90%) of the registered breeds of cattle, buffalo, sheep, goat, equines, camel and poultry; identification of more than 1600 SNPs for various major candidate genes related with production, reproduction, environmental adaptation and disease resistance traits in different species; cytogenetic analysis revealing the Manipuri buffaloes of NEH region as swamp buffaloes (2N=48). This premier institute is dedicated to work with its mandate of identification, evaluation, characterization, conservation and utilization of livestock and poultry genetic resources of the country.

2.0 Characterization of Cattle and Buffalo

Characterization of a cattle and buffalo population should be done primarily on phenotypic basis (*phenotypic characterization*). However, molecular level (*genetic characterization*) may be carried out further to complement the phenotypic characterization of a population.

2.1. Phenotypic characterization

Phenotypic characterization of a population is intended to document the detailed information of newly identified population. It should take account of geographical distribution of the population, collection of data on production systems in which the breed/population is found, morphological traits, phenotypic attributes (physical features, performance levels and any unique features), reproductive status, historical development of the breed/population, upgrading and selection, socio-economic status of the communities rearing the breed, utility of the breed/population in their typical production environment and relevant gender-specific knowledge of management strategies used by communities to utilize the genetic diversity in their animals.

Questionnaires for survey of cattle and buffaloes genetic resources developed by NBAGR, Karnal can serve this purpose. As per their guide line, Information should be recorded on 3000 animals covering 3 districts of the breeding tract. Within each district, select 4 strata randomly. From each stratum, 5 villages should be randomly selected. Thus, there should be 1000 animals in a district, which should be randomly selected from 4 randomly selected zones. In each district, 200 animals under each of the categorized group should be studied for aspects given against the group. The duration of the survey may be 24 months for cattle and buffalo. During the first 3 months the data on general information viz. population enumeration, management practices, and socio-economic status of the farmers should be completed. During this phase, the households and animals for detailed data recording should be identified. Subsequently, the enumerators should continue recording information on morphological characteristics, performance and utility traits as per the questionnaires developed by NBAGR. Collected data is then analyzed and compiled in the form of breed descriptors. Data should be analyzed on the basis of districts, animal classes and user-defined strata. As phenotypic characterization involves the collection of a large volume of data so it needs to be processed and analyzed carefully in designed database of a flexible computer package. ICAR-NBAGR has developed a Data Processing System for Animal Genetic Resources (DPSAnGR) for general and flexible applicability for management of field survey data of any domestic animal species. Other commercially available general statistical software for data analysis could also be used. After phenotypic characterization, it should be clear that if the population is found distinct, then only it should to be registered as breed.

2.2. Genetic characterization

Molecular characterization should ideally be done along with phenotypic characterization. Genetic characterization assesses the genetic constitution of a breed/population of a species. It is also helpful in providing insights into breed formation, informing about closest wild ancestral species and localization of the site of domestication. Phylogenetic relationships of populations based on genetic analysis unravel the evolutionary history of the breeds/populations of a species. DNA based microsatellite markers analysis methodologies are advantageous and most preferred for genetic characterization. With the automation in sequencing and genotyping technologies, it has now become much easier to genotype microsatellite loci in large number of samples within a short span of time.

Samples should be collected preferably from the breeding tracts that are closest to the site of the development of the breed. Typically not more than 10 percent of any one herd or village population should be sampled and in any case not more than five animals should be sampled from any herd. Always avoid sampling from animals with common ancestors at least for three generations. For genetic characterization, it should be ensured that samples are drawn in such a way that it should cover most of the genetic variability in the population. For the sample collection, consider the structure of the production system, geographic locations and pedigree relationships.

Blood sample is most preferable tissue for sampling. Generally 10-15 ml of blood should be collected as a sample from an individual. Other samples like semen, hide, bone, tissue (e.g. ear tissue), faeces, fossils, plucked hair with root cells and feathers can also be used for genetic characterization. For reliable estimation of allele frequencies, at least 25 and preferably 50 animals per breed should be typed for genetic characterization. More than 50 animals should be collected in view of possible losses, mistyping or missing.

Standard protocol should be followed for DNA extraction from blood or any other tissue. Standard polymerase chain reaction (PCR) procedure should be followed to amplify small amount of DNA, which should be sequenced further, using set of primers designed to amplify the fragment of DNA region. Obtained nucleotide sequences should be analyzed further for sequence alignment, identification of nucleotide variations, generation of haplotypes, estimation of population indices, such as, gene diversity, nucleotide diversity and pair-wise nucleotide differences, calculation of within breed and among breed differences through AMOVA, determination of demography, population expansion, estimation of phylogenetic relationship among different breeds of a species, identification of ancestral and descendent haplotypes and estimation of coalescence age using estimator (rho) for time divergence by using various software programme. Comparative analysis of data should be performed essentially to define the new breed.

3.0 Registration of Cattle and Buffalo Genetic Resources

India is the first country to set up National Bureau of Animal Genetic Resources (NBAGR) with a view to developing suitable documentation, evaluation, conservation and management measures of our indigenous germplasm. In this programme scientists of NBAGR as well as other institutes are actively involved to develop data banks and gene banks and for genetic characterization and evaluation of indigenous germplasm resources on modern scientific lines. ICAR-National Bureau of Animal Genetic Resources (ICAR-NBAGR), Karnal is a nodal Institute for the registration of animal germplasm of the country. The proper guide line for registration and documentation of cattle and buffalo genetic resources are described by ICAR-National Bureau of Animal Genetic Resources (Indian Council of Agricultural Research), G.T. Road By-Pass, Near Basant Vihar, Karnal-132 001 (Haryana) India are now presented below:

3.1 General Criteria

Population: Any population of cattle and buffalo found in India can be registered in the form of breed but they must fulfil the criteria laid down for the registration standard. The cattle and buffalo population to be registered for breed recognisation should have some definable and identifiable external characteristics that enable them to be separated by visual appraisal from other similarly defined groups within same species or geographical and/or cultural separation from phenotypically similar groups has led to acceptance of its separate identity.

Nature of material: Breeds/populations/strains of domesticated cattle and buffalo having unique, stable and uniform, and has potential attributes of academic, scientific or commercial value are entitled for breed registration. Material without accompanying documentary evidence for the claim made in the application or material for which any form of protection has been sought elsewhere, shall not qualify for breed registration.

Eligibility Criteria: At least 1000 animals in a population will be considered for registration as a breed. These animals may be maintained by the applicant/ breed society/ NGO/ Govt. Agency/ farmers in field conditions. All claims concerning the material submitted for registration should accompany scientific evidence for uniqueness, reproducibility and value in the form of: Publication in standard peer reviewed journal (a copy of reprint to be submitted) and/or Evaluation data for at least three years under research programmes like All India Coordinated Research Project (AICRP), Network Project, Adhoc Schemes, etc. supported with relevant extracts of the documents or verification by concerned Director/Project Director (PD)/Project Co-ordinator and/or Publication of information on potential value of germplasm in institute annual report or any other such reports. Recommendation of the State Animal Husbandry Department/ Livestock Development Board regarding the novelty and uniqueness of the breed claimed.

Nodal Agency: The application should be addressed to the Director, ICAR-NBAGR, along with the required information as ICAR-National Bureau of Animal Genetic Resources (ICAR-NBAGR), Karnal is the nodal Institute for registration of breeds. The prescribed application format for cattle and buffalo breed registration is readily available at NBAGR website. Any citizen of India or any registered breed society as per constitution of India/NGO/Govt. agency is eligible for its applicant. The period for validity of registration shall be 25 years.

De-notification: Registration Committee can call for de-notification in case of false claim(s) or disputed IPR claim. Appeal for counter claim, if any, should reach the Registration Committee within a period of three months of the publication of Notification in Indian Journal of Animal Sciences - published by the ICAR.

3.2 Submission Procedure

- Applicant should submit 3 copies of the application along with relevant documents, literature, no matter how small (even one page), for the proper evaluation of the breed.

- Application must be signed by the applicant and countersigned by Director, Department of Animal Husbandry of the concerned state(s) or his representative with rubber seal.
- Application must be accompanied by complete description of the breed using standard descriptors.
- A detailed history of the breed should be submitted.
- Difference, distinction and details that are specific for that breed in comparison to other breeds in the vicinity or elsewhere should be listed.
- Representative photographs of the breed (male, female, young ones and herd) should be submitted.
- List of registered animals of the breed that are conforming the breed standards laid out by applicant or organization should be submitted.
- Breed should complete a minimum of 10 generations.
- Letters from at least three different breeders/owners of the breed should be submitted, explaining: Why they believe it should become a recognized breed? How long they have been breeding the breed? Spell out the reasons for reorganization of the breed as a separate identity. What has been done to establish this breed-breeding strategies, parental stock etc.? What are the suggestions to further improve this breed in a long term perspective? What makes this breed clearly different and distinctive from all other breeds?

3.3 Breed Accession Numbers

ICAR-NBAGR will provide the unique accession number to each breed after registration. Accession numbers of existing breeds of cattle and buffaloes are given in Annexure of their website. The animal germplasm registration needs to be carried out at breed/type/strain/variety level within a species. Species-wise national animal germplasm registration shall be maintained at NBAGR, Karnal. The known breeds of various species shall be registered to begin with. The registration shall be carried out using a well laid breed descriptor which has been evolved by the Bureau. An alpha numeric code has been designed for all the breeds in the following format.

INDIA_SPECIES NAME_ABCD_BREED NAME_XYEFG

AB = Two Digit Numeric Code for State One (Major Tract)

CD = Two Digit Numeric Code for State Two

XY = Two Digit Numeric Code for Species (as given by NBAGR)

EFG = Three Digit Numeric Code for the Breed (as given by NBAGR)

3.4 Animal Genetic Resources of India-Information System

ICAR-NBAGR has developed Information System on Animal Genetic Resources of India (AGRI-IS) that covers all the indigenous breeds of domestic livestock and poultry species in India. AGRI-IS database contains descriptors of various breeds of livestock and poultry, information on farms, semen production, vaccine production; and district-wise information on population, animal breeding, animal health infrastructure, animal products like milk, meat, egg, wool, etc. Photographs of male and female animals of breeds are also stored in it. Information on newly registered breed is also incorporated for documentation purpose.

A total of 30 cattle breeds were registered as existing breeds and accession numbers were allotted to them in the year 2008. Since then another 11 new cattle populations were also registered as recognized breeds and accession numbers were allotted. The new cattle breeds were Binjharpuri (Odisha), Ghumsuri (Odisha), Motu (Odisha), Khariar (Odisha), Pullikulam (Tamilnadu), Kosali (Chhattisgarh), Gangatiri (Uttar Pradesh and Bihar), Malnad Gidda (Karnataka), Belahi (Haryana and Chandigarh), Badri (Uttarakhand) and Lakhimi (Assam). If any individual/organization feels that there is a new population in a particular area, they may contact NBAGR, Karnal and request the Bureau for its characterization so that it may later be registered as new breed of cattle. As on today, there are altogether 13 buffalo breeds are registered and their accession number were allotted by NBAGR, Karnal, Haryana.

4.0 Monitoring of Cattle And Buffalo Genetic Resources

It is very much essential to monitor the cattle and buffalo population in the country for a time interval to know the present status as well as to take necessary measure for their proper conservation. Here the proper guide line for monitoring the cattle and buffalo as per ICAR-NBAGR, Karnal is presented briefly.

The generation interval of cattle and buffalo is about five years. Breed wise livestock census throughout country in every five years interval can be best utilized to monitor the population status and trend of the breeds. DAHDF, Government of India is presently conducting Breed wise census in every 5 years interval. But, breed-wise census should be required for providing number of breeding males and females in the population.

Baseline survey of any breed can provide a starting reference point for the monitoring of the population in future. So, population size of available breed needs to be recorded at the time of breed survey. This will help to record the population trend in minimum time duration. Recognized breeds which are very much important can also be monitored in their own breeding tract by conducting such monitoring surveys. The important aspects need to be remembered during breed monitoring survey as follows: present population size, geographical distribution, breeding males and females size, geographical and temporal changes, increasing or decreasing trend, increasing trend relative to other Breed in vicinity, possible reasons in increasing or decreasing trend and recognized threats to Breed.

Questionnaires for monitoring survey should be developed in such a way that it can identify and analyze threats to survival of the breed. Maintenance of a database containing all relevant information's on breeds is essential to keep watch on the breed and further for designing and implementing conservation strategies.

The demographic parameters should be collected during monitoring survey, based on these parameters the risk status of a breed can be assessed. These are (i) Size of population of a breed (ii) Population of breed in country, specifically in breeding tract of the breed (iii) Registered animals in breed inventories (iv) Number of breeding males and breeding females and (v) Distribution of population

Breed wise sample survey can be conducted for identifying total number of animals of a particular breed according to their age and sex. For this purpose about 15 percent of villages in every block of the each district of the breeding area of that breed should be selected randomly. The assigned survey should be completed within one month of commencement of breed survey.

5.0 Determining Risk Status of Cattle and Buffalo

The assessment of risk status of breeds or populations is a prime factor in planning of Cattle and Buffalo Genetic Resources management, conservation and finally for their genetic improvement. Pertaining information help the policy planner and stake holders whether, and how urgently, actions need to be taken for conservation. The following Breed Risk Classification for our country as described by ICAR-NBAGR, Karnal, Haryana are now presented below:

5.1 Breed not at risk

In this category, total population is more than 20,000 and total number of breeding females is more than 10,000 and total number of breeding males is more than 40 in cattle and buffalo.

5.2 Vulnerable Breed

Total population is 20,000 or less but more than 10,000 or total number of breeding females is 10,000 or less but more than 5,000 or total number of breeding males is 40 or less but more than 20 in cattle and buffalo are considered under this vulnerable category.

5.3 Endangered Breed

Under this category, total population is 10,000 or less, but more than 1,000 or total number of breeding females is 5,000 or less but more than 500 or total number of breeding males is 20 or less but more than 5 in cattle and buffalo. Attention for conservation of cattle and buffalo is very much essential in this stage.

5.4 Critical Breed

Total population is 1,000 or less; or total number of breeding females is 500 or less or total number of breeding males is 5 or less in cattle and buffalo. Extensive conservation and preservation program need to be taken with elapsing any more time to avoid the extinction of valuable country's cattle and buffalo germplasms.

5.5 Extinct Breed

In this situation, there is no breeding males (or stored semen) or no breeding females (or oocytes) or no embryos remaining left. They lost perpetually from the earth. So there is no chance to regain them.

The classification of the risk status considering above population criteria, the number of animal must be present in less than 75 sq. km area and 10 percent or more degree of introgression per generation is required. At least in 5 years interval, routine conduct of monitoring survey for particular breed is required to know the update of risk status of breed. Any breed under high risk status should be given higher weightage or priority for conservation. Under the same risk category, priority should be given to the most genetically diversed breed, likewise genetically superior for economically important and unique traits.

Cattle and Buffalo breeds or populations categorized under any category of risk will require urgent action. It will be essential to develop strategic plan for conservation and implement these conservation/ development programmes so that population may further expand and can be prevented from reaching any severe categories.

❑❑❑

APPENDIX-I

Questionnaries for Survey of Cattle and Buffaloes Genetic Resources

Questionnaire-1. General information about the householder and animals maintained by him (only once) *Source:* NBAGR.

Date of visit	**District/ Stratum**	
Code :	Tehsil/Taluka/Zone :	Village :
Code :	Household Number :	

Name & Address:
Name of Enumerator :

GENERAL INFORMATION

Ag. Holding (acres):
Irrigated (acres):
Unirrigated (acres):
Fodder Grown
(1)/ Not (2): Winter: Summer:
Profession:
Annual Income (Rs.):
No.of family members:
No. of literate members:
No. of members engaged in dairying: Male: Female:
Sale/purchase of animals:

1. Animal Fair:
2. Middle man:
3. Any other:

UTILITY

	Cattle	Buffalo
1. Milk production		
2. Agricultural operation:		
3. Breeding:		
4. Religion:		
5. Any other:		

MANAGEMENT PRACTICES

Housing

during day(1)/ night(2)both day & night(3)/ none(4) :

a) Open(1)/closed(2):
b) Kutcha(1)/ Pucca(2):
c) Separate)/ part of residence(2)
d) Flooring Kutcha(1)/ Pucca(2):
e) Full walled(1)/ half walled(2):
f) Well ventilated Y(1)/ N(2):
g) Sanitary condition of the stall: very clean Y(1)/ N(2):
h) Pucca drain for urine to drain out Y(1)/ N(2):

WALLOWING

Morning: Y(1)/N(2)	Noon: Y(1)/N(2)	Evening: Y(1)/N(2)

Fodder Grown (Yes / No)

Green Fodder	Dry Fodder
Winter:	Winter:
Summer:	Summer:
Chaffed(1)/Unchaffed(2):	Chaffed(1)/ Unchaffed(2):

FEED

Seeds/ Grains:

Cakes/ Concentrate:

Others:

Feeding: Soaked/ Cooked/Raw:

Feeding: Mixing with fodder/ alone:

At milking time/ other times:

Cleaning of milking utensiles Y(1)/ N(2):

Udders washed before milking Y(1)/ N(2):

Breeding method: Natural(1)/ Artifical Insemination(2):

Species /Breeds	**Upto 1 year**		**1-3 years**		**3 Years and above**					
	Male	**Female**	**Male**	**Female**	**Male**			**Female**		
					Used for breeding	**For breeding and work**	**For work only**	**In milk**	**Dry**	**Not calved even once**
Cattle										
(Breeds)										
Buffalo										
(Breeds)										
Others										
(Species/										
Breeds)										
Disease				Treatment			Herbal(1)/ Allopathic(2)/ Local(3)			
Vaccination:										

Questionnaire-2. Feed and feeding practices (Individual animals)

District/Stratum : **Code :** **Tehsil/ Taluka/ Zone :**

Date of visit :

Village : Code : Household Number :

Address :

Name of Enumerator :

Allotted No.: Breed : (name/ code) Classification : (name/ code)

Date of Birth : Age :

Dam No.: Sire No.:

FEEDING

a) Grazing Distance(km) Time(hrs)
   Morning(1)
   Evening(2)

b) Individual(1)/ Group feeding(2):

c) Feed:

Feed	**Morning**		**Noon**		**Evening**	
	Name	**Qty (kg)**	**Name**	**Qty (kg)**	**Name**	**Qty (Kg)**
Green fodder						
Dry fodder						
Concentrate						
Minerals						

d) Water: Adequate(a)/ inadequate(b): Quantity:
   Water source(Name):

e) Feeding (Green Fodder/ Dry Fodder)
   i) Green Fodder mixed in Dry fodder:
   ii) Drying method of fodder:
   iii) Silage making:

Questionnaire 3. Physical and qualitative traits (Individual animals)

Date of visit :

District/ Stratum : Code : Tehsil/Taluka/ Zone :

Village : Code : Household Number :

Name & Address :

Name of Enumerator :

Allotted No : Breed : (name/code) Classification : (name/code)

Date of Birth : Age :
Dam No.: Sire No.:
Purpose of breeds: milk(1)/ meat(2)/ draugth(3)/ others (specify):

Hair characters

a) Length Short(1)/ medium(2)/ Long(3):
b) Sheen Glossy(1)/ Dull(2):
c) Curl Curly(1)/ straight(2):

Colour Name

a) Coat (hair):
b) Skin:
c) Muzzle:
d) Eyelids:
e) Hoofs:
f) Tail switch:

Horns : Present(1)/ Absent(2)

a) Colour/ Black(1)/ Brown(2)/ White(3)/, others(specify):
b) Size(cms):
c) Shape: Straight (1)/ Curved(2):
d) Orientation:

Lateral pointing tips(1)/ inward pointing tips(2)/ Upward pointing tips(3)/ downw pointing tips(4)/ Forward pointing tips(5)/backward pointing tips(6):

Ears

a) Length (cms):
b) Orientation: horizontal (1)/ Dropping (2):

Head

a) Length (cms):
b) Poll prominent(1)/ Not prominent(2):
c) Any other peculiar character (specify):

Body

a) Hump: large(1)/ medium(2)/ small(3)
b) Dewlap: large(1)/ medium(2)/ small(3)
c) Naval flap: large(1)/ medium(2)/ small(3)
d) Penis sheath flap: large(1)/ Medium(2)/ small(3)/ absent(4)
e) Basic temperament: docile(1)/ moderate(2)/ tractable(3)/ wild(4)

Udder

a) Shape: bowl(1)/ round(2)/ trough(3)/ pendulous)
b) Fore udder size: large(1)/ medium(2)/ small(3)
c) Rear udder size: large(1)/ medium(2)/ small(3)
d) Teat shape: cylindrical (1)/ funnel(2)/ pear(3)
e) Teat tip: pointed(1)/ round(2)/ flat(3)
f) Milk vein: large(1)/ medium(2)/ small(3)

Body size: Massive/ large/ medium/ small

Weight(kg)

a) Birth weight:
b) 6 month weight:
c) 12 month weight:
d) 24 month weight:
e) Weight at Ist mating:
f) Weight at Ist calving:

Measurements

a) Chest girth(cm):
b) Body length(cm):
c) Height at withers:
d) Tail length (Above hock/at hock/below hock touching the ground)

Reproduction (Females)

a) Age at 1 oestrous (months):
b) Oestrous cycle duration(days):
c) Oestrus duration (hrs):
d) Age at 1 mating (months):
e) Age at 1 calving (months):
f) Interval from calving to Ist conception (days):
g) No. of services/ conception:
h) Calving interval (days):
i) Gestation length (days)
j) No. of calvings :

Reproduction (Males)

a) Age at training of bull:
b) Age at first ejaculation/ mounting (days):
c) Age at first mating (N.S.):
d) Age at first collection of quality semen(AI) :

Abnormalities

a) Twinning:
b) Dystocia:
c) Placental retention:

d) Abortions:
e) Still births:
f) Postgestational mortality:
g) Others(Specify):

Type of Work

a) Drought tolerance
(Allocate grades 1 to 5, 1=high)
b) Heat tolerance
(Allocate grades 1 to 5, 1=high)
c) Purpose: ploughing(1)/ threshing(2)/ power(3)/ etc
d) Capacity for work : hard(1)/ medium(2)/ light(3)
e) Average duration of work per day (hrs):

Questionnaire 4. Milk Recording

Name :	s/ o :	Village :
Block :	District :	Milk recorder :
Animal No :	Breed :	Date of Birth/Age

Homebred/purchased

1. Age at first service:
2. Order of lactation
3. Age of first conception:
4. Date of calving:
5. Age/date at first calving:
6. Sex of calf & No : weaned/unweaned
7. Date of conception:
8. No. of services: Natural/A.I
9. Date of drying:

S.No.	Date of Recording	Milk Yield Morning	Milk Yield Evening	Total Fat%	SNF	Remarks/ Sign.

❑❑❑

APPENDIX-II

Application for Registration of Cattle and Buffalo Breeds

(To be submitted to The Director, NBAGR, Karnal-132001, Haryana) Please refer to guidelines for filling the application form appended and Codes (*Source:* NBAGR)

1. Application status (Code) : N R
2. Species name
3. Breed name
4. Origin: IN EX CR SY OT
5. Criteria for registration [Distinct feature(s)]
6. Documentary evidence

For Use of NBAGR

i) Application number
ii) Date of application
iii) Whether new or revised?
iv) If revised, Date of 1st Application
v) Action taken
   a) Forwarded for registration
   b) Sent for validation
   c) Incomplete, sent for revision
vi) Whether registered or rejected
vii) Date of registration or rejection
viii) Registration Number
ix) Notified on:
x) Remarks

7. Particulars of community/agency/scientist(s)/breeders/farmers who evolved and maintained the breed
8. Name and address of the corresponding person
   Name (Dr./Ms/Mr.)
   Designation
   Address
   Tel- Fax- E-mail
9. Passport information of the breed
   Place of origin (Tehsil/Distt/Province) Present area of distribution
   Utility

Approximate population No. of Breedable Males
No. of Breedable females

Remarks

(Farmers/community contributions, if any)

Parent Stock/Pedigree involved in breed development Method of development

SB CB UG OT

Organised Herd/Breed Society, if any

10. Salient Characteristics (attach detailed description as per Breed Descriptor performa)
11. Additional Information/ Remarks (if any)

UNDERTAKING

I/We undertake to ensure long term conservation of the aforesaid breed in its natural habitat and to provide required germplasm/genetic stock to NBAGR; its sustainable use by maintaining appropriate numbers and providing access as appropriate on prior informed consent and on mutually agreed terms. I/We also agree to provide any further information or data pertaining to the description and unique characteristics to the ICAR/NBAGR in a transparent manner.

COUNTERSIGNED by Director
Department of Animal Husbandry
of the concerned state or his
representative

Signatures
Full Name
Designation & Address
Ph Fax
E-mail
SEAL

SIGNATURES of the Applicant (s)
Name
Designation & Address
Ph Fax
E-mail

Guidelines for filling Application and description of Codes

1. Use capital letters or write legibly. All items are self-explanatory. Give explanation for a particular item in "Remarks" wherever needed.
2. Use Codes for filling in *Item 1, 4, 6 and 9*. In case of the code "Other" fill in specific details.
3. For filling species and breed name (*Item 2 & 3*) give English or Hindi name, if known. In case a local name is given then also specify in parenthesis the language or dialect in which this name is used.

4. Be to the point for *Item 5*, give only the distinct features, traits or products/ bye-products, considered suitable for consideration of registration.
5. Give particulars of organisation associated with development of the breed in *Item 7*. Attach separate sheet for additional names along with address and phone/fax/email, etc.
6. Give particulars of developers in *Item 7* and that corresponding person in Item 8 as the applicant and developer may not be always the same.
7. Item 9 has passport information of the breed. Give clearly place of origin, present area of distribution (state, district), utility ((milk, egg, wool, meat, draught power, etc.), Approximate population including number of breedable males and females, Parent stock/Pedigree involved.
8. in development of the breed, Also give breeding method used.
9. Give detailed description of traits & characteristics of the material in Item 10. Follow the format of descriptor for the respective species.
10. Undertaking to the effect ensuring conservation and maintenance of the breed for facilitating access and sustainable use has been given, which may be read and implied before putting signatures.
11. Furnish the application form complete in all respects along with requisite documents to *The Director, NBAGR, P O Box 129, Karnal* – 132 001 (*Haryana*)

Codes for filling information in Col. 1, 4, 6 and 9

Item 1 : Application Status

N	New
R	Revised

Item 4 : Origin in Indigenous

EX	Exotic
CR	Crossbred
SY	Synthetic
OT	Others (Specify)

Item 6 : Documentary evidence

PR	Published literature
IR	Institute annual report
OR	Any other report

Item 9 : Method of development

SB	Selective breeding
CB	Crossbreeding
UG	Upgrad ing
OT	Others (Specify)

❑❑❑

APPENDIX-III

Breed Descript or Format for Cattle & Buffalo Breeds (*Source:* NBAGR)

I. GENERAL DESCRIPTION

1. Name of the breed
2. Synonyms
3. Background for such a name/ origin
4. Since when the breed is known
5. Strains (or within breed types)
6. Most closely related breeds (in appearance)
7. a) Native tract of distribution in terms of longitude and latitude

   b) Approximate area of distribution

   c) Place(s)   State   District(s)
8. Estimated population

   a) Year of estimation

   b) Population

   c) Source/Reference
9. a) Communities responsible for developing the breed

   b) Description of community (Farmers/nomads/isolated/tribals)
10. Herd Book/ Register established (Yes/ No)
11. Herd: Average size ...

    Composition: Breeding females .... % Replacement females (1-3yrs) .... % Calves .... %

    Breeding bulls .... % Replacement males (1-3yrs) .... % Bullocks .... %
12. Utility of the breed (Milk/meat/draught/manure/other specify)
13. Basic temperament of the breed (docile/ moderate/ tractable/ wild)
14. Any other information

II. PHYSICAL CHARACTERS

1. **Colour** **Male** **Female**
   - a) Coat Colour
   - b) Skin
   - c) Muzzle
   - d) Eyelids
   - e) Tail Switch
   - f) Hooves
2. Horns Male Female
   - a) Colour
   - b) Size
   - c) Shape (Straight/ curved)
   - d) Orientation
3. Ears
   - a) Length
   - b) Orientation (horizontal/ drooping)
4. Head
   - a) Forehead (convex/ concave/ straight)
   - b) General description
5. Body Male Female
   - a) Hump (large/ medium/ small)
   - b) Dewlap (large/ medium/ small)
   - c) Naval flap (large/ medium/ small)
   - d) Penis sheath flap (large/ medium/ small)
6. Udder
   - a) Shape (bowl/ round/ trough/ pendulous)
   - b) Udder size (large/ medium/ small)
   - c) Teat shape (cylindrical/ funnel/ pear)
   - d) Teat tip (pointed/ round/ flap)
   - e) Milk vein (prominent/ not prominent)
7. Any other information

III. PERFORMANCE

1. Body Weight (kg)

Parameter	Male			Female		
	Average	Range	N	Average	Range	N
Birth Weight						
Pre-Weaning Weight						
12 month Weight						
24 month Weight						
Wt. at First mating						
Wt. at First calving						
Adult weight						

2. Body measurements (cm)

Parameter	Male			Female		
	Average	Range	N	Average	Range	N
Chest girth						
Body length						
Height at withers						

3. Dairy performance

Parameter	Male			Female		
	Average	Range	N	Average	Range	N
Daily milk yield (Kg)						
Peak milk yield (Kg)						
Lactation length (days)						
Lactation milk yield (Kg)						
Fat %						
SNF %						

4. Reproduction	Average	Range	N
a) Males			
i) Age at first ejaculation (months)			
ii) Age at first mating (months)			
b) Females			
i) Age at first oestrus (month)			
ii) Oestrous cycle duration (days)			
iii) Oestrus duration (hrs)			
iv) Age at first mating (months)			
v) Age at first calving (months)			
vi) Service period (days)			
vii) Calving interval (days)			

5. Draught performance
   a) Purpose (ploughing, threshing, power etc.)
   b) Physiological parameters   Before work   After work
      Rectal temperature (°F)
      Respiration rate /min
      Pulse rate /min
   c) Fatigue Score
      Frothing
      Leg in-coordination
      Excitement
      Inhibition of progressive movement
      Tongue protrusion
   d) Draught Power (HP)
   e) Average duration of work per day (hrs)
6. Drought tolerance (Excellent/ Very Good/ Good/ Average/ Low)
7. Heat tolerance (Excellent/ Very Good/ Good/ Average/ Low)
8. Any other information specific to the breed

❑❑❑

References

Abbas S., Singh CV., Barwal RS. and Singh CB. (2010). Genetic and phenotypic parameters of first lactation and lifetime traits in Sahiwal cows. Journal of Livestock Biodiveristy. 2(2): 67-70.

Acharya RM., and Bhat PN. (1984). Livestock and Poultry Genetic Resources of India. IVRI Research Bulletin No.1, Indian Veterinary Research Institute, Izatnagar.

Agarwal SP., Menon GN. and Bach NC. (1971). Some aspects of reproductive performance in Kankrej cows. Indian J. Anim. Sci., 41(8): 631-635.

Ahlawat SPS. and Gupta SC. (2006). Domestic animal biodiversity and breeding policy-issues and perspectives. National symposium on Conservation and Improvement of Animal Genetic Resources under low input system: Challenges and Strategies. NBAGR, Karnal. 1-7.

Ahmad B. (1998). Productive and reproductive performance of Red Sindhi cattle under hot humid environment of Balochistan Province of Pakistan. M.Sc. (Hons) thesis, Dept. Anim. Breed. Genet. Uni. Agri. Faisalabad, Pakistan.

Alderson L. (2009). Breeds at risk: Definition and measurement of the factors which determine endangerment. Livestock Science, 123: 23-27.

Ambardekar DV. (2000). Studies on body measurement and qualitative traits in Pandharpuri buffaloes. M. Sc. (Agri.) Thesis submitted to Mahatma Phule Agricultural University, Rahuri, M. S., India

Ambhore GS., Singh A., Deokar DK., Gupta AK., Singh M. and Prakesh V. (2017). First lactation production and reproduction performance of Phule Triveni cattle in hot arid region of Maharashtra. Indian J. of Animal Sciences. 87(1): 105-108.

Anonymous (2002-03). Annual Report of the National Bureau of Animal Genetic Resources, Karnal, Haryana, pp:16-36.

Anonymous (2003-04). Annual Report of the National Bureau of Animal Genetic Resources, Karnal, Haryana, pp: 8-15.

Anonymous (2004). Cattle and Buffalo Breeding Policy of the State. Recommendation of National Seminar on Cattle and Buffalo Breeding

Policy- Perspective-Indigenous non-descriptive held on 23rd and 24th December 2004 at Great Eastern Hotel, Kolkata, West Bengal.

Anonymous (2004-05). Annual Report of the National Bureau of Animal Genetic Resources, Karnal, Haryana, pp: 1-4.

Anonymous (2007). Research Achievements AICRPs on Animal Sciences (2002-07). Indian Council of Agricultural Research, Directorate of Information and Publications of Agriculture, Krishi Anusandhan Bhavan, New Delhi-110012.

Anonymous (2009). Guidelines for registration of livestock and poultry breeds. National Bureau of Animal Genetic Resources, Karnal (www.nbagr.res.in) ICAR guidelines for intellectual property management and technology transfer/commercialization (2006), Indian Council of Agricultural Research, New Delhi.

Anonymous (2012). Annual Report 2011-2012. National Bureau of Animal Genetic Resources. Karnal, Haryana.

Anonymous (2012). The 19th Livestock Census-2012. All India Report. Ministry of Agriculture, Department of Annual Husbandry, Dairying and Fisheries, Krishi Bhawan, New Delhi. Pp 12, 49-52.

Anonymous (2015). Estimated livestock population Breed wise based on breed survey 2013, Government of India Ministry of Agriculture & Farmers Welfare, Department of Animal Husbandry, Dairying & Fisheries (Animal Husbandry Statistics Division), Krishi Bhawan, New Delhi.

Anonymous (2013-14). Annual Report of the National Bureau of Animal Genetic Resources, Karnal, Haryana, pp: 11.

Anonymous (2014-15). Annual Report of the National Bureau of Animal Genetic Resources, Karnal, Haryana, Pp:16.

Anonymous (2015-16). Annual Report of ICAR-Central Institute for Research on Cattle, Meerut Cantt-250 001, Uttar Pradesh.

Anonymous (2015). Basic Animal Husbandry and Fisheries Statistics. Ministry of Agriculture, Department of Animal Husbandry, Dairying and Fisheries, Krish Bhawan, New Delhi, Pp 35-36.

Anonymous (2016). Guidelines for Management of Animal Genetic Resources of India. ICAR-National Bureau of Animal Genetic Resources (Indian Council of Agricultural Research) G.T. Road By-Pass, Near Basant Vihar, Karnal-132 001 (Haryana) India

Balain DS. (1999). Inflow and outflow of buffalo germplasm resources and their global contribution. Invited papers presented in short course on characterization and conservation of domesticated livestock and poultry resources. 10-19 May, 1999, National Bureau of Animal Genetic Resources (ICAR) Karnal.

Banerjee AK. (2013). Principles of Animal Genetics and Breeding. Kalyani Publishers.

Banerjee GC. (1996). A Textbook of Animal Husbandry. Seventh Edition. Oxford & IBH Publishing Co. PVT. LTD.

Basu SB. (1996). Genetic Improvement of Buffaloes. Kalyani Publisher.

Basu SB., Bhatnagar DS., Taneja VK. and Rao VP. (1979). Comparative performance of Indian Dairy Breeds. Indian Journal of Dairy Science. 32: 497-499.

Bawre VK. (1989). Survivability and reproductive effiency of Gir herd. M.V.Sc. & A.H. Thesis, JNKVV, Jabalpur.

Bera PK., Saha D., Ghosh SK. and Das S. (2016). Phenotypic characterization of different colour variants of endangered Siri cattle in West Bengal and Sikkim. Indian J. Anim. Hlth. 55(2): 149-156.

Bhadoria HBS., Khan FH., Tomar SS. and Yadav MC. (2002). Sources of variation in some of the reproductive traits of Gir cows. Indian J. of Animal Sciences. 72(2): 157-160.

Bhinchhar BK., Paswan VK., Yadav SP. and Singh P (2016). Physical and morphometric characteristics of Gangatiri cattle. Agricultural Research Communication Center Journals. Article ID: B-3167.

Bhutkar SS., Thrombre BM. and Bainwad DV. (2014). Effect of non-genetic factors on production traits in Deoni cows. IOSR Journal of Agriculture and Veterinary Science (IOSR-JAVS). 17(12):9-14.

Birthal PS. (2008). Linking smallholder livestock producers to markets: Issues and approaches. Indian Journal of Agricultural Economics. 63(1): 19-37.

Birthal PS. and Jha AK. (2005). Economic losses due to various constraints in dairy production in India. Indian Journal of Animal Sciences. 75(12): 1470-1475.

Borghese A. (2011). Situation and Perspectives of Buffalo in the World, Europe and Macedonia. Macedonian Journal of Animal Science. 1(2): 281–296

Chakravarthi MK., Ekambaram B. and Nasik BR. (2017). Growth and production performance of Sahiwal cattle in Andhra Pradesh. International Journal of Science, Environment and Technology. 6(2):1140-1142.

Chakravarthi MK., Sasidhar PVK. and Reddy YR. (2002). Productive and Reproductive Performance of Deoni Cattle. Indian J. of Dairy Sci., 55(1): 56-57.

Chand T. (2011). Genetic evaluation of lifetime productivity in Tharparkar cattle. M.V.Sc. Thesis. Rajasthan University of Veterinary and Animal Sciences. Bikaner, India.

Chandran PC., Dey A., Pandian J., Barari SK. and Kaushal DK. (2012). Red Purnea cattle- an unexplored indigenous germplasm. Indian J. of Anim. Sci., 82(12): 1594-1597.

Chandran PC., Dey A., SK Barari., Kamal R., Bhatt BP. and Prasad RE. (2014). Characteristics and Performance of Bachaur cattle in the gangetic plains of North Bihar. The Indian Journal of Animal Sciences. 84(8): 872-875

Chantalakhana C. and Skunmun P. (1999). Long-term Breeding Strategies for Genetic improvement of buffaloes in developing countries: review. Asian-Aus. J. Anim. Sci., 12(7): 1152-1161.

Chauhan DS. and Ghosh N. (2015). Estimates of Genetic Parameters and trends of Lactation performance traits of Deoni cattle. Theriogenology Insight. 52(2): 69-79.

Chowdhary MS. and Barhat NK. (1980). Age at first calving and its influence on important economic traits of Nagauri and Malvi cattle. Indian Vet. J., 57: 811-815.

Dangar NS. and Vatatliya PH.(2014). Factors affecting age at first calving in Gir Cattle. Indian Vet. J., 92 (7): 71-73.

Das AK., Sharma D. and Kumar N. (2008). Buffalo genetic resources in India and their conservation. Buffalo Bulletin. 27: 265-268.

Das GC., Zaman GU. and Nahardeka N. (2016). A monograph on local cattle of Assam. A Monograph, 2017. DRV/PUB-801/2016-17/59.

Dasari S. (2013). Breeding policy strategies for genetic improvement of cattle and buffaloes in India. Vet World. 6(7): 455-460

Dash SK., Sethi BP. and Rao PK. (2013). Evaluation of Binjharpuri cattle of India in the native tract. International Journal of Livestock Production. 4(7):102-105

Dash SK., Sethi BP., Rao PK. and Prakash B. (2010). Evaluation and cytogenetic profiling of Binjharpuri cattle of India in its native tract. Journal of Livestock Biodiversity. .2:59-63.

Dhaka CS. (2013). Performance oF Rathi cattle under organized farm management conditions. Krishikosh. Thesis(/handle/1/79578).

Dhaka CS., Kachwaha RN. and Bais B. (2015). Study of milk production traits of Rathi cattle under organized farm management conditions in Rajasthan. Research and Reviews: Journal of Veterinary Sciences. 2(1):75-78.

Dhal BK. (2007). Genetic performance of Khariar cattle in its native tract. M.V.Sc. Thesis, OUAT, Bhubaneswar.

Dhal, BK., Patro PK., Rao BK. and Panda P. (2007). Khariar cattle- An indigenous germplasm of Nuapada in the undivided Kalahandi district of Orissa. The Indian Journal of Animal Sciences. 77(9): 889-893.

Dhaware SA., Deshpande KS., Thombre BM., Deshmukh DS. and Chauhan DS. (2008). Factors affecting productive and reproductive traits in Khillar breed of cattle in Maharashtra. Indian J. of Anim. Res., 42(1): 57-59

FAO (2011). Developing the institutional framework for the management of animal genetic resources. FAO animal production and health guidelines. No. 6. Rome.

FAO (2011). Surveying and monitoring of animal genetic resources. FAO animal production and health guidelines. no. 7. Rome.

FAO (2012). Draft guidelines on in vivo conservation of animal genetic resources. FAO. Rome. http://www.fao.org/docrep/meeting/026/me879e.pdf.

FAOSTAT(2008). Animal genetic resources. Strategies for improved use and conservation. FAO.1987. www.faostat.org http://www. fao.org/docrep/ 010/ah806e/ah806e00.htm pp.336

Gahlot GC., Pant KP. and Kachawaha RN. (2000). Variation in production performance of Tharparkar cows in north-western Rajasthan. Indian J. of Anim. Sci., 70(7):718-722.

Ganapathi P., Kumar V. and Rajesh NV. (2013). Production and Reproduction performance of endangered Bargur cattle under the field condition in Tamil Nadu. International Journal of Food, Agriculture and Veterinary Sciences. 3 (1): 207-209.

Ganapathi P., Rajendran R., Subramanian A. and Meenakshisundaram S. (2013). Bargur Cattle: Characterization and Management Practices. *The Indian Veterinary Journal,* 90 (11): 9–10.

Gandhi RS., Gurnani M. and Singh A. (1995). Influence of non-genetic factors on some of the economic traits of Sahiwal cattle. Indian J. Dairy Sci., 48: 605-606.

Gaur GK., Singh A., Singh PK. and Pundir RK. (2015). Morphometric characteristics and present status of Ponwar cattle breed in India. National Bureau of Animal Genetic Resources, Post Box 129, G T Road Bypass, Karnal 132 001 (Haryana), India.

Gaur GK., Kaushik SN. and Garg RC. (2002). Ongole cattle status in India. Animal Genetic Res. Information, 32: 27-34.

Gaur GK., Kaushik SN. and Garg RC. (2003). The Gir cattle breed of India-Characteristics and present status. AGRI, 33:21-29.

Gaur, GK., Garg RC and Singh K (2005). Experiences of Crossbreeding in Cattle in India. Proceedings of VIII National Conference on Animal Genetics and Breeding (National Livestock Breeding Policy) March 8-10, 2005, CIRG, Makhdoom, Farah-281 122 Mathrua (UP) India by Indian Society of Animal Genetics and Breeding. Page: 38-49.

Gokhale SB., Bhagat RL., Singh PK. and Singh G. (2009). Morphometric characteristics and utility pattern of Khillar cattle in breed tract. Indian Journal of Animal Sciences. 79(1):47-51.

Gurtu BN. (1973). Studies on the birth weight and gestation length in Nagori cattle. M.V.Sc. Thesis, College of Veterinary and Animal Science, Bikaner.

ICAR (1997). Hand Book of Animal Husbandry. Published by Publications and Information Division. Indian Council of Agricultural Research. New Delhi.

Iype S., Venkatachalapathy T., Santosh PK. and Behera A.(2016). Characterization of Kasargod cattle of Kerala. IOSR Journal of Agriculture and Veterinary Science (IOSR-JAVS). 9(11): 26-32.

Jadhav BS. and Patange DD. (2009). Effect of lactation order and stage of lactation on fat, TS and SNF content of milk of Phule Triveni cow. https://www.researchgate.net/publication/268264321_Effect_of_ lactation_order_and_stage_ of_lactation_on_fat_TS_and_SNF_content_of_milk_of_Phule_Triveni_cow

Joshi BK., Tantia MS., Vij PK., Kumar P., Gupta N., Nivsarkar AK. and Sahai R. (1996). Performance of Hariana cows under farmer's herd condition in the breeding tract. Indian J. of Animal Sciences. 66(4):393-397.

Joshi NR. and Phillips RW. (1953). Zebu Cattle of India and Pakistan, FAO Agriculture Studies No. 19, Publ. by FAO, Rome, pp256.

Kanakaraj P., Natarajan N., Balasubramanian D. and Krishnan AR. (1993). A study on the performance of Umblachery breed of cattle. Cheiron 22: 209-210.

Karthickeyan SMK., Saravanan R. and Thangaraju P. (2006). Characterization of Krishna Valley breed of cattle (*Bos indicus*) in south India using microsatellite markers. Livestock Research for Rural development. 18(12):2006.

Khan UN. (1992). Sahiwal breed development in Pakistan. Journal of Animal Production and Rural Development. 974:171-178.

Khatri P., Baksh KM and Samo U. (2004). Productive Performance of Red Sindhi Cattle. Journal of Animal and Veterinary Advances. 3(6): 353-355.

Kierstein G., Vallinoto M., Silva A., Schneider MP. and Iannuzzi L. (2004). Analysis of mitochondrial D-loop region casts new light on domestic water buffalo (Bubalus bubalis) phylogeny. Molecular Phylogenetic Evolution. 30: 308-324.

Krovvidi S., Panneerselvam S., Thiruvenkadan AK., Rajeswar JJ., Sivakumar K. and Vinoo R. (2013). Lactation performance and milk constituents of Ongole cattle in its Breeding tract. Research and Reviews: Journal of Veterinary Science and Technology. 2(2): 2319-3441.

Kumar S. and Bhat PN. (1979). Reproductive performance of Hariana cattle. Indian J. of Anim. Sci., 49:1001-1008.

Kumar S., Gupta J., Kumar N., Dikshit K. and Navani N. (2006). Genetic variation and relationships among eight Indian riverine buffalo breeds. Molecular Ecology. 15: 593-600.

Kumar S., Nagarajan M., Sandhu J.S., Kumar N. and Behl, V. (2007). Phylogeography and domestication of Indian river buffalo. BMC Evolutionay Bioliogy. 7: 186.

Kumar S., Nagarajan M., Sandhu, J.S., Kumar N. and Behl, V. (2007). Mitochondrial DNA analyses of Indian water buffalo support a distinct genetic origin of river and swamp buffalo. Animal Genetics. 38: 227-232.

Kuralkar SV., Bankar PS., Chopade MM., Kuralkar P. and Dhaware SA. (2014). Phenotypic characteristics, production and reproduction performance of Deoni cattle in its native tract. Indian Journal of Animal Sciences. 84(1): 75-77.

Kushwaha S., Khan FH., Singh A. and Qureshi MI. (2002). Economic traits in Sahiwal cattle. Indian Vet. Med. Jour., 26:193-196.

Lal M.(1996). Studies on breed characteristics, managemental practices and utilization pattern of Nagori cattle. Ph.D. Thesis, National Dairy research Institute, Karnal, Haryana-132001.

Lasley JF. (1972). Genetics of Livestock Improvement. Second Edition. Prentice-Hall, Inc. Englewood Cliffs, New Jersey. London

Lush JL. (1956). Animal Breeding Plans. 3rd Edition.

Malhotra PK. and Singh RP. (1980). Estimation of lifetime production in Red Sindhi cattle using ridge trace criterion. Indian J. Anim. Sci., 50(3):215-218.

Mane AG., Despande AD. and Keshpamde KS.(1998). Study of some of the economic characteristics of Khillar breed of cattle. Indian J. of Dairy Sci., 52(6):380-382.

Mason IL. (1996). A world Dictionary of Livestock Breeds, Type and Varieties. Fourth edition. CAB International. pp-273.

Mathur AK. and Chahal RS. (1997). Performance of Hariana cows in their breeding tract. Indian J. of Anim. Sci., 67(10):882-889.

Mathur AK. and Khosla SK. (1994). Gir cows in their breeding tract. Indian J. of Anim. Sci., 64:1207-1218.

Mruttu HA. (2013). Studies on performance of Deoni cattle at MAU Dairy Farm, Parbhani, doctoral diss., Marathwada Agriculture University, Parbhani(MS), 2013.

Muhammad MUD. (2014). Buffalo genome research - a review. Animal Science Papers and Reports. 32(3): 187-199.

Mukherjee DP. and Banerjee GC. (1995). Genetics and Breeding of Farm Animals. Oxford & IBH Publishing Co. PVT. Ltd.

Okantah SA. (1992). Partial milking of cattle in smallholder herds on the Accra Plains: some factors affecting daily partial milk yield and milk composition. Animal Production. 54:15-21.

Panneerselvam S., Natarajan N., Thangaraju P., Iyue M. and Rahumathulla PS. (1990). Genetic studies on productive and reproductive traits in Tharparkar cattle. Cheiron. 19:1-6.

Pareek NK., Ankuya KJ., Patel MP., Joshi NA., Rathod BS., Prajapati KB. and Patel JB. (2016). Factors affecting age at first calving in Kankrej cattle. Journal of Animal Research. 6(2): 61-63.

Parekh HKB., Srivastava PN. and Sarkhel B.C. (2010). Text Book on Animal Genetics and Breeding. Kalyani Publishers.

Pasha TN. and Hayat Z. (2012). Present situation and future perspective of Buffalo production in Asia. The Journal of Animal and Plant Sciences. 22(3): 250-256

Patel AK., Mathur BK., Mathur AC., Mittal JP. and Kaushik SK. (2000). Production and reproductive performance of Tharparkar cattle in hot arid region. Indian J. of Anim. Sci., 70(5): 530-532.

Phanchung RJA. (1996). Characterisation of the Siri breed and Mithun cross Siri in Bhutan. Animal Genetic Resources Information. 20:1996.

Prajapati KB., Ashwar BK., Patel JP., Patel JB. and Singh DV. (1995). Size and shape of udder and teats in Kankrej cows. Indian J. Anim. Management. II(1): 43-48.

Pundir PK., Singh PK., Dangi PS. and Singh B. (2016). Siri cattle- An endangered breed of Sikkim, India. Indian Journal of Animal Sciences. 86(8):947-949.

Pundir PK., Singh PK., Sharma D., Saini A., Singh CV. and Prakash B. (2012). Hill cattle of pithoragarh district of Uttarakhand. Indian Journal of Animal Sciences. 82(12):1591-1593.

Pundir RK. and Singh PK. (2008). Status, characteristics and performance of Red Kandhari cattle breed in its native tract. The Indian Journal of animal sciences. 75(1): 56-61

Pundir RK. Sahana G., Navani NK., Jain PK., Singh DV., Kumar S. and Dave AS. (2000). Characterization of Mehsana Buffaloes in India. Animal Genetic Resources Information Bulletin. 28: 53-62.

Pundir RK., Kathiavaran P., Singh PK. and Mudaliar M. (2009). Bargur cattle: Status, characteristics and performance. The Indian Journal of Animal Sciences. (7):681-685

Rahman SM. and Rahman MM. (2006). Productive and reproductive performances of native cows under farm conditions. Asian J. of Animal and Veterinary Advances. 1:65-69.

Rajendran R. (1995). Distribution and Characteristics of Kangayam Cattle. M.V.Sc., Thesis submitted to Tamil Nadu Veterinary and Animal Sciences University, Chennai, Tamil Nadu, India.

Rajendran R. (2007).Lactation performance and milk constituents of Umblachery breed of cattle (Bos indicus) in its native coastal ecology of Tamilnadu, India. Livestock Research for Rural Development. 19 (5):2007

Rao SJ., Rao BVR. and Rao GN. (2000). Performance of crossbred cows and buffaloes under village conditions of Vishakhapatnam district of Andhra Pradesh. Indian J. of Dairy Sci., 53:222-226.

Report (2010). Basic animal husbandry statistics-AHS Series -12. Ministry of Agriculture, Dairying and Fisheries, Government of India, New Delhi

Resali DP. (2000). Recent trends in buffalo production in Nepal: A review, Buffalo News letter. Bulletin of the FAO Inter-Regional cooperative Research Network on Buffalo Europe-Near Estate, 14: 6-10.

Robertson A., Waite R. and White JCD. (1956). Variation in the chemical composition of milk with particular reference to the solids-not-fat:The effect of heredity. Journal of Dairy Research. 23(1):82-91.

Sadana DK. (2010). Buffalo Diversity in India: Breeds, Defined Populations, Production Systems and Avenues. Proceedings of the 9th World Buffalo Congress Buenos Aires, Argentina, pp. 1032-1035.

Sahoo NR., Srivastava PN. and Parmar SNS. (2003). Estimation of genetic parameters for some of the economic traits of Malvi cattle. Indian J. of Dairy Sci., 56(1): 59-60.

Sahoo SP. (1989). Characteristics and performance of Ghumsari cattle. M.V.Sc. Thesis OUAT, Bhubaneswar.

Samantray KC., Rao PK., Panda P. and Dash SK. (2009). Ghumsar cattle- an indigenous germplasm of Ghumusar tehsil in Ganjam district of Orissa. Indian Journal of Animal Sciences. 79(10): 1069-1070.

Sangwan ML. (2012). Analysis of Genetic Diversity of Indian Buffalo Breeds by DNA Markers. *Journal of Buffalo Science,* 1: 91-101

Sarkhel BC. (2001). Characterization of Nimari breed of cattle. J.N.K.V.V. Technical Bulletin: DRS/2001/09 1-46.

Sarkhel BC., Parmer SNS., Arora JS., Srivastava PN. and Pillai PVA. (2001). Characterization of Nimari breed of cattle. JNKVV Research bulletin. Jabalpur, India.

Sastry NSR., Thomas CK. and Singh RA. (1994). Livestock Production Management.Third Revised Edition, Kalyani Publisher.

Saxena HK. and Gupta AK. (1990). Economics of Gangatiri cow: an analytical approach. Livestock Adviser.15(6) : 41-44

Sethi RK. and Kala SN. (2005). Buffalo wealth and genetic improvement programmes in India. VIIIth National Conference on Animal Genetics and Breeding, 8-10 March, 2005, New Delhi pp 51-59.

Sharma A. and Pundir RK.(2015). Indigenous Breeds of Cattle In India. Dairy Year Book (2014-15). National Bureau of Animal Genetic Resources, Karnal 132 001 Haryana, India, Page no. 68-75

Sharma A. and Tantia MS.(1999). The Buffalo: A valuable genetic resource that needs more attention. Livestock International, 3(3): 9.

Sharma H., Tomar SS. and Kumar A. (2015). Effect of genetic and some other sources of variation on dry period in Malvi cows. The Indian Journal of Veterinary Sciences and Biotechnology. 10 (3): 32–35.

Sharma R., Pandey AK., Singh PK., Maitra A., Mukesh M., Singh SR. and Singh B. (2012). Characterization of Sahabadi cattle of Bihar-phenotypic and molecular approaches. Indian Journal of Animal Sciences. 82 (3): 318-322.

Sharma R., Singh PK., Maitra A., Pandey AK., Mukesh M., Singh SR. and Kumar B. (2013). Molecular characterization, body parameters and management practices of Red Purnea cattle. Indian Journal of Animal Sciences. 83(5):536-541.

Shingare VM., Chauhan, DS., Bhise BR. and Ghosh N. (2015). Estimates of genetic parameters and trends of lactation performance traits of Deoni cattle . Theriogenology Insight. 5(2): 69.

Shrestha SK. and Shrestha NP.(1998). Genetic improvement of buffalo. In Proc. First Nat. workshop on Anim. Genet. Resources Conserv. Genet. Improvement of Domest. Anim. NARC, Kathmandu, pp 98-102.

Singh D. and Singh RZ .(1991).Principles of Animal Breeding (Pashu Parjanan Ke Sindhant). 1st edition. p. 234.

Singh G., Gaur GK., Nivsarkar AK. and Patil GR. (2002). Deoni cattle breed of India. A study on population dynamics and morphometric characteristics. Animal Genetic Resources. 32:35-43.

Singh PK., Gaur GK., Pundir RK. and Singh A. (2007). Characterization and evaluation of Gangatiri cattle breed in its native tract. Indian Journal of Animal Sciences. 77(1): 66-70.

Singh PK., Pundir RK., Kumarasamy P. and Vivekanandan P. (2012). Management and physical features of migratory Pullikulam cattle of Tamil Nadu. Indian J. of Animal Sci., 82(12): 1587-1590.

Singh R. and Singh N. (1999). Effect of socio-economic variables on management of milking practices under different farming systems. Indian J. Anim. Prod. Mgmn., 15(1): 31-32.

Singh RR., Dutta T., Kumar A., Tomar AKS. and Singh M. (2011). On-farm characterization of Vrindavani cattle in India. Indian Journal of Animal Sciences. 81(3): 267-271.

Singh RR., Dutta T., Singh M. and Kumar A. (2010). Association of Udder and Teat dimensions with production traits in Vrindavani cattle. Indian J. of Dairy Sciences. 63(6): 65-69.

Singh RV. and Nivasarkar AE. (1998). Status of Gangatiri cattle in Uttar Pradesh. Indian J. of Anim. Prod. And Mgmt., 14:148-149.

Singh RV., Sachdeva GK., Garg RC., Kaushik SN. and Singh K. (2004). Conservation and Genetic improvement of important indigenous cattle breed of India. In Preceeding of National Symposium on Conservation and Propagation of indigenous breeds of Cattle Buffaloes 26-28 Feb, 2004.

Singh U., Kumar A. and Khanna AS. (2011). Performance of Hariana cattle in its native tract. The Indian Veterinary Journal, 88(02):40.

Singh, A., Gaur, GK. and Singh, PK. (2005). Characterization, evaluation and current status of Kherigarh cattle breed of Uttar Pradesh. Indian Vet. Med. Journal. 29: 21-26.

Singh, CB. and Gurnani, M. (1997). Cattle and Buffalo Breeding Policy in India-Present Status and Strategy for Future. National Dairy Research Institute (I.C.A.R). Karnal - 132001 (Haryana). March,1997

Sreenivas D. (2013). Breeding policy strategies for genetic improvement of cattle and buffaloes in India. Vet World., 6(7): 455-460

Srivastava PN., Parmer SNS., Sarkhel BC. and Tomar SS. (2002). Characterization of Malvi cattle. JNKVV Research bulletin. Jabalpur, India.

Swain KT. (2003). Performance and conformation of Motu cattle found in Malkangiri District of Orissa. M.V.Sc. Thesis, OUAT, Bhubaneswar.

Tamizhkumaran J. and Radhakrishnan R. (2016). Role of livestock in Indian Economy. Livestock Technology. 5(9): 14.

Tantia MS., Rajeev AK., Aggarwal R., Singh K. and Sodhi M. (2016). Guidelines for Management of Animal Genetic Resources of India. ICAR-National Bureau of Animal Genetic Resources, Karnal (Haryana) Publication at: https://www.researchgate.net/publication/312626319

Thiruvenkadan AK., Rajendran R. and Muralidharan J. (2013). Buffalo Genetic Resources of India and Their Conservation. Buffalo Bulletin. 32(1): 227-235.

Thomas PV. (1995). Breed Characteristics and Performance of Umblachery Cattle. Ph.D. thesis submitted to Tamil Nadu Veterinary and Animal Sciences University, Chennai, Tamilnadu, India.

Tomar SS. (2005). Text Book of Animal Breeding. Kalyani Publisher.

Uthaman PK. (2005). World's smallest cow rescued from extinction. Press Information Bureau Govt. of India.

Venkatachalapathy RT. and Iype S. (1998). Fat, total solids and solids-not-fat percentage of milk in Vechur cattle. Indian Journal of Animal Sciences. 68(6):570-573.

Vij PK., Nivsarkar AE., Tantia MS., Vijh RK., Kumar P. and Joshi BK. (1995). Performance characteristics of Nagori cattle. Indian Journal of Animal Sciences. 65(8):59-65.

Vij PK., Nivsarkar AK., Tantia MS., Vij R.K., Kumar P., Joshi BK. and Sahai R. (1994). Rathi cattle of Rajasthan. Research Bulletin No.2. NBAGR, Karnal, India.

Vohra V., Mishra AK., Niranjan SK., Chopra A., Kumar M. and Joshi B.K. (2016). Phenotypic characterization, management and performance of Belahi cattle. Indian J. of Animal Sciences. 86(3): 355-358.

Wakchaure R., Ganguly S., Ahmad PP., Kumar PP., Kumar A. and Sharma S. (2015). Development of Crossbred Cattle in India: A Review. International Journal of Emerging Technology and Advanced Engineering, 5(10): 65-69

Woolliams J. (2004). Criteria to assess the degree of endangerment of livestock breeds in Europe. Livestock production science. 91: 173-182.

Yadav AS. and Rathi SS. (1991). Genetic evaluation of some performance traits in Hariana cattle. Asian Journal of Dairy Research. 10: 103-110.

Yadav BP., Tripathi GS. and Singh A. (2003). Genetic study of gestation period in Gaolao breed. Indian Vet. Med. Jour., 27:359-360.

Yang DY., Liu L., Chen X. and Camilla FS. (2008). Wild or domesticated: DNA analysis of ancient water buffalo remains from north China. Journal of Archaeological Science, 35: 2778–2785.

□□□